The Practitioner Guide to
Skills Training for Struggling Kids

The Practitioner Guide to
Skills Training
for Struggling Kids

Michael L. Bloomquist

THE GUILFORD PRESS
New York   London

To my wife, Rebecca

© 2013 The Guilford Press
A Division of Guilford Publications, Inc.
72 Spring Street, New York, NY 10012
www.guilford.com

Printed in the United States of America

This book is printed on acid-free paper.

Last digit is print number: 9 8 7 6 5 4 3 2 1

The author has checked with sources believed to be reliable in his effort to provide information that is complete and generally in accord with the standards of practice that are accepted at the time of publication. However, in view of the possibility of human error or changes in behavioral, mental health, or medical sciences, neither the author, nor the editor and publisher, nor any other party who has been involved in the preparation or publication of this work warrants that the information contained herein is in every respect accurate or complete, and they are not responsible for any errors or omissions or the results obtained from the use of such information. Readers are encouraged to confirm the information contained in this book with other sources.

Library of Congress Cataloging-in-Publication Data

Bloomquist, Michael L.
  The practitioner guide to skills training for struggling kids / Michael L. Bloomquist.
       p.   cm.
  Includes bibliographical references and index.
  ISBN 978-1-4625-0736-8 (pbk. : alk. paper)
  1. Problem children—Behavior modification.   2. Behavior disorders in children—Treatment.
  3. Problem children—Education.   4. Problem children—Services for.   5. Parenting.   I. Title.
  HQ773.B55 2013
  618.92′89—dc23
                                                                                2012028855

About the Author

Michael L. Bloomquist, PhD, is Associate Professor in the Department of Psychiatry at the University of Minnesota, and he provides psychological services and program consultation at PrairieCare Medical Group (a University of Minnesota affiliate site), both in Minneapolis. In his practice, he specializes in parent and family skills training for youth with behavioral–emotional problems. As a researcher, he is a coinvestigator at the Center for Personalized Prevention Research in Children's Mental Health, University of Minnesota, and a principal investigator on several studies examining the effects of comprehensive community-based prevention programs for high-risk youth and families. Dr. Bloomquist has written extensively about effective intervention methods, and he trains children's mental health professionals in evidence-based practice.

Acknowledgments

Many people helped me in writing the "Struggling Kids" books, and I am most indebted to them. I am forever grateful for the love and support of my wife, Rebecca Syverts, who is always there for me. I thank Steve Schnell and Marcia Jensen for early helpful ideas and comments that shaped the focus of the books. I am very appreciative of the feedback and guidance of Kitty Moore, Executive Editor, and Christine Benton, Developmental Editor, both at The Guilford Press. Lastly, to the many families with whom I have had the privilege to work over the years and who have taught me so much, I want to express my sincere gratitude.

Contents

Introduction

As a clinical child psychologist involved in clinical practice in a children's mental health setting, I see children and families with a wide variety of presenting problems. On a typical day, my caseload might look like this:

- 8:00 A.M.—9-year-old Tony has a diagnosis of attention-deficit/hyperactivity disorder (ADHD). He has few friends, is picked on, teased and rejected by other children, and often says, "Nobody likes me."
- 9:00 A.M.—13-year-old Jennifer has depression, and her stressed-out single father says she is increasingly irritable, moody, and argumentative, and her grades are declining.
- 10:00 A.M.—A busy single mother who owns a restaurant has a 7-year-old son named Carlos with ADHD/oppositional defiant disorder (ODD). He is very argumentative at home and school. He has just been suspended, which is increasing family stress as the mother tries to arrange child care. The boy and his mother are growing apart.
- 11:00 A.M.—15-year-old Franklin is on the path of a conduct disorder. He smokes cigarettes, breaks curfew, skips school, and occasionally smells of alcohol. His mother thinks that he is hanging out with the "wrong crowd" in their low-income neighborhood. He is flunking out of school.
- 1:00 P.M.—11-year-old Dominique has posttraumatic stress disorder (PTSD) related to his stepfather's physical abuse. He appears to be increasingly sad, irritable, and withdrawn. His mother says he is argumentative and fights with his sister nearly every day.
- 3:00 P.M.—15-year-old Melissa has bipolar disorder. Sometimes she "explodes," destroys property, and is violent in the home. There is frequent family conflict, and her father admits losing his temper and verbally abusing his daughter, which causes marital strife. In the session Melissa's mother stated, "I have failed as a parent," and her father noted, "I give up!"
- 4:00 P.M.—Parent group for children with a variety of diagnoses and presenting problems participating in a partial hospital program.
- 5:00 P.M.—Parent group for teens with a variety of diagnoses and presenting problems participating in a partial hospital program.

Finding the most effective ways to help children with such a broad range of behavioral–emotional problems (and their parents) can be challenging, even with extensive experience in intervention-focused research as well. My colleagues and I have dedicated our efforts to developing and testing child- and family-focused prevention interventions to use in school and community settings (see Bloomquist, August, Lee, Berquist, & Mathy, 2005), and as a "scientist-practitioner" I always strive to use research-informed methods in practice. But there are very few practical texts available to guide this endeavor.

Over many years I have gradually developed practice guidelines for skills enhancement that are informed by solid research in an attempt to fill this gap. The resultant *Struggling Kids* books are my attempt to bring it all together for myself and now for other practitioners. This practitioner volume is part of a two-book package that includes a corresponding parent volume. Together these books offer a toolkit to help families with a child who is delayed in, or struggling with, psychological development, as evidenced by broadly defined behavioral–emotional problems.

The ideas and methods in the "Struggling Kids" program are derived from proven behaviorally anchored practices, but they also integrate my 25 years of experience in providing skills-training interventions to families, training aspiring practitioners, and conducting applied research. The program is a practical distillation of the essential intervention ingredients observed across research-validated programs, and it is organized to allow for flexible use. The resulting specific methods have also been field-tested and refined extensively with families.

The "Struggling Kids" program can be applied with children and families in clinics, schools, community agencies, juvenile court–affiliated settings, and faith centers. It can be used by practitioners licensed to work with children and families in various professional capacities, as long as they are well trained in child and family behavior intervention methods. Together the two manuals can increase the effectiveness of parent and family skills training.

The strategies for building skills included in the "Struggling Kids" program are appropriate for children ages 5–17 years, and both books describe how to adapt the strategies for different ages in this span. In these books the term *parent* means any adult assuming a caregiver role, and *family* refers to any primary living arrangement(s) for a child.

How This Book Can Help the Struggling Child and Family

Struggling children display a wide variety of symptoms and functional problems, including disrupting the classroom, arguing with adults, fighting with siblings, mood swings, excessive worrying, difficulty making and keeping friends, and falling behind at school. At the root of these problems may be a variety of psychiatric disorders and symptoms, including externalizing difficulties such as ADHD, ODD, and conduct disorders, as well as internalizing emotional concerns such as mood and anxiety disorders. Not all children who are struggling will, however, qualify for a psychiatric diagnosis. What all struggling children, as defined in this program, have in common is difficulty progressing and mastering psychological development-related tasks in behavioral, social, emotional, and/or academic domains. As practitioners know, the comorbidity of psychiatric diagnoses and multiple symptom presentation are more the rule than the exception. Therefore, most struggling children need help in more than one domain. The "Struggling Kids" program is designed to target multiple problems in a way that often is impossible for service providers focusing on one area of need, such as academics or behavior.

The primary goal of the "Struggling Kids" program is to facilitate parents' and practitioners' efforts in collaborating to help a struggling child and his or her stressed family get back on track. The program provides a platform from which the practitioner and the parent can agree on the child's and parent/family's difficulties and then collaborate to create and execute an effective and tailored intervention. The child can be trained in developmentally related skills to make gains in behavioral, social, emotional, and academic domains. The parent and/or family can also be trained in skills to enhance well-being that will boost the child's development, reduce behavioral–emotional problems, and result in a more competent child.

The Importance of Parents

Although families typically seek help for problems exhibited by a child, the parent is the primary focal point of the skills-building approach espoused in the "Struggling Kids" program. Research, experience, and knowledge of child development confirm that a focus on the parent is effective in getting a struggling child back on track. Therefore, many of the ideas and procedures described involve either parents changing their own behavior or parents assisting their child to make behavior changes, with the practitioner teaching skills-building methods, guiding practice, and providing coaching and support. The child is still ultimately impacted by the intervention but often through the parent's efforts. Although the practitioner should target the child more and more directly as the child matures into adolescence, the parent should always be in the loop and actively involved.

The Importance of Evidence-Based Practices

The primary theoretical and procedural models that are often applied with a struggling child include parent management training, social competence skills training, cognitive-behavioral therapy, and behavioral family skills training. The content and delivery procedures across these and other emerging intervention models are integrated within the "Struggling Kids" program via principles of evidence-based practice. The evidence-based practice framework incorporates research-validated procedures that are applied using practitioner experience and tailoring to the characteristics and preferences of the client(s). Likewise the methods in the "Struggling Kids" program are informed and derived from research-validated models, but are presented in a manner that relies on the practitioner's judgment, the use of shared decision making to fit the specific skills-building interventions to each unique family, and teamwork to carry out the plan. This is arguably the best approach for "real-world" practice where children and families have a wide variety of presenting problems and differ in their level of motivation.

How to Use the Practitioner Manual and Parent Handbook

This book and the parent book are based in part on a revision of *Skills Training for Children with Behavior Problems*, published in 2006. That volume presented the skills-building training methods and then included information for practitioners in a single chapter. To make the program more widely usable for a variety of needs and settings, and to reflect recent advances in the field of child-focused intervention, I divided the material into two books. In the process the work was significantly updated and reorganized, and there is much more skills-training content. The books also reflect a greater emphasis on preparing and motivating the parent and child to follow through in using skills. In addition, the new practitioner manual allows for much more guidance in applying the training methods for greater success with families, including:

- Up-to-date information on behavioral–emotional problems in children and corresponding effective methods for intervention
- Conceptualization of children's problems as developmental struggles and of parent/ family difficulties as setbacks in coping with stress
- Suggestions for tailoring skills-building efforts to the unique needs and preferences of each family
- Ideas for getting families to attend sessions and motivating them to use what they are being trained in at home
- Instructions for training a family in skills-building strategies to develop a child's behavioral, social, emotional, and academic skills and to improve a parent's coping and broader family interactions

Each of these topics is briefly summarized in Chapters 1 and 2 and then elaborated on throughout the practitioner book. Chapters 3–10 provide step-by-step instructions on how to deliver the skills-training methods to families. Chapter 11 shows application of the methods through carefully described case studies. The Appendix briefly outlines an implementation and quality assurance protocol that can be used to train practitioners and help them maintain fidelity or integrity in applying the methods.

The following suggestions are intended to maximize success with this book and the "Struggling Kids" program.

1. ***Read the parent handbook in addition to the practitioner manual. The two books are best used in tandem.*** The parent book contains step-by-step instructions for each skills-building strategy in layperson's language. It is imperative that you, as the practitioner, also read and fully understand all of the content in the parent book in order to apply the delivery methods described in the practitioner book. You can use the appropriate chapters or sections in the parent book to teach parents the strategies and the corresponding chapters in the practitioner book for additional suggestions, troubleshooting, and customizing ideas. Worksheets, checklists, and other hands-on materials to be used by parents are included in both books.

2. ***Use the parent book and/or forms during sessions with families and as an at-home reference for parents. The parent book is best used by parents with the guidance of a practitioner.*** Parent and practitioner can literally be "on the same page" when you give parents the parent book at the beginning of your work with them and then refer to it throughout training sessions. With their own book to serve as a reminder of how to apply the skills-building methods and what the goals are, parents are less subject to misunderstanding and more likely to persevere with practicing and applying the strategies as intended at home. The combination of effective training by the practitioner and the availability of a user-friendly reference book for the parent to use at home can have a significant impact on progress.

3. ***Use the "Struggling Kids" program in either individual family or parent group meetings.*** If you are working with just one family, you have many options for organizing the intervention. For example, you can first train the parents, who then work with the child by themselves. You could also teach the child new skills alone and then bring the family in to teach the other members the same strategies. Another possibility is to work with the entire family at once. Finally, you can also conduct parent groups, which involves teaching the same skills to a small number of parents at once. The practitioner book illustrates some such applications, and the program is easy to adapt for your specific purposes. In any of these intervention approaches, provide the parent book to parents and use the practitioner book to guide the skills-training process.

The Author's Hope

I hope you find the "Struggling Kids" books a valuable aid in your work. They should assist you in carefully planning and carrying out a collaborative and effective skills-building intervention with a child and family. This broad-based intervention will ultimately get the struggling child and his or her family back on track. Good luck!

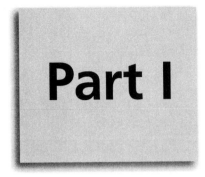

Part I

Background Information

Behavioral–Emotional Problems and Developmental Struggles in Children

The "Struggling Kids" program is designed to help parents who have children with behavioral–emotional problems. What usually prompts parents to seek help, however, and what may prompt a referral to a practitioner from a school or other agency is that the child is having trouble functioning in everyday life. Most parents interpret these troubles overtly as behavior difficulties, but they are as easily caused by emotional frustrations or acting out. A child could be exhibiting aggressive behavior because of an underlying problem with regulating anger or due to a deficit in social skills. A child who is throwing tantrums when it is time to go to school might be suffering from anxiety. A child who is withdrawing or behaving irritably at home might be struggling with depression. It is important for practitioners to identify the child's problems as specifically as possible so that the appropriate skills can be built. This chapter provides an overview of the array of behavioral–emotional problems and developmental challenges that can be addressed with the "Struggling Kids" program.

Common Diagnoses and Characteristics of Youth with Behavioral–Emotional Problems

Often, but not always, youth with behavioral–emotional problems manifest formal **DSM-IV diagnoses.** The common presenting concerns that can be addressed with the "Struggling Child" program include, but are not limited, to the following:

- **Attention-deficit/hyperactivity disorder (ADHD).** Hyperactivity/impulsivity with or without inattention. Usually the child exhibits an onset of symptoms prior to age 7.
- **Oppositional defiant disorder (ODD).** Oppositional/defiant actions that are much more than normative for the age of the child or teen. Research suggests two primary

dimensions (Burke & Loeber, 2010) of ODD: **emotion dysregulation** (symptoms of anger) and **defiant behavior** (willful oppositionality).

- **Conduct disorder (CD).** Behaviors include aggression, destruction of property, deceitfulness/lying/stealing, and/or violation of rules such as truancy, running away, etc. The onset of CD can occur in childhood, with symptoms typically observed prior to age 11, or during adolescence, after age 12.

- **Major depressive and dysthymic disorders.** Presenting with sad mood and/or irritability. These children also are likely to have physical symptoms (e.g., sleep disturbance, headaches) and experience anhedonia or lack of pleasure. Dysthymic disorder is characterized by chronic and less intensive depressive symptoms.

- **Bipolar disorder.** Episodic or persistent and severe irritable, sad, and/or euphoric moods. Unpredictable and sometimes "explosive" behavior can occur.

- **Generalized anxiety disorder (GAD).** Experiencing high levels of anxiety in multiple situations.

- **Social anxiety disorder (also known as social phobia).** High level of distress when thinking about, or being in, certain social situations.

- **Posttraumatic stress disorder (PTSD).** Diagnosed when a child has been exposed to significant traumatic events (e.g., child maltreatment, war, accidents) and is manifesting ongoing distress and anxiety afterward.

A recent comprehensive review showed that comorbidity is more the rule than the exception (Ollendick, Jarrett, Grills-Taquechel, Hovey, & Wolff, 2008). Table 1.1 shows the comorbidity rates between common externalizing and internalizing disorders for children. As can be seen, a child with one externalizing disorder is highly likely to manifest another externalizing disorder and/or an internalizing comorbid diagnosis.

Another way to describe the behavioral–emotional difficulties of children is by specific

TABLE 1.1. Comorbidity Rates for Most Common Childhood Psychiatric Diagnoses

Externalizing diagnoses	Comorbid externalizing and/or internalizing diagnoses
ADHD	• ODD and/or CD (43–93%) • Anxiety and/or mood disorder (13–51%)
ODD	• ADHD (35%) • Anxiety and/or mood disorder (46–62%)
CD	• ADHD (80%) • Anxiety and/or mood disorder (40–50%)

Note: Data culled from Ollendick et al. (2008).

characteristics. **These characteristics often cut across different diagnoses and are often the direct target of skills training interventions.** The characteristics most commonly observed in children with behavioral–emotional problems include the following:

- **Hyperactivity**—can't sit still and constantly in motion
- **Impulsivity**—not thinking before acting; exhibiting behavior such as blurting out, shoving in line, or even stealing something that is too tempting to resist
- **Inattention**—distracted, hard time focusing, and low effort and motivation to complete tasks and stay focused
- **Defiance**—argues or disregards adult directives
- **Rule-violating behavior**—violates commonly accepted standards of behavior, such as breaking curfew, stealing, vandalizing, running away from home, skipping school, etc.
- **Aggression**—displays actions that harm or intimidate others; can take the form of **physical aggression,** like punching, hitting, and kicking, or **relational aggression,** such as spreading rumors or excluding someone from a group. Both forms of aggression can be expressed **reactively** (spur of the moment) or **proactively** (planned out)
- **Moodiness**—depression-like sadness, discouragement, and hopelessness and/or euphoria-like excitability, mania, or irritability
- **Anxiety**—worries, physically tense, and avoidant of certain places, people, or events because of feeling nervous
- **Emotionally overreactive**—aroused, agitated, and "ready" for action
- **Emotionally underreactive**—calm with low guilt and/or concern for others (sometimes with lower empathy)
- **Underachievement**—delays in reading, arithmetic, written language, and other areas of academic proficiency
- **Social difficulties**—hard time with friendships and peer interactions; may include being socially troublesome to others and/or withdrawn and shy

Of course no one child will have all of these characteristics, but they are among the range of possible foci when working with children presenting with behavioral–emotional problems. A practitioner will undoubtedly be more effective for having considered them so that interventions can expressly address each one. For example, a child with CD manifesting proactive aggression and emotional underreactivity would require a different intervention from a child with CD exhibiting reactive aggression, anger, and mood dysregulation. Indeed Chapter 2 in the parent book (and Chapter 4 in this volume) helps the parent and practitioner identify and prioritize specific dimensions to focus on and then create a plan for helping the parents and child build compensatory skills one by one.

Development of Common Behavioral–Emotional Problems

The "Struggling Kids" program is founded in the idea that children's behavioral–emotional problems are rooted in developmental lags or deficits. **Struggling children are trying, but failing for a variety of reasons, to meet normative developmental expectations, and the goal is to get them back on track.** How individual children may have gotten off track, what risk and protective factors are at work in their lives, which specific dimensions characterize their problems, and which diagnoses they have received or may qualify for are all factors that practitioners should take into account if they hope to design the most effective intervention for a child's specific circumstances.

Developmental Processes in Children

It is generally accepted that children gradually develop skills, or "competencies," in different domains. These domains pertain to intrapersonal (emotional), interpersonal, behavioral, sexual, and physical development (Urquiza & Winn, 1999). Most children successfully negotiate the successive tasks within these domains and follow a path of typical development. Some children get off track, however. In these cases the developmental psychopathology perspective can be used to examine different development pathways within each of the domains (Cicchetti & Toth, 2009; Cummings, Davies, & Campbell, 2000). Most children follow the so-called normal pathway, along which they successfully negotiate a sequence of developmental tasks within a developmental domain. Some children have difficulties negotiating early developmental tasks, which then snowball, creating greater problems over time. Other children have successfully negotiated earlier developmental tasks but falter at some point and end up off course. Finally, resilient children may be off track, or are at risk to get off track, but nonetheless achieve a satisfactory outcome. It is possible for a child to be on track in one domain (e.g., intrapersonal development) and off track in another domain (e.g., behavioral development). It is the balance of risk and protective factors (reviewed below) that determines the pathway. Understanding each child's unique path in different domains of development helps practitioners personalize interventions for him or her.

Developmental Pathways for Children with Behavioral–Emotional Problems

Recent research reveals two separate but overlapping developmental pathways of **early-onset** behavioral–emotional problems (see Baker, Raine, Liu, & Jacobson, 2008; Frick & Nigg, 2012; Hubbard, McAuliffe, Morrow, & Romano, 2010; Ostrov & Crick, 2007; Patterson, Capaldi, & Bank, 1991). One is a **primarily reactive/impulsive pathway,** which is characterized by children who are easily activated emotionally and physiologically. They are often diagnosed with comorbid ADHD, anxiety disorders, and/or bipolar disorders. The other, much less common, is a **primarily proactive/callous–unemotional pathway,** in which children exhibit low levels of guilt, anxiety, and empathy and may be fearless or thrill seekers. These children are less likely to be diagnosed with comorbid ADHD, anxiety, and/or bipolar disorders. Children on both pathways are at risk for a host of mental health and functional problems in later life. Children on the primarily proactive/callous–unemotional pathway are most at risk for continuing and increasingly severe antisocial behavior into adolescence and adulthood. Of course, not all children with behavioral–emotional problems fit cleanly into these two developmental pathways, and some may exhibit elements of both. Nonetheless, the two pathways offer a framework for thinking about the development of children with behavioral–emotional problems. Practitioners would be wise to consider which path a child might be on and develop a responsive intervention accordingly.

There is also a **late-onset pathway** of behavioral–emotional problem development (i.e., late-onset CD; see Moffitt & Caspi, 2001; Odgers, et al., 2008; Van Lier, van der Ende, Koot, & Verhulst, 2007). These children tend to be less aggressive but still engage in antisocial behaviors such as breaking rules at home, at school, and in their communities. They are more likely to eventually desist in their antisocial behavior but can still have functioning problems at home, at school or on the job, and/or within the community. These problems can be quite serious and continue to impact the child negatively into the adult years.

Gender differences in the development of behavioral–emotional problems have been described (Moretti, Catchpole, & Odgers, 2005; Silverthorn & Frick, 1999; Van Lier et al., 2007). Boys tend to more often display disruptive, defiant, and aggressive behavior leading to antisocial outcomes. Girls show more differentiation in their maladaptive behaviors. Some girls are similar to boys in showing comparable levels of early physical aggression and a similar developmental course. Other girls show less aggressive or coercive behavior than boys, but nonetheless are at risk because of oppositional and hyperactive/inattentive behavior. Still other girls go down pathways similar to those of boys but may develop problems somewhat later. It is noteworthy that the girls most similar to boys are more severely disturbed and more at risk (Schaeffer et al., 2006). In addition, externalizing girls have more internalizing problems and relational aggression than do externalizing boys (Crick, Ostrov, & Werner, 2006; Pepler, Jiang, Craig, & Connolly, 2010).

Risk Factors Associated with Development of Behavioral–Emotional Problems

Whether behavioral–emotional problems develop early or late, children may end up on these pathways as a result of a variety of risk factors.

Child Biological/Neurological Risks

The central nervous system of children with behavioral–emotional problems may differ from that of typical children due to genetic vulnerability, early brain "assaults" (e.g., drug/alcohol/

cigarette use during pregnancy, birth complications, malnourishment), exposure to environmental toxins, head injury, and/or experience of psychological trauma (Barkley, 2006; Connor, 2002; Crowe & Blair, 2008; Ishikawa & Raine, 2003; Moadab, Gilbert, Dishion, & Tucker, 2010; Nigg & Huang-Pollock, 2003; Rubia et al., 2008; Tuvblad, Zheng, Raine, & Baker, 2009). These factors may adversely affect the central nervous system of children in a number of ways. Children with a wide variety of behavioral–emotional problems may have frontal lobe–based **executive functioning deficits** (Loeber & Pardini, 2008; Nigg & Huang-Pollock, 2003; Raaijmakers et al., 2008; Seguin & Zelazo, 2005). These include problems with "cold" executive functions, which are mostly cognitive in nature and involve working memory, sustained attention, and organization; or "hot" executive functions, which involve emotions and response inhibition (Zelazo & Müller, 2002). Another risk factor in this area is **stress reactivity,** having to do mostly with emotional regulation (Crowe & Blair, 2008; Hawes, Brennan, & Dadds, 2009; Moadab, Gilbert, Dishion, & Tucker, 2010; Rubia et al., 2008; Ruttle, Shirtcliff, Serbin, Ben-Dat Fisher, & Schwartzman, 2011). Reactive/impulsive behavior is related to overarousal stemming from higher or blunted cortisol hormone (depending on stress exposure), an overresponsive amygdala, and an underresponsive ventromedial prefrontal cortex; whereas stress reactivity underarousal that is observed in the proactive/callous–unemotional pattern is associated with lower cortisol and reduced amygdala and ventromedial prefrontal cortex input. The cited research shows that executive functioning and child stress reactivity dimensions overlap but are also distinct mechanisms that uniquely predict behavior problems.

Child Cognitive and Academic Risks

It is well known that many children with behavioral–emotional problems have **cognitive and/or academic delays** (Brownlie et al., 2004; Fergusson & Lynskey, 1997; Frick et al., 1991; Nigg & Huang-Pollock, 2003). These are most often expressed as speech/language delays, limited verbal abilities, and/or poor reading proficiency. These problems are most evident for those who are diagnosed with ADHD. Many studies show that children with CD have lower full-scale or verbal IQ scores than other children; however, this effect largely disappears when socioeconomic factors are controlled, suggesting this may have more to do with lower income than CD per se.

Executive functioning problems, especially cold executive functioning, can also negatively impact a child's **self-directed academic behavior skills** (Barkley, 2006; Dawson & Guare, 2010). Skills necessary for time management, organization, planning, reviewing, and staying on task obviously affect academic productivity and therefore deficits in them impede learning, leading to increased difficulties down the road.

Child Social and Information-Processing Risks

A child's social skills competency is obviously impeded by the development of behavioral–emotional problems in children (Dumas, Blechman, & Prinz, 1994; Hinshaw & Melnick,

1995; Rubin, Hymel, & Mills, 1989; Snyder et al., 2008). **Social skills deficits** are frequently seen in children who have difficulty making and keeping friends. Children with externalizing behaviors exhibit aggressive, bothersome, and intrusive behaviors while interacting with others. Internalizing children are inclined to be withdrawn and have a hard time getting into the social mix.

Information processing refers to the ability to take in new data about the environment and then use that effectively. Those at risk in this area will show problems in how they think about themselves and their understanding of their social context (see Crick & Dodge, 1994, 1996; Luebbe, Bell, Allwood, Swenson, & Early, 2010). Children encode, interpret, and reason out information in a sequential fashion that is influenced by existing beliefs, and this in turn influences emotional, behavioral, and physiological responses to ongoing events. **Social information-processing aberrations** are observed in many aggressive/externalizing and internalizing children. Aggressive/externalizing children lean toward a hostile intent bias, which means that they often assume others did mean things to them on purpose. In addition, they generate more aggressive solutions to problems (especially reactive aggressive) and expect more positive outcomes from their aggressive actions (especially proactive aggressive). Then they behave according to how they process ongoing social information. For example, when bumped in the hallway by a peer, a reactively aggressive child might assume that the person bumped him or her on purpose and respond with aggression.

Internalizing children exhibit a pessimistic (especially those who are depressed) and/or worrisome (especially those who are anxious) view of themselves, their world, and the future. These children exhibit a negative information-processing style wherein they attend to and evaluate information to "confirm" their pessimistic and/or worrisome views. This in turn exacerbates these children's emotional symptoms and reduces productive coping. It is worth noting that the aforementioned maladaptive ways of thinking are exacerbated when a child is acutely upset or agitated (Lemerise & Arsenio, 2000).

Parent- and Family-Related Risks

Of course the family environment influences a child's functioning, and many parent- and family-related factors have been linked to behavioral–emotional problems in children (Dodge, Coie, & Lynam, 2006; Erath, El-Sheikh, & Cummings, 2009; Hoeve et al., 2009; Miller, Loeber, & Hipwell, 2009; Moffitt & Caspi, 2001; Seng & Prinz, 2008). **Parent-related personal factors** correlated with child behavioral–emotional problems include a high frequency of psychopathology, relationship problems, low social support, and stressors within the parent. **Parents' cognition** also has an indirect influence on children. In particular, parents' unhelpful beliefs about their child and a tendency to make negative, internal, stable, dispositional attributions about their child's misbehavior can result in harsh and/or inconsistent discipline methods. **Coercive parent–child interactions** have a powerful influence on the child. These are ongoing negative interchanges between a difficult child and a sometimes volatile/harsh parent between whom "escape conditioning" occurs. In other words, the parent and child have learned coercive tactics over the years to cause the other to "give in." This tendency could overlap with "overreactive" parents who are easily angered and have a tendency to respond harshly (de Haan, Prinzie, & Dekovic, 2010; Prinzie et al., 2004). A lower level of **family routine**, as in predictable and organized daily family functioning, is related to behavior problems in low-income, urban, ethnic-minority children (Lanza & Drabick, 2011). **Other family variables** related to children with behavioral–emotional problems include marital/relationship problems, family conflict, domestic abuse, single-parent status (mixed evidence), and family instability such as mobility, homelessness, etc.

Peer Risks

Peer risks are potent in maintaining and exacerbating behavioral–emotional problems (Dodge et al., 2006; Dishion, Nelson, & Yasui, 2005; Miller et al., 2009). Children with behavioral–emotional problems often suffer from low **social acceptance status.** Frequently rejected or neglected by positive-influence peers, they lose out on opportunities to learn from and have development-enhancing experiences with positive peers. Children with significant behavioral–emotional problems also tend to affiliate with like peers during the preschool, school-age, and teen years. Such **peer affiliations** can influence a child in subtle and direct ways to engage in aggressive, antisocial, and/or risky behaviors. Such "**deviancy training**," or negative reciprocal peer influence, is associated with problem behaviors and depression-related symptoms in childhood and adolescence (Dishion & Tipsord, 2011).

Contextual Risks

A distal influence on youth is a myriad of contextual risks (Kohen, Leventhal, Dahinten, & McIntosh, 2008; Mrug & Windle, 2009). **Low socioeconomic status** is linked to many behavioral–emotional problems in children. The association is mediated by parent-related factors. In a low-income context there are more distressed parents, such parents are more likely to use harsh and/or lax discipline with their children, and this in turn is associated with child behavioral–emotional problems. In addition, children in families that live in low-income supportive housing exhibit significant externalizing, internalizing, and school adjustment problems (Lee et al., 2010). **Neighborhood disadvantage** is another indirect risk. In such neighborhoods there are more "deviant peers" with whom to associate, and antisocial role models are more prevalent. **Stressful events** are more common in a low-income context due to family/community violence, everyday hassles, etc. Such events compromise parenting and are related to emotional reactivity in children. In addition, child outcomes related to family/community violence exposure include PTSD and aggression (Allwood & Bell, 2008; Fowler, Tompsett, Braciszewski, Jacques-Tiura, & Baltes, 2009).

Cumulative Risks

Not every child with behavioral–emotional problems will be exposed to all of these risks. There is a linear effect of risk, however. The more risk factors present, the more likely a child will exhibit behavioral–emotional problems (Deater-Deckard, Dodge, Bates, & Pettit, 1998; Moffitt & Caspi, 2001; Trentacosta et al., 2008). Research reveals that children who persist with behavioral–emotional problems over time have an earlier onset of problems, comorbid ADHD, lower intelligence, and greater family adversity (Loeber & Pardini, 2008). By identifying and targeting these risk factors, it may be possible to lessen their influence via intervention so that a child can achieve a better developmental outcome.

Protective Factors Associated with Development of Resilience

Protective factors are attributes and resources within the child, parent/family, peer group, and larger community that can "shield" the child from risks (Luthar, Cicchetti, & Becker, 2000; Masten, 2001; Vanderbilt-Adriance & Shaw, 2008) and help a child go down a more adaptive or resilient pathway. Table 1.2 lists the protective factors found in studies of populations of children who emerge resilient within the context of risk (see Bloomquist & Schnell, 2002; Masten & Coatsworth, 1998; Masten & Wright, 2009, for further discussion).

TABLE 1.2. Protective Factors That Influence a Child's Development

Area of influence	Specific protective factors associated with successful development
Child	• Behavioral and emotion regulation skills • Social skills • Intellectual ability • Academic skills and success • Positive self-perception and self-efficacy • Faith, hope, and a sense of meaning in life
Parent/family	• Close relationship with a stable adult • Supportive and authoritative parenting • Family with predictable routines and rituals • Positive parent–child interactions • Positive and stable family environment
Peer	• Accepted by positive-influence children • Associations with positive-influence children
Contextual	• Attends and is bonded to school • Lives in safe and organized neighborhoods • Opportunities for positive-influence school, religious, and community activities

Protective factors are associated with resilient outcomes in at-risk children, though the association is not necessarily one of cause and effect. Different protective factors can exert direct or indirect effects on children's development and are more or less effective as a buffer in the face of varying levels of risk. By identifying and targeting these protective factors, it may be possible to increase their influence via intervention so that a child can achieve a better developmental outcome.

How the "Struggling Kids" Skills-Building Model Addresses Behavioral–Emotional Problems in Children

The "Struggling Kids" approach addresses the heterogeneous population of children with behavioral–emotional problems. It can be applied to children manifesting the diagnoses and characteristics associated with behavioral–emotional problems described above, while also attending to developmental processes and considering risk and protective factors within a comprehensive skills training model. The overarching goals are to provide a useful and efficient way to plan and carry out skills-building interventions and to offer a platform on which practitioners and parents can work together to enhance a child's functioning.

Enhancing the Child's Development

The program conceives of behavioral–emotional problems in children as manifestations of lags in their psychological development, with the purpose of intervention being to get them back on track. Four domains of psychological development that can be targeted include the following:

- **Child behavioral development.** Learning to follow reasonable external directions and rules and to internalize a moral and honest code of conduct.
- **Child social development.** Bonding with others and learning social skills.
- **Child emotional development.** Learning to understand/express feelings, think rationally, and regulate stress-related emotions.
- **Child academic development.** Learning self-directed academic behaviors and pursuing educational opportunities.

In Chapter 1 of the parent book, the struggling child and successful child are contrasted in each of these domains. The parent and practitioner then use Chapter 2 of the parent book to collaborate in fashioning a plan to help get the struggling child back on track.

Enhancing the Parents' and Family's Well-Being

As seen in the discussion of risk and protective factors above, parent and family functioning and capacities are also important in helping a child with behavioral–emotional problems. Therefore, the "Struggling Kids" program targets these two areas as well as the domains in which the child develops and operates:

- **Parent well-being:** Parents' personal functioning
- **Family well-being:** Family relationship functioning

In Chapter 1 of the parent book, the stressed parent/family and the coping parent/family are compared. The parent and practitioner then employ Chapter 2 of the parent book to develop a plan to enable the stressed parent/family to also get back on track.

The "Struggling Kids" program provides an opportunity for the parent and practitioner to share the same understanding of the child's and parent's family's difficulties and collaborate in ways to turn those around. This conceptualization of the struggling child leads to a developmentally informed intervention approach. The struggling child can be trained in developmentally related skills to transition to an adaptive or resilient pathway within the domains of behavioral, social, emotional, and academic functioning. The parent and/or family unit can be trained in skills that enhance well-being and that will ultimately improve the developmental status of the child.

The "Struggling Kids" skills-building intervention framework, which also serves to organize the parent book, is elucidated in the remainder of this practitioner book.

2

Skills-Training Methods Used in the "Struggling Kids" Program

As described at the end of Chapter 1, the "Struggling Kids" program uses child- and parent-family-focused methods to help children with behavioral–emotional problems build the specific skills they need to master essential developmental tasks and to help parent and family enhance well-being. How the program in this book accomplishes these goals is discussed in the following pages. This chapter is the foundation for the practice-oriented chapters in Part II, which provide details, practical suggestions, and examples of the methods introduced here.

Research-Validated Child and Parent/Family Skills Models

In the "Struggling Kids" program **skills training** is defined as a method of assisting children and parents to acquire the knowledge and behaviors that enhance day-to-day functioning. Skills training involves education, practice, and homework. Ideally, the recipients of skills-training efforts would also be required to demonstrate skill knowledge and proficiency in the training context and in their natural family environment. The skills-training methods used in the "Struggling Kids" program are composed of a variety of interventions that have been proven effective in helping children with behavioral–emotional problems.

Primary Intervention Models and Methods

Four theoretical and procedural models have been shown to be particularly effective for children with behavioral–emotional problems: parent management training, social competence skills training, cognitive-behavioral therapy, and behavioral family skills training. The content and delivery procedures across these models are integrated within the "Struggling Kids" program.

Parent Management Training

Behavioral parent training methods are based on social learning theory and use behavior analysis and operant-based change strategies. Its goals are to reduce problem child behaviors, increase positive alternative child behaviors, and improve parent–child interactions by teaching parents strategies that alter the child's home environment (Barkley, 1997; Barkley, Edwards, & Robin, 1999; Eyberg & Boggs, 1998; Kazdin, 2005; McMahon & Forehand, 2003; Patterson, Reid, Jones, & Conger, 1975; Sanders, 1999; Webster-Stratton & Hancock, 1998; Weisz, 2004). Techniques include shaping and reinforcing desired behavior, ignoring and punishing undesired behavior, reducing coercive parent–child interactions, enhancing parental monitoring and supervision, and building the parent–child bond.

Social Competence Skills Training

Social competence skills training refers to the use of operant, modeling, coaching, and social–cognitive techniques that enhance children's social skills and capacity (Beelmann, Pfingsten, & Losel, 1994; Bierman, Greenberg, & Conduct Problems Prevention Research Group, 1996; Larson & Lochman, 2002; Lochman, Boxmeyer, Powell, Barry, & Pardini, 2010; Prinz, Blechman, & Dumas, 1994). Many programs that focus on social competence also incorporate techniques of cognitive-behavioral therapy (discussed next). Under this umbrella are behavioral social skills training, social–cognitive training, and emotional skills training, as well as environmentally based strategies that support children's social skills development. Techniques include direct teaching of social behaviors such as sharing, cooperating, communicating, ignoring, and asserting; fostering perspective taking, accurate attributions, and solving of social problems; as well as administering contingencies to shape specific social behaviors and competencies.

Cognitive-Behavioral Therapy

Cognitive-behavioral therapy focuses on changing maladaptive thoughts, feelings, and behaviors that underlie behavioral–emotional problems (David-Ferdon & Kaslow, 2008; Sauter, Heyne, & Westenberg, 2009; Silverman, Pina, & Viswesvaran, 2008; Weisz, 2004). Procedures derived from stress inoculation training, which emphasizes the teaching of stress-coping techniques (Meichenbaum, 1977), also fall into this category of intervention. Techniques for children include affective education, the teaching of helpful thinking habits, and stress (anger/anxiety) management skills training. Cognitive-behavioral therapy aimed at parents can enhance their engagement in parent-focused skills training (Hoza, Johnston, Pillow, & Ascough, 2006; Mah & Johnston, 2008; Morrissey-Kane & Prinz, 1999) and also help them manage anger and change hostile attributions about their child, which in turn reduces unrealistic and negative expectations of the child and increases the program's over-all effectiveness (Sanders et al., 2004; Wiggins, Sofroonoff, & Sanders, 2009).

Behavioral Family Skills Training

Behavioral family skills training enhances the parent–child relationship and facilitates broader family interactions. Strategies from behavioral parent training, family systems, and family interaction skills training are often integrated within this intervention (Alexander, Pugh, Parsons, & Sexton, 2000; Dishion & Stormshak, 2007; Robin & Foster, 1989; Szapocznik & Williams, 2000; Weisz, 2004). Techniques include shoring up parenting strategies, enhancing family connections and organization, and improving family interaction skills related to communication, problem solving, and conflict management. Several family therapy approaches blend behavioral methods with systemic interventions for adolescents (Henggeler, Schoenwald, Borduin, Rowland, & Cunningham, 2009; Liddle & Hogue, 2000).

Motivational Enhancement Methods

Increasingly attention is being paid to preparing and motivating clients to learn and use the methods they are taught. Such efforts are typically rooted in stages of change theory (Prochaska & DiClemente, 1986) and in motivational interviewing procedures (Miller & Rollnick, 2002). This approach often begins with determining the degree of clients' readiness to change. Then motivational enhancement intervention can range from brief strategies such as reviewing goals and providing information on how the program may help achieve them (Sterrett, Jones, Zalot, & Shook, 2010) to more elaborate approaches such as weighing the pros and cons of making change, examining discrepancies between current status and goals, and encouraging commitment to change (Chaffin, Funderburk, Bard, Valle, & Gurwitch, 2011). Accordingly, the application of motivation-oriented strategies to get clients to actually use the skills they are learning is essential, as evidence as to their effectiveness is accumulating (Chaffin et al., 2009, 2011; Dishion & Stormshak, 2007; Nock & Kazdin, 2005; Sterrett et al., 2010; Winters & Leitten, 2007).

Similar Training Methods across Models

The approaches mentioned above often overlap in focus and methods. The "Struggling Kids" program incorporates the many commonalities found in the above models (see Bloomquist & Schnell, 2002; Chorpita & Daleiden, 2009, for more discussion). Specifically:

- An emphasis on engaging children and parents so that they are fully capable of using and following through with skills-building strategies

- The use of behavioral training methods, including psychoeducation, didactic instruction, modeling, role playing, behavioral rehearsal, goal setting, and homework
- Encouragement of clients to monitor their progress in skills acquisition, skills implementation, and daily functioning

Emerging Models and Methods

Other models are accumulating evidence of efficacy in treating children with behavioral–emotional problems and their families. One model teaches mindfulness skills to children (Biegel, Brown, Shapiro, & Schubert, 2009; Semple, Lee, Rosa, & Miller, 2010) and to parents (Coatsworth, Duncan, Greenberg, & Nix, 2010; Duncan, Coatsworth, & Greenberg, 2009) to help them focus their attention and awareness in the present moment, which promotes emotional well-being. Another model enhances children's school-related executive functioning skills, such as getting organized, staying on task, checking work, planning, and so forth (Dawson & Guare, 2010; Meltzer, 2007), so a child can achieve his or her potential. Since at the time of this writing, these emerging interventions are not as well established as the primary approaches, they may be best considered an augmentation to them.

What the Research Tells Us about Skills-Training Models

Literally hundreds of randomized controlled research trials conducted over decades have evaluated the utility of child- and parent/family-focused intervention for behavioral–emotional problems. Taken as a whole, this research shows that children, parents, and families do benefit from structured, empirically tested interventions (Weisz & Kazdin, 2010). These interventions effect behavioral change in children and their families and promote child development and day-to-day parent/family functioning. Practitioners armed with specifics about how and where the interventions have been seen to work best will find it easiest to integrate them successfully into real-world practice settings. The literature is too voluminous to discuss in full here, but important points culled from reviews of the literature (narrative reviews and meta-analyses) will help readers feel confident in the methods used in the "Struggling Kids" program:

General Benefits

- Variations of the primary intervention models discussed above have been shown to be effective for the treatment of ADHD (Pelham & Fabiano, 2008), oppositional behavior and conduct problems (Eyberg, Nelson, & Boggs, 2008), depression (David-Ferdon & Kaslow, 2008), anxiety disorders (Silverman et al., 2008), and exposure to trauma (Silverman, Ortiz, et al., 2008). Parent and family skills programs have shown outcomes of both statistical and clinical significance for problematic child behavior after intervention (de Graaf, Speetjens, Smit, De Wolf, & Tavecchio, 2008; Kaminski, Valle, Filene, & Boyle, 2008; Kazdin, 2003; Serketich & Dumas, 1996; Thomas & Zimmer-Gembeck, 2007).

- Programs with a parenting component yield a broad range of positive youth and family outcomes that extend into long-term follow-up assessments (Drugli, Larsson, Fossum, & Mørch, 2010; Forgatch, Patterson, DeGarmo, & Beldavs, 2009; Sandler, Schoenfelder, Wolchik, & MacKinnon, 2011).
- Individuals from different cultural groups benefit from a standard parent and family skills approach (Huey & Polo, 2008; McCabe & Yeh, 2009).
- Child-focused skills training achieved a small to moderate effect size and parent/family-focused skills training obtained a moderate effect size in a meta-analysis of 71 child- and parent/family-focused skills training studies for youth with behavior problems (McCart, Priester, Davies, & Azen, 2006).
- Parents' own personal adjustment improved with parent/family skills training in the same meta-analysis (McCart et al., 2006), an effect that extended earlier meta-analysis findings of the positive effects of parenting-focused programs on mothers (Barlow, Coren, & Stewart-Brown, 2002).
- Cognitive-behavioral therapy for child depression and anxiety produced moderate effect sizes for symptom reduction in a meta-analysis of studies for internalizing disorders (Chu & Harrison, 2007).
- Behavioral family therapy models for treatment of conduct problems and substance abuse in teens derived modest effect sizes in a recent meta-analysis (Baldwin, Christian, Berkeljon, & Shadish, 2012).
- Parental involvement with the child in intervention has inherent benefits, whether the parent is trained to train the child, the parent and child are trained in the same skills in concurrent sessions, or other variations are applied (DeRosier & Gillione, 2007; Dowell & Ogles, 2010; Frankel, Myatt, Cantwell, & Feinberg, 1997; Griffin, Samuolis, & Williams, 2011; Mikami, Lerner, Griggs, McGrath, & Calhoun, 2010).

Important Limitations

- Preschool/school-age children with behavior problems evidence somewhat better outcomes from parent/family skills training than teens (McCart et al., 2006).
- Effect sizes of cognitive-behavioral therapy in the meta-analysis for internalizing disorders were larger for adolescents than elementary school-age children (Chu & Harrison, 2007).
- There is mixed evidence as to the efficacy of child- and family-focused interventions for children with callous–unemotional traits. Some studies show that such children are less responsive to interventions (Hawes & Dadds, 2005; Lewis et al., 2008; Stadler et al., 2008; Waschbusch, Carrey, Willoughby, King, & Andrade, 2007), whereas

other research shows that these children can benefit from intervention (McDonald, Dodson, Rosenfield, & Jouriles, 2011).

- Mothers benefit to a greater extent than fathers (Lundahl, Tollefson, Risser, & Love-joy, 2008).

Bridging the Research-to-Practice Gap

The research evidence for the efficacy of child- and parent/family-focused skills-training programs indicates that they hold great promise for children with behavioral–emotional problems. Yet using these programs in real-world settings has proven to be fraught with challenges (Jensen-Doss, Hawley, Lopez, & Duvivier Osterberg, 2009; Rohrbach, Grana, Sussman, & Valente, 2006; Weisz, 2004). At the practitioner level, there is often poor understanding and substandard implementation of practice parameters. As a result many research-validated programs are revamped to such an extent that they bear little resemblance to the evidence-based model. In addition, there is often a poor fit between what was validated in a research context and what works in real-world practice. Research-validated programs are often designed for homogeneous populations and used as a "one-size-fits-all" approach. That doesn't work in most applied settings, where heterogeneity of clients is the rule and there is a need for an individualized approach. Finally, at the community and organizational level, there is often limited funding and insufficient buy-in by administrators and/or practitioners of research-validated models. What transpires in practice has to conform to realistic funding constraints and must be feasible or it is of little use. The following suggestions for bridging the research-to-practice gap are all incorporated into the "Struggling Kids" program.

Using Evidence-Based Practice Methods

Evidence-based practice (EBP) is the integration of research with clinical expertise while considering patient characteristics, culture, and preferences (American Psychological Association, 2006; Kazdin, 2008; Mitchell, 2011). In other words, EBP is the intersection of research, practitioner experience, and client variables (see Figure 2.1). In EBP, practitioners integrate their knowledge of current research, rely on their accumulating experience-based expertise, and use shared decision making with clients (Spring, 2007).

Using Research to Guide Practice

Keeping current with research to determine the best interventions means gathering information on well-established and probably efficacious intervention methods, with an eye to effect sizes, statistical and clinical significance, and an accumulating body of supporting evidence.

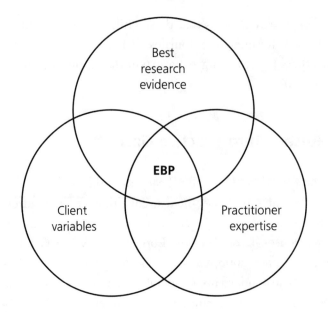

FIGURE 2.1. Components of evidence-based practice (EBP).

Using Clinical Expertise

Practitioners need to have the skills and competencies involved in assessing, diagnosing, conceptualizing, and implementing an intervention, as well as the savvy to tailor the evidence-based protocols to individualized interventions for clients. Such practitioner expertise emerges from training and education, an awareness of mistakes and successes, and accumulated experience in working with clients.

> Of course, basic practice skills are critical to intervene effectively. These include forming a therapeutic alliance, the capacity to monitor progress, and an awareness of the influence of individual, cultural, and contextual factors on client acceptance and use of the intervention.

Considering Client Variables

Practitioners must take into account the unique characteristics, preferences, and circumstances of each client. This includes involving clients in collaborative decision making to ensure that an intervention fits with their perceptions. Such an approach is consistent with a central goal of EBP, which is to maximize client choice among effective alternative interventions. It is also in keeping with a call to personalize or tailor interventions (Insel, 2009).

Interventions can be personalized based on needs and/or preferences (August, Gewirtz, & Realmuto, 2009). **Needs** are based on client characteristics (e.g., age, behavioral risk status, severity) and family risk status (e.g., parenting skills, family psychiatric history, family adversity). Respecting **preferences** entails guiding clients to make decisions about intervention options that are consistent with their values, cultural background, and immediate goals. A combination of needs and preference-based tailoring may be best. Then it is up to the practitioner to apply the evidence-based procedures with which he or she has experience to achieve the best outcomes for clients. The "Struggling Kids" program emphasizes tailoring the intervention for each child and family. The rest of this practitioner book provides a "toolbox" of many intervention methods that can be applied in relation to child and parent needs and preferences.

Using Common Practice Elements

As mentioned before, interventions developed and evaluated in idealistic research circumstances need to be adapted for real-world clinical practice. Some have suggested that one way to accomplish this adaptation is to extract "practice elements" (i.e., common content and delivery procedures) from research-validated interventions for use in practice (Chorpita & Daleiden, 2009; Kaminski et al., 2008). Such practice elements could then be tailored according to the needs and/or preferences of the families presenting for intervention.

Chorpita and Daleiden (2009) examined practice parameters across 322 studies and protocols in an effort to extract practice elements. They coded studies for the presence of practice elements and then matched those elements to disorders (i.e., including observed problem, age, gender, and ethnicity). Table 2.1 shows the practice elements observed most often in effective interventions for common behavioral–emotional dimensions (practice elements observed in a smaller percentage of effective interventions have been omitted from the table). In essence, Table 2.1 presents a synthesis of intervention approaches that could be used in EBP with these types of presenting problems.

Engaging Families

It is imperative that practitioners motivate families to show up, to keep showing up, and to actively participate in the learning process. Indeed, studies show that there is a relationship between "dosage," or amount of services received, and outcome. Generally there is more progress when families (particularly parents) receive a higher dosage of the program (August, Bloomquist, Lee, Realmuto, & Hektner, 2006; August, Lee, Bloomquist, Realmuto, & Hektner, 2004; Maher, Marcynyszyn, Corwin, & Hodnett, 2011). In addition, just showing up is insufficient to make any meaningful progress. Research shows that parents and children who make an effort to learn and use skills achieve good outcomes (Chu & Kendall, 2004; Nix, Bierman, McMahon, & Conduct Problems Prevention Research Group, 2009; Podell & Kendall, 2011). The "Struggling Kids" program emphasizes parent and child engagement. This is accomplished by addressing "external" barriers such as where and when services

TABLE 2.1. Percentage Frequency of Practice Element Codes in Interventions for Children and Adolescents by Common Behavioral–Emotional Problem Dimension

Externalizers

Attention-deficit/hyperactivity	Oppositional/aggressive	Delinquent
• Praise: 45	• Praise: 53	• Tangible rewards: 51
• Tangible rewards: 36	• Time out: 51	• Problem solving: 56
• Psychoeducation—parent: 36	• Tangible rewards: 46	• Praise: 49
• Time out: 32	• Commands: 43	• Social skills training: 46
• Problem solving: 32	• Problem solving: 41	• Cognitive: 46
• Modeling: 32	• Differential reinforcement: 40	• Monitoring: 46
• Monitoring: 23	• Modeling: 37	• Response cost: 46
• Commands: 23	• Cognitive: 35	• Communication skills: 41
• Relaxation: 23	• Psychoeducation—parent: 34	• Goal setting: 41
• Stimulus control/antecedent management: 21	• Monitoring: 26	• Therapist praise/rewards: 41
	• Communication skills: 26	• Maintenance/relapse prevention: 38
	• Goal setting: 24	• Psychoeducation—parent: 38
	• Response cost: 21	• Family therapy: 26
	• Behavioral contracting: 21	• Natural/logical consequences: 26
	• Attending: 21	• Parent coping: 23
		• Commands: 23
		• Time out: 21
		• Differential reinforcement: 21
		• Education support: 21

Internalizers

Anxiety	Traumatic stress	Depressed mood
• Exposure: 80	• Exposure: 91	• Cognitive: 75
• Relaxation: 42	• Cognitive: 91	• Psychoeducation—child: 71
• Cognitive: 38	• Psychoeducation—child: 82	• Maintenance/relapse prevention: 67
• Modeling: 33	• Relaxation: 64	• Activity scheduling: 58
• Psychoeducation—child: 27	• Psychoeducation—parent: 45	• Problem solving: 54
• Therapist praise/rewards: 25	• Maintenance/relapse prevention: 45	• Self-monitoring: 54
• Self-monitoring: 24	• Assertiveness training: 27	• Goal setting: 46
• Self-reward/self-praise: 20	• Modeling: 27	• Social skills training: 46
	• Problem solving: 27	• Relaxation: 42
	• Personal/safety skills: 27	• Self-reward/self-praise: 42
		• Behavioral contracting: 38
		• Communication skills: 38
		• Psychoeducation—parent: 38
		• Guided imagery: 29
		• Talent or skill building: 29
		• Therapist praise/rewards: 29
		• Modeling: 25

Note. Data culled from Chorpita and Daleiden (2009). See article for definition of practice element terms.

are offered and "internal" barriers such as thoughts about the presenting problems and proposed intervention(s), as well as motivation to do some work.

Making Cultural Adaptations to Research-Based Models

In real-world settings practitioners often find that cultural adaptations have a way of knocking down internal barriers to a family's engagement, and it makes the intervention a better match for the family. Making cultural adaptations involves (1) gathering information from the cultural group being served, (2) initially adapting the program based on that information, (3) preliminarily testing the adapted program to see how it is accepted by clients and whether it works, and (4) based on feedback, continuing with refinement as needed (Barrera & Castro, 2006). The prevailing wisdom about how much to adapt is to make some alterations while retaining the essential elements related to change (Castro, Barrera, Holleran Steiker, 2010). This could involve changes in **surface structure,** such as making the program's materials or activities take into account observable variables such as language, music, foods, and cultural events; and/or changes in **deep structure** that focus on culturally based historical and current beliefs and traditions about child rearing, families, and help seeking (Resnicow, Soler, Braithwait, Ahluwalia, & Butler, 2000). Such cultural considerations and adaptations should be incorporated into everyday practice with the "Struggling Kids" program whenever possible.

Delivering Interventions with Fidelity

It goes without saying that research-validated intervention models are meant to be applied as designed and tested. Nonetheless, fidelity to the original design is often neglected, even though it is critical in translating research to practice (Dane & Schneider, 1998; Durlak & DuPre, 2008; Henggeler & Schoenwald, 1999; Lee, August, Realmuto, Horowitz, Bloomquist, & Klimes-Dougan, 2008; Weisz, 2004). The general goals of fidelity are to provide a rough approximation of:

- **Exposure,** which is the number of sessions/contacts that are provided
- **Adherence,** which pertains to using the specified content and delivery methods
- **Quality of delivery,** which has to do with preparation, enthusiasm, asking guiding questions, or what can be construed as general practice competence

One way to ensure fidelity is to provide implementation support to practitioners. This support typically entails the use of manuals, training/supervision, fidelity monitoring, and continuous performance feedback (Durlak & DuPre, 2008; Henggeler & Schoenwald, 1999; Weisz, 2004). The more implementation support provided, the better in terms of achieving more positive gains (Lochman, Boxmeyer, et al., 2009). Implementation support, which is a standard of research-validated programs, can also be used in the practice context (Beidas & Kendall, 2010). One could argue that implementation support is critically important because it enhances fidelity, which should result in better services being provided. One study supports this very assertion. Researchers found that implementation support predicted fidelity, which in turn predicted better outcomes for adolescents in multisystemic therapy (Schoenwald, Sheidow, & Chapman, 2009). Thus the use of implementation support methods might be considered a basic and necessary feature of EBP (Carroll, Martino, & Rounsaville, 2010). The "Struggling Kids" program has an implementation support protocol. This practitioner book (and the companion parent book) can be considered "the manual," and there is also a training/supervision, fidelity monitoring, and continuous performance feedback protocol described in the Appendix.

Principles of the "Struggling Kids" Program as an EBP Model

This section integrates the conceptual framework, procedural methods, and overarching practice parameters described thus far in Chapters 1 and 2, essentially summarizing the foundation of the "Struggling Kids" model. The specific related practice guidelines are then detailed in the remainder of the practitioner book.

Focus on Coping Skills and Self-Regulation to Promote Competence in Child and Parent

As discussed in Chapter 1, whether a child develops along a typical or a maladaptive pathway has much to do with mastering age-related developmental tasks (Masten & Coatsworth, 1998; Masten, 2001). In other words, mastering of earlier tasks helps a child succeed with later tasks, and vice versa, for children with problems (Masten, 2001). A **coping competence model** of intervention (Blechman, Prinz, & Dumas, 1995; Dumas, Arriaga, Begle, & Longoria, 2010) can be used to get a child back on track by teaching him or her specific coping skills designed to enhance developmental competencies. In accordance with the coping competence model, the "Struggling Kids" program aims to help children develop social, emotional, and instrumental (or behavioral) skills to enhance competencies in those and related developmental domains. The coping competence model further posits that it is the family setting where most children will learn social, affective, and instrumental skills, provided there is support and guidance from parents. Therefore, parents should be given tools to help a struggling child become more competent in everyday life.

One of the tenets of the "Struggling Kids" program is that parental self-regulation be a central focus in working with parents of children with behavioral–emotional problems (Sanders, 1999, 2008). Parental self-regulation is addressed in several concrete ways. First, parents are taught to plan, set goals, and monitor progress. Second, parents are given concrete ideas and specific strategies to solve a wide variety of everyday problems with their child. Finally, some methods directly teach parents to stop, think helpful thoughts, and stay calm. The result will be improved parenting behaviors and increased confidence and self-efficacy. These will result in turn in calmer and more productive parent–child interactions and in the parent's being a good role model, which will facilitate development of self-regulation by the child.

Adapt the Strategies to the Child's Age

Skills-building strategies must obviously be delivered in a developmentally nuanced manner to meet the needs of different age groups (Holmbeck, Devine, & Bruno, 2010; Ollendick, Grills, & King, 2001). With a defiant child, for example, gaining compliance is attempted by a procedure in which the parent presents an effective command, a warning with a consequence, and then follows through if the child remains obstinate. With a younger child this process may end with him or her in time-out, whereas an older child or teen might face removal of a privilege. Another example is with a child-focused skills-building effort such as social skills training, in which adaptive social behaviors are targeted, directly trained, and then guided for use in social settings. With a younger child the skills will be basic, such as taking turns, using eye contact, and starting conversations, whereas an older child or teen might work on age-appropriate skills such as resisting peer pressure, negotiating, and resolving conflicts. In designing the best possible intervention for a family, the child's developmental age must always be used to customize the skills-building strategies. Practitioners and parents will also find that the broad range of skills-building strategies in the parent book makes it usable across the whole child age range of 5–17 years, as the child's behavioral–emotional problems wax and wane and evolve, requiring different strategies to be employed.

Collaborate with Parents

Although the "Struggling Kids" program consists of a parent book and a practitioner book, they are meant to be used in concert. By design the parent book is the centerpiece of the program because its primary purpose is to provide the content of skills training. The forms and charts provided in the parent book to be used by parents are, however, also presented at the ends of Chapters 5–10 in this practitioner book. The practitioner book is designed to help practitioners deliver that content to families, in part by providing numerous ideas and procedures for collaborating with parents and families. Parent–practitioner collaboration in fashioning and using a skills-building intervention for the family is essential to the success of implementation. Parents who buy into a particular intervention plan will be much more engaged with training, will be motivated to stick with skills-building practice, and will feel acknowledged for their critical role in helping their child get back on track developmentally.

Use Modular Components to Make Interventions Flexible and Effective

The "Struggling Kids" program integrates many helpful skills-building approaches derived from parent management training, social competence skills training, cognitive-behavioral therapy, behavioral family skills training, and other modalities and presents them as different modules. These modules are the "containers" of research-validated practice elements, procedures for making decisions on how to use them, and methods needed to deliver them (Chorpita, 2007; Chorpita, Taylor, Francis, Moffitt, & Austin, 2004). A modular approach is effective in ensuring flexibility to match the needs and preferences of each family as long as fidelity within the module is maintained. In addition, a modular approach is preferred over a manualized intervention by many practitioners (Borntrager, Chorpita, Higa-McMillan, & Weisz, 2009).

It is noteworthy that modular approaches have precedence for intervening with externalizing (Kolko, Baumann, Bukstein, & Brown, 2007; Kolko et al., 2009) and anxious internalizing (Chorpita et al., 2004; Chorpita, 2007) problems in children. A recent study (Weisz et al., 2012) determined that a modular intervention with elements for behavioral and emotional problems was superior to manualized programs and usual care treatment. These results suggest that a modular approach may be a promising way to deliver evidence-based interventions in practice settings (i.e., evidence-based practice).

The seven skills-training modules within the "Struggling Kids" program can be viewed as "toolboxes," each containing different "tools" for the "job." Just as there are unique toolboxes and tools for plumbing (pipe wrench, tube cutter, drain snake, etc.), carpentry (saw, hammer, screwdriver, etc.), and fixing a car (socket wrench, caliper, pliers, etc.), to name a few, there are unique modules for addressing the presenting problems of children with behavioral–emotional problems and their parents/families. The module-like toolboxes contain unique strategies or tools with which to address specific areas of child and parent/family functioning. The modules have their own separate sections within the parent book. Many, but by no means all, of the practice elements reviewed in Table 2.1 are included in the chapters within each module. The "Struggling Kids" modules and accompanying chapters are listed below:

Module 1: Getting Started and Staying with It

1. The Struggling Child: Understanding Your Child's Behavioral–Emotional Problems
2. Getting Back on Track: Coming Up with a Skills-Building Plan for Your Child and Family
3. Taking Care of Business: Getting Going and Following Through

Module 2: Enhancing Your Child's Behavioral Development

4. Doing What You're Told: Teaching Your Child to Comply with Parental Directives
5. Doing What's Expected: Teaching Your Child to Follow Rules

6. Doing the Right Thing: Teaching Your Child to Tell the Truth and Behave Honestly
7. Staying Cool under Fire: Managing Your Child's Protesting of Discipline and Preventing Angry Outbursts

Module 3: Enhancing Your Child's Social Development

8. Making Friends: Teaching Your Child Social Behavior Skills
9. Keeping Friends: Teaching Your Child Social Problem-Solving Skills
10. That Hurts!: Helping Your Child with Bullies
11. Hanging with the "Right Crowd": Influencing Your Child's Peer Relationships

Module 4: Enhancing Your Child's Emotional Development

12. Let It Out!: Teaching Your Child to Understand and Express Feelings
13. You Are What You Think: Teaching Your Child to Think Helpful Thoughts
14. Staying Calm: Teaching Your Child to Manage Stress

Module 5: Enhancing Your Child's Academic Development

15. Surviving School: Teaching Your Child to Manage Time, Organize, Plan, Review, and Stay on Task
16. Teaming Up: Collaborating and Advocating for Your Child at School

Module 6: Enhancing Your Well-Being as a Parent

17. You Parent the Way You Think: Thinking Helpful Thoughts to Enhance Parenting
18. Cool Parents: Managing Your Own Stress to Enhance Parenting

Module 7: Enhancing Your Family's Well-Being

19. Let's Get Together: Strengthening Family Bonds and Organization
20. We Can Work It Out: Strengthening Family Interaction Skills

The practitioner, based on an assessment of the family's needs, and the parent, based on personal preferences, collaborate on which modules are eventually used. The practitioner uses engagement strategies and decision aids within the first module, "Getting Started and Staying with It," to guide the collaborative process. This process is elaborated on in Chapters 3 and 4 in this practitioner book.

Use Consistent Training Procedures

Behavioral procedures are used throughout training of these modules. All of the parent book chapters incorporate psychoeducation, motivation enhancement, and skills procedures. Parents are asked to set and work toward specific goals and monitor progress. Didactic instruction, modeling, role playing, behavioral rehearsal, and homework are used throughout. There are consistent suggestions for making developmental adjustments. Specific training procedures for all of the modules are elaborated on throughout the rest of this practitioner book.

Delivering a Comprehensive Intervention

Effective interventions must reduce risk and promote protection to enhance children's development. To accomplish these objectives, an intensive model of intervention may be needed. For some, the child and parent/family skills-building interventions will be only one piece of the puzzle. Table 2.2 summarizes other interventions that are considered evidence-based options for these children. Integrating parent/family skills-building interventions with different combinations of the interventions in Table 2.2 may be the best way to reduce problem behaviors and promote competencies in children with behavioral–emotional problems.

Most children will not need all these interventions, and one practitioner could not possibly provide them all. It is also beyond the scope of this practitioner book to review them (see Bloomquist & Schnell, 2002, for a detailed discussion). Table 2.2 is intended only to organize the "big picture" to put child and family skills-building interventions such as those in the "Struggling Kids" program into perspective. It is the responsibility of the practitioner to assist families in accessing and using additional interventions, as needed, to bolster a skills-building approach.

TABLE 2.2. Evidence-Based Interventions for Children with Behavior-Emotional Problems

• Child skills training	• Schoolwide interventions
• Parent/family skills training	• School-based peer mediation
• Psychiatric medications	• Classroom management
• Outpatient and restrictive mental health services	• Mentoring/after-school programs
• Academic skills building	• Family support case management
	• Multicomponent interventions (two or more of above)

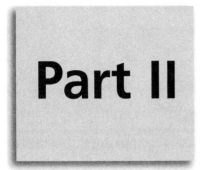

Part II

Practice Guidelines for the "Struggling Kids" Program

3

Procedures to Use with All Families Receiving the "Struggling Kids" Program

This chapter provides a framework and presentation of fundamental methods for using the "Struggling Kids" program. **As such, it serves as a procedural foundation and base from which the personalized and module-oriented interventions in Chapters 4–10 of this book can be implemented.** These methods apply regardless of which modules are chosen for a given family. The chapter covers topics related to engagement (especially with parents), motivational enhancement, conducting a functional assessment to determine a tailored focus for skills training, administering skills training via family or parent group training formats, techniques for delivering interventions, and augmenting skills training with case management.

Engaging Families in Skills-Training Intervention

Research shows that dropout rates are high for externalizing youth and especially for multiproblem families (Johnson, Mellor, & Brann, 2008; Kazdin, 1996). Indeed about half of families enrolled in an intervention for child behavior problems drop out prematurely (Kazdin, 1996; Miller & Prinz, 2003), and rates are higher for low-income, minority families (Fernandez & Eyberg, 2009; Lavigne et al., 2010). Even paying families to show up has limited effect (Dumas et al., 2010).

One reason research-validated programs succeed is that much effort is put into getting families to show up for sessions and to work hard learning the skills. Understanding the engagement process and using best practices for maximizing it are essential components in effectively delivering any intervention.

A central theme of the "Struggling Kids" program is that engagement-related activities must be used throughout the intervention to facilitate both **attendance** (showing up) and

participation (doing the work). This engagement is accomplished by minimizing external barriers/obstacles that might derail the intervention and by using procedures to enhance the parent's and child's internal motivation to successfully complete an intervention. It is important to stress as well that engagement is a **collaborative process** between the family and the practitioner and that facilitating the task of engagement is often revisited throughout the intervention. These fundamental assumptions are at the root of the engagement strategies presented next (see also Bloomquist & Schnell, 2002, and Ingoldsby, 2010, for reviews).

Characteristics of an Engaging Practitioner

The practitioner is obviously a critical variable in the equation for any effective intervention and has much to do with whether or not family members engage. Strong child–practitioner and parent–practitioner alliances are associated with better engagement and positive changes in children, improvements in parenting, fewer barriers perceived by parents, and higher treatment satisfaction (Kazdin, Marciano, & Whitley, 2005; Kazdin & Whitley, 2006; Kazdin, Whitley, & Marciano, 2006). Key ingredients for establishing a good alliance include practitioner attributes such as warmth, authenticity, optimism, and humor. The practitioner also must facilitate alliance building through active listening, collaborating, providing information, and assisting in solving family-identified problems. Finally, practitioner personality characteristics of conscientiousness, agreeableness, low neuroticism, and extraversion are associated with parent and family engagement (Bloomquist et al., 2009; Lochman, Powell, et al., 2009). This suggests that practitioners who are willing to go the extra mile for families, do good work, and present an outgoing and positive tone are best at garnering engagement. The engaging practitioner must also directly tackle the many client variables that impact engagement and respond accordingly with specific engagement-enhancing strategies (described below).

Conceptualizing and Monitoring Engagement

A family's readiness to engage is determined by two family dimensions. One dimension is **family problem severity,** which includes the nature of the child's difficulties, the stress within the parent–child relationship, and the family's day-to-day functioning difficulties (Armbruster & Kazdin, 1994; Bloomquist et al., 2009; Kazdin, 1996; Kazdin, Holland, & Crowley, 1997; Snell-Johns, Mendez, & Smith, 2004). The other dimension is **parent capacity,** which pertains to the parent's thoughts about child, self, and the program; the parent's personal problems, strengths, aptitudes, and motivation; and potential obstacles faced by the parent such as transportation difficulties, limited time, and other life stressors (Hoza et al., 2006; Kazdin, 1996; Mah & Johnston, 2008; Miller & Prinz, 2003; Morrissey-Kane & Prinz, 1999; Nock & Ferriter, 2005; Reyno & McGrath, 2006). Figure 3.1 organizes the family's problem severity and the parent's capacity into four quadrants that point to how much

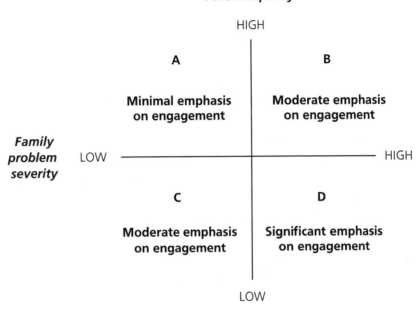

FIGURE 3.1. Family readiness to engage and corresponding emphasis on engagement.

emphasis or effort will be needed from the practitioner to actively engage the family. With an "A" family it is possible to get right in there and begin skills training. The "B" and "C" families may require some effort in engagement before or during skills training. The "D" families require much attention to strategies to enhance their ability to attend and participate (described below).

To monitor engagement and estimate potential progress in skills building, the practitioner should observe the family during training sessions to routinely assess how attentive, cooperative, and involved the child and parent are. The practitioner should also use the strategies and tools in Chapter 4 of this book to determine how much progress the family has made toward any skills-building-related activities between meetings. Any indication of limited participation during meetings and/or little momentum between meetings signals a need to halt direct skills-building activities and refocus on boosting engagement temporarily (see below).

Overcoming Access Barriers and Providing Practical Assistance

A common reason for not attending meetings is that services are not accessible (Kazdin, Holland, Crowley, & Breton, 1997; Lee, August, Bloomquist, Mathy, & Realmuto, 2006; Mendez, Carpenter, LaForett, & Cohen, 2009). Commonsense strategies have been identified to overcome access barriers (Bloomquist, August, Lee, Piehler, & Jensen, 2012; Henggeler, Pickrel, Brondino, & Crouch, 1996; McCay, Stoewe, McCadam, & Gonzales, 1998; Snell-Johns et al., 2004):

- Offering transportation and/or child care (if needed).
- Utilizing flexible scheduling so that services are offered at times convenient for families.
- Using the phone to call or text prior to a session, to call or text after a session, and then as a tool to be available for consultation on an as-needed basis.
- Offering home- and/or community-based services (as opposed to clinic or institutional setting).
- Assisting the family in accessing other practical and needed services (e.g., financial, housing, school-based, medical).

Sharing Information

Making sure the intervention is understood and the family knows the practitioner can be of use right off the bat in promoting attendance and participation (McCay et al., 1998; McCay, Nudelman, McCadam, & Gonzales, 1996). This includes:

- Allowing family members to tell their story.
- Fully explaining and "selling" the intervention to family members, especially the parents.
- Identifying any burdens or barriers that might affect attendance and/or participation and then brainstorming to resolve them.
- Offering practical and concrete information and assistance for any immediate needs or crises.

This method is in line with the suggestion to delay the technical aspects of skills training until the parents have had time to adequately express their concerns (Patterson & Chamberlain, 1994). This information sharing likely creates goodwill and optimistic expectation of positive effects from the training.

Matching Parent Expectations

Since the parent is typically the catalyst for intervention, full engagement also depends on whether the parent's expectations are being met. Procedures for matching the parent's expectations include the following (Bloomquist et al., 2012; Mah & Johnston, 2008; Miller & Prinz, 2003):

- Determining who the parents think is the focus of the intervention and proceeding accordingly. This may mean emphasizing working more with the child (with parent involvement), or the parents, or the family, depending on what the parents want.
- Determining parents' goals and addressing them. Collaborate with parents to understand their preferences for areas of focus and intervention.
- It is worthwhile to specify the length of an intervention. Generally speaking, short-term programs are better for promoting engagement, so it may be wise to break the intervention into small steps. For example, tell the family it is useful to work for six sessions and then evaluate progress to ascertain whether additional meetings are needed.

Modifying Unhelpful Parent Thoughts about the Intervention

The way the parent thinks about an intervention influences how well he or she will engage with it (Hoza et al., 2006; Johnston, Mah, & Regambal, 2010; Mah & Johnston, 2008; Morrissey-Kane & Prinz, 1999; Nock & Ferriter, 2005). Parent cognitions or thoughts that may be related to poor engagement include the following:

- **Parent's attribution about the cause of "the problem":** The parent excessively blames the child, self, or others (teacher, other parent, etc.).
- **Parent–practitioner mismatch in expectations for intervention:** The parent has child-focused expectations (e.g., the parent wants the practitioner to "fix" the child), but the practitioner offers parenting-focused services, or vice versa.
- **Parent acceptance of and motivation about intervention:** The intervention is not thought to be relevant and/or is a low priority for the parent (i.e., the parent doesn't buy into it).
- **External parental locus of control:** The parent views the child's behavior and family circumstances as out of the parent's control and that nothing will help.

These ways of thinking by a parent can be modified by the practitioner. Several informal strategies include the following:

- **Dialoguing about parents' beliefs, attributions, and expectations:** Engage in back-and-forth discussion with the goal of trying to understand the parent's point of view, but also educate the parent about interventions broadly and specific skills-building strategies narrowly.
- **Reframing problems within a child development and/or parent/family well-being context:** Discuss how the child's problems indicate "developmental struggles" in behavioral, social, emotional, and academic development and that the goal is to figure out where the child is struggling and then use skills training to get the child "back on track" and

"successful." Further, discuss how the parent's or the family's problems indicate "stress" and that the goal is to figure out the sources of those stresses and then use skills training to get the parents/family "back on track" and "coping." Explain the central role of the parent in helping a struggling child become more successful and helping a stressed family cope better (see Chapter 4 in this volume for more on this topic).

   • **Reframing problems within an interactional context:** Discuss how the child and parent mutually affect one another and how intervening on either side will change the other.

   • **Reframing solutions as shared responsibility:** Help parents realize that no matter what caused the family's problems in the past, it is likely going to take the whole family working together to produce solutions going forward.

Finally, it can be useful to expose parents to more formal cognitive restructuring activities such as those presented in Chapter 17 of the parent book. This chapter guides parents to evaluate their thoughts and change them to be more "helpful." Included in this discussion are the parents' thoughts related to intervention.

Assisting in the Completion of Homework

Homework is designed to facilitate real-world utilization of the skills being learned in the training context, and its completion indicates a form of engagement. It provides between-session practice and heightens awareness of skills. There is no question about it: Skills training is much more effective if homework is prescribed (Kazantzis, Whittington, & Dattilio, 2010) and if it is actually completed (Kling, Forster, Sundell, & Melin, 2010). Yet surprisingly few child- and family-focused practitioners use this important implementation strategy (Garland, Brookman-Frazee, & Chavira, 2010). The best practice models cited earlier apply different strategies to facilitate this process.

In the "Struggling Kids" program, completion of homework is critical to family members' learning and using new skills. First, **homework assignments need to be very easy to understand and implement**. The information in the parent book and the charts and forms in each chapter there will hopefully assist in the homework process. The chapters and charts/forms provide easy-to-use step-by-step instructions. Second, when homework noncompliance occurs, it is useful to **discuss obstacles interfering with homework completion.** The practitioner and family members could discuss whether or not the chosen skills-building parenting strategy is a good "fit" now that it has been tried. If it still is, then brainstorm strategies to deal with obstacles related to forgetting, not having enough time, feeling discouraged, etc.

Even with practitioner efforts to encourage homework completion, some parents may not do the homework. In that case, pushing it too much might cause them to drop out. It may be that the family is still unsure or unable to use the skill (e.g., time-out or family cool-down), so it is important to check for comprehension of the method and perhaps do modeling and role playing to make sure everyone really knows how to implement the skill. Additionally, it might be effective to allow parents to implement homework more informally, such as setting general goals or implementing skills at their own pace and in their own way. At a minimum, it is a good idea to ask parents to self-evaluate using one of the many *Parent Checklist* forms (at the end of Chapters 4–20 in the parent book) to get a rough idea of skills implementation progress.

Being Sensitive to Cultural Differences

Cultural adaptations might result in better engagement of families with skills-building programs (Dumas, Arriaga, Begle, & Longoria, 2010; Kumpfer & Alvarado, 2003). It is beyond the scope of this practitioner book to thoroughly review concepts and procedures involved in delivery of culturally sensitive services, but several suggestions are offered (Brondino et al., 1997; Castro et al., 2010; Dumas, Arriaga, Begle, & Longoria, 2010; Dumas, Rollock, Prinz, Hops, & Blechman, 1999; Resnicow et al., 2000):

- It is important that practitioners increase their **understanding** of how ethnicity, culture, acculturation, and minority status impact family functioning. Practitioners should also take into account differences in language, information processing, stressors experienced, and help-seeking behaviors of families from different cultural groups.
- Practitioners should encourage parents to make **modifications** of ideas and skills presented to fit their beliefs, values, and goals as shaped by their cultural background. For example, all families value social skills in their children, but there may be subtle differences in exactly what social skills are important for a particular cultural group.
- Interventions might be more effective if **augmentations** are provided in accordance with "racial socialization" practices (Coard et al., 2004). This includes providing an intervention while also assisting children in developing "racial pride," valuing "racial equality," enhancing "racism preparation," and striving for "racial achievement."
- It is important to make necessary **language translations,** especially for new immigrant populations who do not know the English language.
- It is also effective to **reduce practical access barriers** (see earlier section) with culturally diverse families (Morawska et al., 2011).

Making cultural adaptations is a significant step to take because children and families from diverse cultural groups **do** benefit from evidence-based skills training interventions if they engage with them (Huey & Polo, 2008; McCabe & Yeh, 2009).

Using Motivational Enhancement Strategies

The preceding engagement strategies are good ways to encourage a family to show up and to set the stage for them to do some work. Making meaningful changes and progress over the long haul, however, requires motivation. **In the "Struggling Kids" program, all families can benefit from motivational enhancement strategies that incorporate stages of change theory (Prochaska & DiClemente, 1986) and motivational interviewing methods (Miller & Rollnick, 2002).** To briefly summarize, practitioners can use psychoeducation and discussion to facilitate change and to work on motivating the parent and the child individually. The basic idea for getting parents and children (especially teens) motivated is to help them set goals, prioritize what to work on, and commit effort. In addition, with children, a "family teamwork" approach and possibly "jumpstarting" the child's motivation by offering rewards can promote trying new things and cooperating. **Methods for using motivational enhancement methods in a personalized manner for a specific family are elucidated further in Chapter 3 of the parent book and are emphasized in Chapter 4 of this volume.**

Conducting a Functional Assessment and Tailoring Skills

As mentioned in Chapter 1 of this book, children with behavioral–emotional problems are very heterogeneous in their problem presentation, and so it makes sense that interventions be tailored to their unique needs. **Using methods of shared decision making, a functional assessment should be conducted with all families to identify specific areas of focus and to tailor a skills-building plan.** To summarize briefly, the practitioner guides the parent to evaluate his or her child's current functioning in terms of behavioral, social, emotional, and academic development and to consider the degree of well-being in the parent/family. Next the practitioner coaches the parent in selecting responsive choices from intervention options. **How to work through the functional assessment and tailoring process with a family is described in parent book Chapter 2, with a focus on the two worksheets included there (and also at the end of Chapter 4 of this book), and is elaborated on in Chapter 4 of this volume.**

Delivering Skills Training to Individual Families or Parent Groups

Most of the primary models of intervention, as reviewed in Chapter 2 of this volume, provide skills training through 45- to 60-minute individual family or parent group sessions. The one-family-at-a-time delivery allows the practitioner to match skills content to each family's needs and preferences, whereas a parent group may elicit more common themes related to consensus of group members (Bloomquist et al., 2012). The group delivery also promotes emotional support among parents. The practitioner is encouraged to consider these pros and cons when delivering skills-building interventions.

Individual Family Delivery

There is an underlying assumption that the parent and child will be involved one way or another in a skills-training intervention, and perhaps other family members too. There are four ways to configure who is involved and when in family delivery:

Train the Parents, Who Then Train the Child

This entails meeting with the parents to instruct, model, role-play, plan, and so forth. Once the practitioner has trained the parents, the child is invited in to plan and learn skills. The parent-focused approach can be used with all of the "Struggling Kids" modules but is particularly useful when working on the behavioral development module, because the parent is being taught how to "manage" the child's behavior (practitioner book Chapter 5), and is very appropriate for working on the parent well-being module (practitioner book Chapter 9), because the focus is on the parent.

Train the Child and Then Parents to Guide the Child

This involves meeting with the child to instruct, model, role-play, plan, and so forth. After the child has been trained by the practitioner, the parent is invited in to plan and learn skills. This mode of skills training is most applicable when teaching the child skills modules (practitioner book Chapters 6–8), because the child's own personal skills are the focus, and this mode of delivery may be preferred by some teens.

Train All Family Members Simultaneously

The practitioner meets with family members to instruct, model, role-play, plan, and so forth. This delivery strategy can be used with all modules but is especially well suited for the family well-being module (practitioner book Chapter 10). In that module all family members are a focus, so working with them all together usually is the best approach.

Consider Inviting Other Family Members

Generally speaking, siblings who are affected by, or affect, the child in a significant manner and are over the age of about 5 or 6 years can benefit, to varying degrees, from the family sessions. The sibling could learn similar skills, and the parents could guide the child and the sibling together in their application. There may be situations also in which a child spends a lot of time with extended family members (e.g., grandparents). It may be helpful to involve extended family members in the training meetings so that they can better understand the child and be able to guide him or her in skills development.

These methods allow the practitioner to be flexible in accommodating the preferences and expectations of the parents and child (especially teens) about who gets what and when. The practitioner should reflect on the reasons for different configurations, as outlined above, when determining how to involve family members. Of course, it is a good idea to fully explore these options with the family and make adjustments as the intervention unfolds.

Parent Group Delivery

Generally it is best to limit the size of the parent group to the parents of 6–12 children and to have a leader (practitioner) and an optional co-leader (another practitioner or trainee). It is ideal to form groups of parents with children in the same age range: roughly 5–11 and 12–17 (teens). Narrowing the age range further, so that the parents have children roughly within 2–3 years of each other, is even better. The exact skills and related parent book chapters presented can be predetermined by the practitioner or determined by group consensus (this approach is elaborated on in Chapter 4 of this book). The notion of providing emotional support for parents cannot be overemphasized in group delivery. Although most of each group session is focused on education and skill acquisition, it is imperative to leave enough time for the parents to discuss their own individual concerns and problems. Many parents comment that the emotional support they receive as part of the group experience is very important and helpful to them.

It is essential to promote a group climate of trust and open dialogue by describing the purpose of the group and some ground rules up front and then reviewing them periodically. Clearly state the *purpose* of the parent group by noting that the group provides a forum in which to discuss parenting challenges, obtain support from other parents, and brainstorm ideas for parenting, and that useful strategies from the "Struggling Kids" program will be taught. It is also important to establish **rules,** including mandating confidentiality about other families' problems, and to suggest that parents be respectful of one another's opinions and take a positive attitude by focusing on solutions to problems rather than just complaining about them. Practitioners are wise to encourage, but not require, parents to talk.

One way to present parent group meetings is as one part of "family nights" event. During these family nights, families come to a center or school to share challenges and successes, support each other, and have fun. The family nights are 90 minutes long: a 15-minute assembly of parents and children with snacks, a 60-minute parent group (with corresponding 60-minute fun, adult-supervised child activity), and a 15-minute parent–child activity at the end of the evening. A recent study with low-income families of early-elementary-age children found that parent-focused skills and support strategies delivered in groups via family nights at a local community center achieved better parent attendance than the same services provided individually with families primarily in their homes (Bloomquist et al., 2012).

Techniques for Delivering Interventions

This section touches on various technical methods for presenting information and training children and parents in skills development. These are practical considerations and strategies that are applicable to every family.

Frequency and Length of Meetings

The research-validated models introduced in Chapter 2 vary in the number of sessions offered and the length of the intervention, though 10–18 sessions seem to be typical (and should vary depending on the family's needs). When working with individual families, it is best to divide the intervention into phases, such as:

- **Intensive phase:** Meet regularly to get things going (six to eight hour-long sessions), and then evaluate progress. Be sure to continue intensive training, if progress is insufficient. The goal is to initially train the skills.
- **Maintenance phase:** Spread out meetings, perhaps at a rate of every other week, and then once per month (four to eight more hour-long sessions). The goal is to maintain the skills and incorporate them into daily family life.
- **Relapse prevention phase:** Meet in several months (make reminder call) and/or be available, as needed, if relapses occur. The goal is to reduce the likelihood that the family will stop using the skills and that problems will reemerge.

The number of sessions in the three phases will vary from family to family. Parents can read about the phases in Chapter 2 of the parent handbook. When working with parent groups, it is wise to provide the 10–18 sessions and then see if more may be needed afterward.

The time allowed for training in specific skills should be tailored to suit each family's needs, but the following broad guidelines are based on a reading of the literature and many years of experience:

- Typically three to six parent book chapters (give or take) are targeted during a round of 10–18 hour-long sessions with the average family. Sometimes only certain skills or sections of chapters are selected, based on needs and preferences of the family.

- It generally takes one or two hour-long sessions to review skills-building strategies within a chapter and provide initial training for a family with a younger child.
- It generally takes two or three hour-long sessions to review skills-building strategies within a chapter and provide initial training for a family with an older child or teen. This extra time is needed because the sections in chapters for older children incorporate more advanced skills.
- It generally takes several more sessions to check progress on skills-building strategies trained earlier. This phase allows for problem solving around internal and external obstacles and barriers to implementation and strategizing to avoid relapses.

Conveying Skills-Building Content

Ideally, the parent chapter selected during the functional assessment and tailoring procedure would be discussed in a session after the parent has read it. The practitioner could also **didactically present the skills-building strategy** while the parent (and sometimes the child) looks at the parent's book or a copy of a specific chart from selected chapters.

When a skill area is introduced, it can be very helpful to refer to the *Parent Checklist* form for a specified chapter (located in Chapters 4–20 in the parent book and at the end of Chapters 5–10 in this book as well). These charts simultaneously ask parents to reflect on key elements of that particular area of skills building and offer a succinct overview of what is involved. Once fully explained and reviewed, it is a good idea to dialogue with parents about their beliefs, attributions, and expectations and whether chosen skills-building strategies will address their concerns about their child. Ask parents something like "Is this what you were looking for?" or "Is this meeting your needs and expectations?"

The practitioner will have to make a judgment based on the child's age and overall cooperation with the intervention to determine whether he or she should be included in a discussion of the chapter or method. Younger children and/or uncooperative children might not profit from review and planning of skills. Additionally, some modules are less appropriate for the child than others. For example, when reviewing the behavioral development module (parent book Chapters 4–7), it may be better to leave the child out of the initial discussion and planning because that module is about behavioral management **of** the child, not building skills **with** the child. Likewise it may be counterindicated to have the child participate in discussions centering on the parent well-being module (parent book Chapters 17 & 18), which focuses on the parents' personal functioning. It is more relevant for the child to participate in discussions of the child skills-building book chapters (parent book Chapters 8–16) and the family-focused chapters (parent book Chapters 19 & 20) in which the child is directly involved. When younger children are included, it is best to convey information via the forms at the end of the chapters. **The practitioner and parents should collaboratively decide whether the child should be present for the information-oriented discussion.**

Adaptations to this procedure have to be made for parents who have limited reading ability. In this case the practitioner could use verbal description and/or emphasize the visually oriented handouts found at the end of many chapters. These forms are, for the most part, fairly easy to comprehend and could be used with less-educated or non-English-speaking parents.

Facilitating Learning and Performing of Skills-Building Strategies

The goal is to advance from a cognitive understanding of the skills to actually applying them. This is usually first accomplished via behavioral rehearsal. The main ingredients of behavioral rehearsal include the practitioner physically modeling the skill, the parent and/or child physically performing and practicing the skill via simulated role playing, and the parent and/or child reflecting and planning on how to use the skill later. Behavioral rehearsal is critical in going from knowledge to action in terms of skills development, and it is a common element used in the delivery of youth- and parent-focused skills-building interventions (Garland, Hawley, Brookman-Fraze, & Hurlburt, 2008).

Sanders, Markie-Dadds, and Turner (2000) provide a good summary of the steps of behavioral rehearsal. These are adapted below as suggested guidelines within the "Struggling Kids" program:

1. Prepare the client and give a rationale ("How about doing some role playing to practice?" "It helps to really learn this if you practice," etc.).
2. Set the scene by eliciting a situation at home, school, with peers, etc., and assigning roles in order to practice a specific skill (e.g., time-out or helpful thinking). This could be a situation derived from the parent and/or child. There are also numerous role-play practice exercises throughout the parent book that can be replicated in sessions. This step could entail discussing or writing a script of the event, that is, what people should say and do.
3. **Model the skill** for the parent and/or child (e.g., time-out or helpful thinking). Usually this involves the practitioner acting as a parent and parent as a child or practitioner as a child and child as a parent or sibling or peer. This can involve any configuration of people in the child's life with the practitioner in the lead role.
4. After modeling, self-evaluate your use of skills for the parent and/or child to see, in order to promote more awareness ("I think I did okay on . . . , but I need to keep working at . . . " "I need to be clearer when I say . . . , " etc.).
5. Check in with the parent and/or child for their reactions and thoughts so far about the skill being rehearsed ("What do you think went okay or not so okay?" "Do you have any questions?" "Do you think you could do that?" "Would you do it any differently?").

6. All participants swap roles and reset the scene (as in step 2 above). Now the parent and/or child is in the lead role as himself or herself.
7. **Guide the parent and/or child to practice the skill** by saying and doing what you said and did in step 3 above (with modifications as determined in step 5 above) using the role-playing method.
8. Prompt the parent and/or child to self-evaluate like you did in step 4 above ("I think I did okay on . . . " "I need to keep working at . . . , " etc.).
9. Guide the parent and/or child to set goals for the next practice and/or for when the skills will be used ("When and where will you practice next?" "Are you ready to try it at home, and if so when?" etc.).

It is a good idea to continue behavioral rehearsal until mastery is achieved. This may take a session or two to accomplish with a particular skill (e.g., time-out or helpful thinking). Usually it is best to recommend using the skills in "real life" only after the parent and/or child are proficient in the training setting.

As an aside, it is not a good idea to require anyone to do role playing if that person is uncomfortable with it or uncooperative. In those cases the practitioner should emphasize modeling of the skills. Sometimes it can be useful to reward a child to motivate him or her to participate in role-play exercises (see parent book Chapter 3 and Chapter 4 of this volume for more ideas on motivation).

Facilitating Generalization and Maintenance of Skills

The next step is to get the parents and child to apply the skills in day-to-day life in their homes, in public, and then to keep it going! Give parents and child specific **homework** assignments to use a corresponding form or chart from a parent book chapter at home. **Graduated homework assignments** can be used to ensure mastery of skills use in real-life circumstances. A three-step process is advised:

1. Ask the family to first replicate role plays done in the training sessions at home to further practice the skill and aid in transfer to the home context (e.g., practice time-out or family cool-down at home with simulated problems just like in training session).
2. Instruct the family to use the skill with a "live" or "in-the-moment" problem at home (e.g., use time-out or family cool-down with real problems at home).
3. Once family members have mastered a skill at home, they can attempt it in public (i.e., the family must be fully proficient with time-out or family cool-down at home before using it in public).

It is also important for parents to prompt, reinforce, and guide the child in using the skill at each of the junctures above. Determine whether the child needs a reward to jump-start motivation to try a strategy at home (see parent book Chapter 3 for ideas).

It is a good idea to dialogue with parents about taking a "long view" in terms of their expectations, noting that progress is typically slow and gradual. Inform parents that it may be necessary to keep using new skills for many weeks, and sometimes months, before progress is seen. It is imperative that parents understand that their progress depends largely on their long-term effort.

It is helpful to include ongoing assessment or ratings of progress over the course of intervention and to provide feedback to parents and plan so that adjustments can be made (Chorpita et al., 2010; Shimokawa, Lambert, & Smart, 2010). Questioning parents about their between-sessions effort increases their follow-through and adherence to the skills they are working on, which in turn leads to better outcomes (Springer & Reddy, 2010). It is also quite useful to help parents and children set goals and measure progress toward attainment. Research shows that skills training that includes a goal attainment method is effective with children (Lochman, Curry, Burch, & Lampron, 1984), adults (LaFerriere & Calsy, 1978), and families (Woodward, Santa-Barbara, Levin, & Epstein, 1978). Procedures for progress monitoring, including goal setting and attainment, are described in Chapter 4 of this volume.

Keeping It Going and Spotting the Signs of Relapse

After a parent and child are trained in skills from parent book Chapters 4–20, it is very important for the parent to periodically review the chapter-specific *Parent Checklists.* Each checklist summarizes the essential methods of the skills in that chapter and can serve as a reminder for the parent.

Another method for keeping it going is to episodically review progress on goals. The *Parenting Goals* form and the *Personal Goals (Basic* or *Advanced)* (described in parent book Chapter 3 and also included at the end of Chapter 4 in this book) allow the parent and older child or teen to set and monitor progress on unique goals. These goals may be related to one skill within a specific parent book chapter or several skills that cut across the skills in parent book Chapters 4–20.

Another valuable way to monitor progress and refine methods is for the parent to conduct occasional **10-minute family meetings** (see parent book Chapter 2 and the sidebar on page 52) at home to review skills. During these meetings the parent should focus on the central themes of the child's and parent's use of specified skills and note efforts toward reaching goals. The parent should encourage the child to keep it going.

It is also helpful to review how to recognize the signs of relapse. Inform the parent that if the original problem(s) resurfaces, the parent should review the specific *Parent Checklist* and the relevant chapter in the parent book as a refresher to get back on track with the strategies.

10-MINUTE FAMILY MEETINGS

A helpful, informal way for parents to monitor progress is to conduct occasional 10-minute family meetings at home. During those 10 minutes, parents review how it's going and troubleshoot any problems that are emerging in using skills-building strategies. Sometimes they will conclude that it would be helpful to do goal setting and more role-play practicing. Emphasize to parents that they keep the meetings positive, review successes more than problems, and be sure to close after 10 minutes (perhaps using a timer). Stress the importance of preparation so that the family can focus on the most important topics and get the child's input for the agenda. These meetings should occur fairly often when the family is getting started and then less frequently once family members are making some progress. Siblings can be involved if they are viewed as part of the problem or if impacted by the child in some way.

TIPS FOR SMOOTH AND SUCCESSFUL SKILLS TRAINING

- Be prepared. The practitioner must be proficient in all parent book chapters to be responsive to the immediate needs and/or preferences of family.
- Use verbal statements and nonverbal gestures (e.g., nodding, eye contact) to reinforce family members' ideas, comments, questions, etc.
- Avoid giving advice and/or directly recommending what family members should do. Instead ask guiding questions to help parents and family members "discover" what they want to work on and the solutions they are seeking.
- Occasionally pause to summarize and/or assess comprehension. Then allow for questions and discussion from the family.
- Make the sessions enjoyable. Use the fun modeling and role-playing exercises that are described throughout the parent and practitioner book chapters.
- Display enthusiasm and a good sense of humor.

Augmenting Skills Training with Case Management

Although the main focus of the "Struggling Kids" protocol is skills building, it is certainly the case that most families require much more than skills training. Indeed the point was made in Chapter 2 that a multicomponent intervention is likely required for many families.

Therefore the practitioner must always be responsive to other needs of the child and/or family. Children and/or family members may need extra help in the domains of child health, child mental health, child school, parent health, parent mental health, and/or basic family needs (e.g., housing, child care, employment assistance), to name just a few. The practitioner should always be cognizant of other needs and provide support and case management to help the family in finding and accessing other needed services.

4

Using the Getting Started and Staying with It Module

This practitioner book chapter corresponds to the parent book section "Getting Started and Staying with It" (Chapters 1–3). The practitioner can use this module to educate the parent about common child and family challenges, enhance motivation of the child and family, form a base for continuing collaboration, and lay a foundation for the parent to effectively implement and use the skills-building strategies. The goal is to help the parent get started and then stay with it for the long haul so that meaningful improvements can be made by the child and family. The ideas and techniques discussed here are often the focus of the first few sessions or meetings, but they are also frequently revisited as the intervention unfolds. **The practitioner should read and fully understand the *content* in parent book Chapters 1–3 before reading and then using the related *procedures* described in this chapter.**

The parent book chapters contained in this module are information focused and need to be reviewed didactically with parents. Sometimes a child can also benefit from this information, depending on his or her age, maturity, and receptivity. Generally children who are at least of elementary school age and are open-minded about meeting with the practitioner can benefit. On the other hand, if a child is very young and/or resistant, it may be fruitful to gear this discussion to the parent only. It is a good idea to collaborate with the parent about whether or not the child should participate in these preliminary discussions.

Overview of the Getting Started and Staying with It Module

The *Overview of the Getting Started and Staying with It Module* chart at the end of this chapter provides a succinct review of the ideas and methods contained in this module. This chart can be used to provide psychoeducation to a parent regarding the challenges of parenting and the "big picture" of what it will take to turn things around through skills building. Verbally summarize each point and note that you will discuss each chapter in greater detail as your work together progresses. Encourage the parent to read all three chapters in the "Getting Started and Staying with It" module. **Note that Chapter 3, on motivation and follow-through, is perhaps the most important chapter in the book since nothing will be gained if the parents don't stick with the program.** Explain to the parent how easy it is to start out motivated but then to lose focus, interest, or commitment. Comparing this work to common adult efforts toward change such as losing weight, quitting smoking, or beginning to exercise can help parents see how easy it is to let efforts slide without making them defensive.

Specific Procedures for Applying Parent Book Chapter 1

This chapter educates the parent about the nature of the child's problems and developmental struggles as well as parent and family stresses. The goals are to get parents to (1) think of their child's behavioral–emotional problems as struggles in psychological development and their parenting and familywide concerns as signs that their own personal well-being or that of their family is not what it should be, and (2) view the skills-building approach as useful in helping their child succeed and the parent/family to better cope.

> **Note.** *The forms and charts referred to in the discussion below are in parent book Chapter 1 and also at the end of this chapter unless otherwise noted.*

Discussing the Child's Behavioral–Emotional Problems

The child's difficulties should be described as observable problematic behaviors that parents can relate to in their day-to-day experiences with their child. Note that the characteristics listed in parent book Chapter 1 are often targeted in skills training. The purpose of this review is to acknowledge the struggles the parents are witnessing every day, problems that are not only impairing the child's functioning but are often also creating problems for the whole family. Don't spend too long discussing these behaviors and characteristics, however. Tell the parents that this is a good beginning, but steer the discussion to translating behaviors into developmental delays that fall into certain categories so the parents start to build a foundation from which they can develop a specific plan of action for the child and family (that plan is presented in parent book Chapter 2).

Discussing the Child's Developmental Status

The parents may have an idea that the child is not keeping up or is behind children of the same age, either from their own observations or because a teacher or other adult working with the child has said the child seems to be behind. It is important to refine the parent's knowledge of the child's development so that specific skills-building strategies can later be identified to get the struggling child back on track. Tell the parent that thinking of the child's problems from a developmental point of view lends itself to a plan of action to improve the child's developmental status. Sum up the four primary domains of psychological development in general terms:

- **Child behavioral development:** Learning to follow reasonable external directions and rules and internalizing an honest code of conduct
- **Child social development:** Bonding with others and learning social skills
- **Child emotional development:** Learning to understand/express feelings, think rational or helpful thoughts, and regulate stress-related emotions
- **Child academic development:** Learning self-directed academic behaviors and pursuing educational opportunities

Then refer to the *Child Psychological Development* chart to review details about these areas of development. Explain that children's behavioral–emotional problems can be thought of as "struggles" in development. In other words the descriptors of a struggling child on the chart are indicators of the child being "behind" in these areas. Ask the parents to think about whether their child is struggling or successful in each of these areas. Suggest that it is possible to teach the child skills to get him or her back on track—which is a primary objective of the "Struggling Kids" program.

Discussing the Parent(s) and Family's Well-Being Status

Most parents readily acknowledge that problems of the whole family affect how an individual child is doing. Explain that the family's well-being can be viewed as having two domains:

1. **Parent well-being:** Parent(s) personal functioning
2. **Family well-being:** Family relationship functioning

Use the *Parent and Family Well-Being* chart to illustrate specific aspects of well-beingness in these domains. Note that some children's struggles are related to the well-being or functioning of the parent and family. This can be a sensitive issue, so tact is sometimes needed to help a parent see how the well-being of the parent and family might need to be a focus. For example, ask the parent if any of the bulleted items on the "Stressed" side of the chart might apply to him or her or the family. For any item the parent endorses, ask what effect, if any, it has on the child. If "Overwhelmed with everyday challenges and problems" and "Distant parent–child relationship" are endorsed, for example, then inquire whether or not, and how, these could impact parenting. Then discuss how this impact on parenting might, in turn, impact the child's behavior or mood, ability to concentrate and learn, etc. Note that it is possible to teach the parents and/or family some skills to reduce stress and improve coping. Learning these skills will also have the extra benefit of helping the child get back on track.

Note: *The **Parent Stress Cycle** chart in parent book Chapter 18 (which also appears at the end of Chapter 9 in this book) can also be used as a psychoeducation tool to help parents understand how their own stress affects parenting.*

Discussing the Power of Protective Factors

Even with a sympathetic, respectful, optimistic practitioner on hand to help, parents seeking assistance for their child and family often feel discouraged, even hopeless. This is a good time to review the protective factors found at the end of Chapter 1 of the parent book and at the end of this chapter. Frame the skills-building approach as one way to build protective factors that will help the child in the long run. Also discuss the child's already existing protective factors from the chart and note that those also bode well for the child's future.

Specific Procedures for Applying Parent Book Chapter 2

Parent book Chapter 2 familiarizes parents with specific intervention targets and helps them collaborate with the practitioner to create a plan that is best for the child and family. The main goals are for the parent to (1) pinpoint the most pressing specific child struggles and parent/family stressors, (2) select corresponding skills-building chapters to address identified areas of concern, and (3) understand the basic ideas and methods of the skills-building approach. This process enables the parent and practitioner to tailor the skills-building effort for that particular family. The skills-building plan for the family is not etched in stone, however, and can be revisited and revised as needed.

Note: *The forms and charts referred to in the discussion below are in parent book Chapter 2 and also at the end of this chapter unless otherwise noted.*

Conducting a Functional Assessment and Tailoring Skills Training

The functional assessment and tailoring of skills training are best conducted within the context of meetings as the practitioner assesses the child and family and then leads the parent to make informed decisions. Similar procedures have been used with families seeking services for youth with behavioral–emotional problems. For example, a "family checkup" (Dishion & Stormshak, 2007; Stormshak & Dishion, 2009) involves meeting with the family to gather information, collaborate, and develop a tailored intervention plan for the family. The meetings focus on assessing family members, discussing goals and concerns with them (especially parents), providing feedback about the practitioner's impression of the family, and discussing options from a menu of family-based interventions. The notion of assessing each child/family and personalizing a plan is also applied in the "Struggling Kids" program.

The functional assessment and tailoring process are also greatly enhanced by the use of **decision aids,** or strategies, that empower the parent to make informed choices about intervention options that fit within his or her views, values, and preferences (Wills & Holmes-Rovner, 2006). Such decision aids facilitate a process of shared decision making as the practitioner provides information and then coaches the parent in making informed choices.

Getting to Know the Family

The practitioner should first meet with and get to know the child and family. This can include a formal diagnostic assessment if the family and/or practitioner is unclear about the specific nature of the child's mental health status (which is beyond the scope of this book), but minimally involves getting acquainted with the family and ascertaining their challenges. The ***Getting to Know You*** form at the end of this chapter can be used to conduct a very basic assessment for the purpose of intervention planning (it is not sufficient for diagnostic assessment). The practitioner simply asks the questions on the form in a semistructured interview. Building rapport and simultaneously getting to know the family, especially from the parent's point of view, enables the practitioner and the parent to put strengths and concerns on the table and begin considering goals to work on.

Leading the Parent to Pinpoint Areas of Focus

After getting to know the family, the practitioner can use the ***Examining How Your Child and Family Are Doing*** form as a decision aid to help the parent better understand the challenges for the child and family. Ask the parent to provide an impression about the child and family from a developmental and well-being perspective, respectively, using the following procedure:

1. Take a few minutes to review the four different areas of child development and the two areas of parent/family well-being.
2. Suggest that the parents consider similar-age children when thinking about their child's development and that some children are behind their peers.
3. Make an observation that how the parent and family are doing also impacts the child. Ask the parents if they agree and if they have any examples.
4. Indicate that some children struggle in multiple areas and that improvement in one area of development might be related to progress in other areas.
5. Make sure that parents understand the 1–6 rating format that indicates **struggling, in progress,** and **successful** for the child; and **stressed, in progress,** and **coping** for the parent/family.

6. Ask the parents to score each area of child development and parent/family well-being and, if possible, to identify specific examples of behaviors from the chart. Offer your input based on what you know about the child and family.
7. Ask the parents to rank-order the child and parent/family areas so that they can focus on one or two areas. Offer your input about which areas might be the best.
8. Answer all questions about development and parent/family well-being.
9. Ask the parents if they would like to work on the areas identified.

The parents should be advised that those areas of focus at **1, 2,** and **3** warrant attention and those at **4, 5,** and **6** might also profit from some "preventive" intervention to give the child a boost to stay on course.

Sometimes parents cannot agree, or they rank multiple areas of child and/or parent/family functioning as significant. When this occurs, keep discussing the issues until the parents can "funnel it down" to a starting place. Explain that by working on **one area of focus,** the chances are good that others may also improve. Subsequently, the child's problems should be framed as **developmental struggles,** and the parents' or family's problems as **difficulties in coping with stress.** The next step is to select corresponding chapters to facilitate any areas of child and parent/family functioning that were identified.

Leading the Parent to Select Skills-Building Strategies

The *Selecting Skills-Building Strategies to Work On* form gives the parent a menu of skills-building options from which to choose. This form summarizes what is described in greater detail in the text of parent book Chapter 2; if the parent seems confused or asks questions about specific skills-building interventions, it can be useful to review the descriptions and related skills-building strategies in that chapter. Collaborate with the parent in choosing chapters that correspond with concerns derived from the discussion of child development and parent/family well-being using the following procedure:

1. Explain that the same six areas on the ***Examining How Your Child and Family Are Doing*** form are also represented on the ***Selecting Skills-Building Strategies to Work On*** form, but the focus now is on selecting skills-building methods to promote child development and parent/family well-being.
2. Ask the parents to concentrate on the sections that correspond to concerns identified earlier (e.g., if child behavioral development was a concern, then they should focus on strategies under the "Enhancing Your Child's Behavioral Development" domain).
3. It can be useful to frame each of the six skills-building areas as a toolbox and the corresponding chapters as tools within the toolbox. The goal in using the tools in each toolbox is to "build" a successful child and a better-coping parent/family.
4. Help the parent narrow his or her focus to one or two skills-building strategies as a starting point.

Ask the parents if they have a better understanding of what areas to focus on and whether the chosen skills-building strategies will help them. As the practitioner, you too can add your observations and inquire about areas to work on that the parents may not have identified. Keep the discussion going until a plan has been identified.

Inevitably, some parents will want to work on multiple chapters. When this happens, the practitioner needs to lead the parent in the right direction through very careful discussion weighing all of the pros and cons. Tell the parent it is best to begin with one or two chapters. Other concerns and corresponding chapters can be focused on later.

At the end of this selection process a broad plan of action should be developed. For example, a parent may be initially most concerned about the child's behavior and select to work on "Doing What You're Told: Teaching Your Child to Comply with Parental Directives," "Doing What's Expected: Teaching Your Child to Follow Rules," and "Staying Cool under Fire: Managing Your Child's Protesting of Discipline and Preventing Angry Outbursts." Because this parent gets so frustrated with the child, the practitioner might also steer him or her to consider focusing on "Cool Parents: Managing Your Own Stress to Enhance Parenting." The parent and practitioner then may also decide that it would be fruitful to eventually work on "Surviving School: Teaching Your Child to Manage Time, Organize, Plan, Review, and Stay on Task" because homework is a frequent trigger for the child's noncompliance and the parent's frustration.

Enhancing Parent Knowledge of the Skills-Building Method

This section of parent book Chapter 2 is essentially about psychoeducation. It involves explaining the fundamentals of the skills-building method. First the "P's to success" (similar to the "keys to success") should be presented to let parents know the "how to" of learning and using new skills. A discussion of the "Phases of Skills Building" should follow to let the parent know how skills building typically unfolds over time. Review the four P's with the parent. Explain that **preparing** entails obtaining knowledge about the skill(s) and planning how the skill(s) will be learned and used. Encourage the parent to read any chapter that corresponds with a chosen skills-building strategy to acquire important information, and suggest that you will assist the parent in coming up with a plan for learning and implementing the new skills.

Note that **practicing** involves physically performing new skills, which usually requires modeling and role playing first. Tell the parent you will guide the family to participate in role-play exercises for any chosen skills-building strategy (see Chapter 3 of this volume for more on behavioral rehearsal). Suggest too that the family consider doing the same role plays at home to make the practice more realistic.

Monitoring progress is consistently shown to be associated with better outcomes in skills-building interventions (Chorpita et al., 2010; Shimokawa et al., 2010; Simpson et al., 2010; Springer & Reddy, 2010), and therefore it should be a major emphasis for the practitioner. Tell the parent that **progress monitoring** involves helping parents periodically review how it's going in implementing skills-building methods and making adjustments. Tell the parents that they have a choice of two monitoring routes offered in the parent book: using the specific *Parent Checklist* forms that correspond to chosen skills **within a parent book chapter** or using the *Parenting Goals* form (found in parent book Chapter 3 and also at the end of this chapter) **to work on specific skills within or across parent book chapters.** In addition, inform parents that it is good to periodically review the *Examining How Your Child and Family Are Doing* form (found in parent book Chapter 3 and at the end of this chapter) to monitor progress of the child's and family's functioning. Tell parents you will help them choose a progress-monitoring method once you get to that point.

Finally, advise parents that real progress typically occurs only through persistent and consistent application of the skills. In the "Struggling Kids" program this is framed as "**PER-CONing**" (i.e., **PER**sistent and **CON**sistent effort). Note that persistence is about using skills over weeks or months and that consistence is about applying the skills the same way each time. Help parents understand that development takes time (hence, need for persistence) and that repetition is best to learn a new skill (hence, importance of consistence). Perhaps analogize that if one begins an exercise and diet program, it can take a while for noticeable changes to be observed.

Explain what happens during the three phases of skills building and why skills building usually transpires in phases: that the initial focused work during the 4- to 8-week "**intensive phase**" is critical to building a solid foundation, that sticking with it during the "**maintenance phase**" will ingrain the skills, and that the "**relapse-prevention phase**" protects against the backsliding that is somewhat common over time. Stress that these three different types of effort are important, and this is why skills building takes 10–18 weeks.

The "P's" and the "phases" should be introduced early on and referred to now and then to promote parent adherence and follow-through with the skills-building methods. As you can imagine, the "P's," although essential, are very difficult for parents to adhere to over all three phases, so reinforcement is crucial. Each later parent book chapter discussed in this book also has specific ideas and examples of how to do the "P's" for each skill in the "Struggling Kids" program.

Specific Procedures for Applying Parent Book Chapter 3

In Chapter 3 of the parent book, goal setting, motivational, and progress monitoring themes are highlighted. It is helpful to review the *Parent Checklist for Getting Going and Following Through* to begin a discussion. It is not the intent that a parent (or practitioner, by extension) do everything in this parent book chapter. Rather, the ideas and techniques could be considered for a family as needed. It is helpful to recall Figure 3.1 in this book (p. 39), which presented a conceptualization of family readiness to engage and corresponding emphasis on engagement. **In terms of using techniques like those in parent book Chapter 3, the "A" families would not need much assistance, the "B" and "C" families might benefit from some, and the "D" families would need the most (along with other engagement methods described in practitioner book Chapter 3).** The practitioner has to collaborate with the family and use judgment to determine how much and which methods from parent book Chapter 3 might be used and then guide the family accordingly.

Note: *The forms and charts referred to in the discussion below are in parent book Chapter 3 and also at the end of this chapter unless otherwise noted.*

Discussing Stages of Change with Parents

Once some skills-building goals have been identified, the best way to begin to work on them is to figure out how ready the family is to make changes in this area. The parent book sums up the five stages that many people go through as they are making changes (Prochaska & DiClemente, 1986) and includes a *Determining Stages of Change* form that parents can fill out as they decide where they are on the readiness-for-change continuum. The discussion of readiness for change is mostly directed to the parent but can involve an older child or teenager if indicated.

First choose a specific problem area and a corresponding goal (from the parents' work in Chapter 2). An example might be child arguments/fighting with a sibling and using the parent-guided social problem solving for sibling conflict mediation in parent book Chapter 9. Then determine the stage of change the parent and family members are at, as it relates to the specified problem area and goal. This process can be repeated with other problems and goals later.

Make sure that the parents have read the description of the stages of change in the parent book. Then, to lead the discussion, sum up each stage, ask which family members might be at that stage, and lead the discussion to move individuals to the next stage, as needed:

Precontemplation (Not Ready for Change)

- Explain that someone in this stage is vaguely aware of a problem or only has an inkling of a need to change.
- Ask who in the family might be at this stage.
- Promote more awareness of problems and challenges to move a parent and/or family member to the contemplation stage. This might entail asking questions or prompting family members to give each other constructive feedback. It is sometimes helpful to revisit the *Examining How Your Child and Family Are Doing* form in parent book Chapter 2 (and also at the end of this chapter) to facilitate further discussion of the problems and challenges.

Contemplation (Getting Ready for Change)

- Explain that a person in this stage is beginning to think that it might be a good idea to make some changes but does not have a specific plan or goal.
- Ask who in the family might be at this stage.
- Examine the pros (benefits) and cons (challenges) of making changes to move to the preparation stage.

Preparation (Ready for Change)

- Explain that a person in this stage has the desire to make changes, has come up with a specific plan, and has articulated some goals.
- Ask who in the family might be at this stage.
- Brainstorm ideas for implementing a plan to get to the action stage. It can be useful to review obstacles/barriers and the parent's priorities for other activities that might interfere with carrying out a plan.

Action (Making Change)

- Explain that a person in this stage is actively working on implementing a plan and is also actively monitoring progress toward goals.
- Ask who in the family might be at this stage.
- Brainstorm ideas to help the parent monitor progress and to be persistent and consistent in using skills-building strategies.
- It can be useful to review obstacles/barriers and the parent's priorities for other activities that might interfere with keeping the plan going long enough to get to the maintenance stage.

Maintenance (Keeping Change)

- Explain that a person in this stage has more or less achieved his or her goals and is doing well over the long term.
- Here the discussion should center on avoiding relapses. At this point it is useful to identify the "signals" that indicate backsliding, such as problems within the child or parent/family reemerging, as before.
- Ask who in the family might be at this stage.
- Brainstorm ideas to help the parent and family get back on track if there should be a relapse.

Explain that a shift to the preparatory or action stage must be accomplished in order to begin making progress. **Keep the discussions going until the parent and/or other family**

members are at the preparation stage or better. Additional strategies in this chapter, designed to motivate the parent and/or child, can also be used to promote progress in the stages of change.

Getting a Parent Going and Following Through

The section in Chapter 3 devoted to motivating the parent is informed by motivational interviewing methods that center on the practitioner's using effective communication and collaboration to facilitate change (Miller & Rollnick, 2002). Key points derived from motivational interviewing methods that are helpful when working with the parent include the following:

- Conveying empathy and positive regard by consistently inquiring how things are going and praising the parent's effort in a nonpatronizing manner.
- Asking open-ended questions to guide the parent in figuring out what to work on.
- Listening and then paraphrasing back to the parent what he or she said.
- Eliciting self-motivational statements from the parent by asking him or her to formulate goals and describe their importance.
- Using collaborative problem solving by working with the parent to define problems and articulate solutions for them.
- Avoiding direct or inadvertent blaming and confronting of the parent.

Typically the parent is at least somewhat motivated to work on goals, since more often than not, the parent initiated contact with the practitioner for this purpose. Coming in for help, however, is only the beginning, and this must be followed by actually doing some work to make progress. Therefore, some examination of the parent's priorities and ability to make a commitment to a skills-building strategy is often necessary and useful. If the parent is truly unmotivated, then it could be helpful to emphasize the stages of change methods above.

Assisting the Parent in Goal Setting

Guide the parent to identify specific target areas and corresponding skills-training strategies (e.g., child noncompliance and protesting/outbursts and using time-out and patient standoff; see parent book Chapters 4 and 7). Then the parent could declare specific goals related to his or her intentions. **Make sure that the parent verbalizes goals that are *dos*, such as "Give effective commands" or "Use brief statements in discussions with [teen]"and not *don'ts*, such as "Stop nagging [son] to comply" or "Quit the long lectures with [teen]."** That way the parent will know what to **do** to replace old unproductive behaviors while working toward using new parenting behaviors. It is helpful to review the stages of change and/or use motivational interviewing procedures, as described above, to help a parent who is having difficulty setting specific goals.

Assisting the Parent in Prioritizing and Making a Commitment

Next ask the parent to denote on a scale of 1 (not important) to 10 (very important) how much of a **priority** it is to work on the proposed skills-related goal(s). Ideally, this rating would be at a **7** or higher, indicating that it is a priority. If not, then further discussion with the parent is needed. The parent has to decide whether this is a priority over other pressing priorities. Tell the parent that skills-building goals that are a high priority lead to the parent's taking action, which leads to child and family progress.

Finally, ask the parent to **pledge effort** (or make a commitment) on a scale of 1 (little effort) to 10 (lots of effort) as to how hard he or she intends to work on a particular skills-building goal. Again it would be ideal for the parent to pledge a level of effort at a **7** or higher, indicating a high level of commitment. If the rating is not a **7** or higher, the practitioner should continue to review concerns and skills-building options until it is. If there is more than one parent, it is important to make sure they are equally motivated. If they are not, keep discussing it until that is achieved. It is a good idea to return to a discussion of the stages of change and/or use motivational interviewing methods to help a "stuck" parent who has difficulty committing effort.

Assisting the Parent in Monitoring Progress on Goals

The parent can informally or formally track progress on goals in the coming days and weeks. The informal process involves verbally reporting in on how it is going in terms of working on previously declared goals. Be sure to assist the parent in recalling precisely what the goal was and ask for examples of progress. This request for specifics will hold the parent more accountable and help him or her to really focus on the identified goal(s).

Of course, formal tracking is preferred, but practical matters need to be considered and discussed (e.g., Is the parent interested?, Does he or she have time?, Will he or she likely remember or follow through?). The *Parenting Goals* form can be used if a parent is interested in a more formalized method of tracking progress. The form can be filled out and just looked at now and then to gauge progress, or copies could be made and filled out on a periodic basis to track progress.

The *Parenting Goals* form uses a goal attainment and progress monitoring methodology. It is important to review the scaling method on the form, which ranges from 1 to 3. There is no right or standardized way to use or interpret the scaling because it is simply a self-evaluation strategy. Ask parents to initially evaluate themselves on whatever goal or step they wrote down as a kind of baseline assessment. Thereafter encourage them to periodically revisit the *Parenting Goals* form, including during sessions with the practitioner, to assess progress via the 1–3 rating.

Brainstorm with the parent as to how often and when the self-evaluation should occur, considering what is optimal and what is practical. There is no right or wrong way to do this, but it is a good idea to have a plan. Whenever the parent is satisfied with his or her own progress, the goal has been achieved (usually several days or weeks of 3 ratings).

Another way to formally track progress is simply by periodically reviewing the *Parent Checklist* forms that are in nearly all of the parent book chapters. The *Parent Checklist* forms provide a brief review of each skill and subskill in that chapter. The parent can review it now and then to measure progress on skills acquisition. Mastery of skills is evident whenever the parent consistently rates his or her own progress as a 3 on the different skills depicted on the *Parent Checklist* forms.

Getting a Child Going and Following Through

It is often the case that a child is much less motivated than the parent when it comes to skills training. Nonetheless, it is essential to cultivate a high level of motivation and commitment in the child, especially to do the work in the more child-focused Chapters 8–15 and the family-focused Chapters 19–20 in the parent book. Motivating the child can be very challenging, so the practitioner has to have many tricks up his or her sleeve to accomplish this phase. This section is derived in part from motivational interviewing methods (like those described in the preceding section) but also incorporates family collaboration and behavioral rewards to motivate a child.

Using a Teamwork Approach

It is very important to emphasize the *teamwork approach* presented in Chapter 3 of the parent book at the outset. First the teamwork notion must be sold to the parent. Since many parents seek out services for their child with the view that the child will be the focus, it is important for the practitioner to spend some time educating parents about why **they** need to be involved and supportive in motivating the child. Emphasizing a developmental approach, as described earlier, can help in this regard. Parents need to understand that they play an important role in promoting their child's development, and they must motivate, teach, and guide their child accordingly. The family teamwork approach helps here.

Next parents must be guided to sell the teamwork approach to the child. This can be difficult at times, especially when working with an older child or teen. Advise parents that it is important to avoid pointing fingers at the child in terms of who needs to make changes. Instead suggest that parents work on skills similar to those the child is working on. For example, *everyone* might work on social skills, stress management skills, or family interaction skills. Another manifestation of the team format is observed when the parent promises to reward the child for using new skills. The bottom line is to communicate to parents that whenever a family works together as a team, there is more motivation and success, and parents should approach their child from this team perspective.

Assisting the Child in Setting Goals and Monitoring Progress

The parent and practitioner should collaborate with the child in identifying specific personal goals to work on from Chapters 8–15 in the parent book. The "team" should encourage the child to think of goals related to skills to work on. Some children will need more assistance than others, since goal setting is a relatively sophisticated cognitive task that requires an ability to reflect on oneself and think ahead. Accordingly, younger children may need overt suggestions for goals from the parent and/or the practitioner, whereas older children and teens can be prompted to set their own goals. Typical goals center on specified target behaviors and/or the use of new social–emotional skills (e.g., getting more sleep, using relaxation techniques, starting conversations, verbally expressing feelings). Tell the parent it is important that the child **buy into, cooperate,** and **commit** to working on goals. The parent (and practitioner) should keep discussing goals, using internal and external motivational methods (described next), until the child is willing to put some effort into them.

One formal method that can be used to structure the child's goal-setting effort is to use one of the many forms provided throughout the parent book. For example, a child could work on stress-coping skills and with the guidance of a parent, complete the ***Staying Calm*** worksheet (see parent book Chapter 14 and Chapter 7 in this book) periodically to monitor progress. Still another child could work on personal communication goals and, along with other family members, fill out the ***My Family Communication Goals*** form (see parent book Chapter 20 and Chapter 10 in this book) as a way to gauge progress. The younger the child, the more guidance he or she will need in being able to use the charts scattered throughout the parent book. The parents and/or practitioner will need to remind, guide, and lead the younger child in this endeavor.

If preferred, the ***Personal Goals (Basic*** or ***Advanced)*** form can be used to customize a child's personal goals and to keep track of progress. If using the ***Personal Goals*** form, it would probably be best not to use the other charts and worksheets and just focus on this broader strategy. Ask the child and parent which method seems to be best suited for them. The ***Basic*** form is best for younger children and the ***Advanced*** form works well with teens. For children in between, it is a good idea to collaborate with parents to determine which will be most applicable.

The ***Personal Goals*** form works best if the **child writes goals that are *dos*, such as "Use relaxation techniques" or "Think helpful thoughts,"** and not *don'ts*, such as **"Stop getting angry" or "No unhelpful thinking."** This goal setting tells the child what to do to replace old, unproductive behaviors. It works best to state broadly defined goals and the individual small steps that will be taken to reach them. With the ***Advanced*** form, ask the child (and parent) to specify specific steps he or she will take to reach the goals. For example, a child may set a goal to work on relaxation skills for stress management. It is good to write down when the child will practice, how often, etc., to reach the goal.

Stress cooperation between the parent and child. Ask if the child will agree to work with the parent on the goal. Seal the deal by asking the child and the parent to sign the ***Personal Goals (Basic*** or ***Advanced)*** form as a kind of contract to hold the child more accountable to following through.

Tell the parent that this form can be referred to occasionally until the child's goals are accomplished. Suggest that it is important to support the child's personal goals by reviewing them periodically. Methods similar to those described earlier for using the ***Parenting Goals*** form can be used to track progress.

Promoting the Child's Internal Motivation to Work on Goals

It is sometimes necessary to elicit the child's internal motivation with methods derived from motivational interviewing. Whereas the preceding discussion of motivational interviewing for the parent was informal, a more formal approach should be used with an older child or teen (this technique may not work with a young child). The ***Thinking about Personal Goals*** worksheet can be used for this purpose. It entails asking the child a series of questions to motivate him or her to work on goals. Explain to the child that the primary reason for filling out the worksheet is to explore whether or not to work on specific goals. Also note that the parent might chime in with impressions and suggestions. The practitioner should be supportive and ask a lot of questions to guide a "self-discovery" process, as follows:

1. Ask the child (and parent) to generate a list of "pros" (positive outcomes) for working on the goal. These pros might be personal benefits (e.g., "I'd have less stress") or relational benefits for the family (e.g., "We'd get along better").
2. Ask the child (and parent) to generate a list of "cons" for working on the goal. These cons typically center on the downside of having to put forth effort, make a commitment, and be accountable (e.g., "This would be a lot of work").
3. Then the child needs to determine which is greater, the pros or the cons. Here the parent might suggest that the child could earn a reward for working on and accomplishing goals (see next section). This might tip the balance to make the pros outweigh the cons and therefore motivate the child.
4. Once the child has identified a goal, ask him or her to rate how important it is and to commit a certain level of effort.
5. Again the parent's input might be helpful. The reluctant child may be more inclined to exert the needed effort if a reward could be earned (see next section). Ask the parent to identify rewards that the child might earn.
6. Ask if the child will agree to work with the parent on the goal. Seal the deal by asking the child and the parent to sign the worksheet as a kind of contract to solidify their intentions to follow through.

At the end of this process, hopefully the child has set some goals and the parent is on board to support the child. If not, then methods for enhancing external motivation (discussed next) could be tried. If yes, then the parent and child can proceed with the execution of the plan.

Promoting the Child's External Motivation to Work on Goals

In spite of the efforts described above, some children will not be all that internally motivated to work on their own skills development. **It is sometimes necessary to jumpstart the child's external motivation with rewards.** Chapter 3 of the parent book provides ideas for rewards for younger children and older children/teens. The practitioner's job is to guide family members to express exactly what the reward is and what the child must do to earn it. The discussion should also touch on the need to gradually fade out rewards once the child's motivation improves and/or he or she has learned the new skill(s).

When using a practice toolbox approach such as the "Struggling Kids" program, it is a good idea to have essential tools nearby for everyday use. It is quite useful and handy to have copies of certain charts and forms available for quick reference during skills-training sessions including the following:

- Chapter-specific **Parent Checklists**
- **Parenting Goals**
- **Personal Goals (Basic** or **Advanced)**
- **Examining How Your Child and Family Are Doing**
- **Selecting Skills-Building Strategies to Work On**

Having these charts and forms at the ready allows a practitioner to quickly help the family learn about new skills, monitor progress, and make adjustments as needed for goals and skills-building strategies to work on. Consider placing copies of these essential charts and forms on a table in the room you are working in so that you and family members are reminded to use them during meetings.

Tailoring the Getting Started and Staying with It Module for Parent Groups

When running a parent group, review the *Overview of the Getting Started and Staying with It Module* chart early on to give the parents a basic idea of what to expect to be successful with parent skills-building efforts. Be sure to prompt group members to talk about the challenges of parenting and making changes.

Reviewing child development and family well-being can generate lively discussion in parenting groups, which gives the practitioner an opportunity to prompt parents to share personal examples that enrich everyone's understanding of child development and parent and family well-being. The result is often a feeling of being "in this together," which promotes openness, enhances motivation, and increases collaboration.

The *Examining How Your Child and Family Are Doing* and *Selecting Skills-Building Strategies to Work On* forms can also be used in parent groups. The parents in the group would take turns reviewing and discussing both charts. When it comes to selecting skills-building strategies in a group format, the practitioner would need to guide members to a consensus on their shared preference for skills-building strategies in later meetings. It can be useful to empower the parents to construct an itinerary for subsequent sessions. Thereafter present one or two topics or chapters per meeting. Over time, the parents can be exposed to several types of skills-building strategies, and each family should be encouraged to pick and choose the ones that best fit their needs and preferences.

The P's to success and the phases of skills building can also be valuable concepts to introduce and refer to now and then. Over time the parents will report their challenges and successes in implementing new skills-building strategies with their families. Guide the parents to encourage each other.

Most of the information and many of the techniques described in parent book Chapter 3 can be used in parent groups. It is often productive to review and discuss the *Parent Checklist for Getting Going and Following Through* form. Facilitate a parent group discussion about the challenges and ideas on the checklist. Inform the parents that they can use the information presented in parent book Chapter 3 to brainstorm ideas and techniques to set goals and get motivated. In particular, the *Parenting Goals* form is important to discuss to set the stage for working toward specific goals.

Overview of the Getting Started and Staying with It Module

Chapter 1. The Struggling Child: Understanding Your Child's Behavioral–Emotional Problems

Understanding Common Behavioral–Emotional Problems in Children

- Hyperactivity
- Impulsivity
- Inattention
- Defiance
- Rule-violating behavior
- Aggression
- Moodiness
- Anxiety
- Emotionally overreactive
- Emotionally underreactive
- Underachievement
- Social difficulties

Understanding Struggling versus Success in Different Areas of Child Development

- Child behavioral development
- Child social development
- Child emotional development
- Child academic development

Understanding Stressed versus Coping in Different Areas of Parent and Family Well-Being

- Parent well-being
- Family well-being

See **Child Psychological Development** and **Parent and Family Well-Being** charts.

Chapter 2. Getting Back on Track: Coming Up with a Skills-Building Plan for Your Child and Family

Pinpointing Areas of Focus for Your Child and Family

- Examine different areas of child development
- Examine different areas of parent and family well-being

Selecting Skills-Building Strategies for Your Child and Family

- Focus on child development skills as needed
- Focus on parent and family well-being skills as needed

Understanding the Skills-Building Method

- *The "P's" to success—Preparing, Practicing, Progress monitoring, and PERCONing*
- *Three phases of skills building—intensive, maintenance, and relapse-prevention phases*

See **Examining How Your Child and Family Are Doing** and **Selecting Skills-Building Strategies to Work On** forms.

(cont.)

Chapter 3. Taking Care of Business: Getting Going and Following Through

Determining Where Different Family Members Are within the Stages of Change

- *Precontemplation*—not too aware of a need to change

- *Contemplation*—beginning to think that there is a need to make some changes

- *Preparation*—coming up with a plan of action and goals

- *Action*—implementing a plan and working on goals

- *Maintenance*—changes are being maintained

Enhancing a Parent's Work on Skills Building

- *Setting parenting-related goals*—identify specific skills-training strategies to work on

- *Prioritizing and committing effort*—determine importance and how much work to put into reaching goal(s)

- *Monitoring progress*—keep track of how it is going in reaching goal(s)

Enhancing a Child's Work on Skills Building

- *Facilitating family teamwork*—communicate that everyone will work on goals together

- *Setting and working on child's personal goals*—identify specific skills-training strategies to work on and tracking progress

- *Promoting a child's internal motivation*—guide child to figure out what he or she wants to work on and the benefits of doing so

- *Promoting a child's external motivation*—provide temporary rewards for working on goals

See **Determining Stages of Change, Parenting Goals, Personal Goals (Basic** or **Advanced),** and **Thinking about Personal Goals** forms.

Getting to Know You

Child Name: _____ **Date:** _____

Parent Name(s): _____

1. Please tell me about your children, including strengths and concerns:

_____

_____

_____

_____

_____

_____

2. Please tell me about your family, including strengths and concerns:

_____

_____

_____

_____

_____

_____

3. Please tell me about you as a parent, including strengths and concerns:

_____

_____

_____

_____

_____

_____

4. Please tell me about any goals you have for your child, family, or yourself as a parent:

_____

_____

_____

_____

_____

_____

Charts from Parent Book Chapter 1

Child Psychological Development

Child Behavioral Development: Learning to follow reasonable external directions and rules and to internalize a moral and honest code of conduct

Age	Struggling child	Successful child
Infant/toddler	Irritable/fussy and/or unresponsive to parent. Often tantrums and whines.	Easygoing and responsive to parent. Manageable "terrible 2's."
Preschool	Often disobeys caregiver's directions. Often violates house rules.	Usually obeys caregiver's directions. Usually follows rules at house.
Elementary school	Often violates school rules; often acts before thinking. Often engages in dishonest behavior.	Usually follows rules at school; can think before acting. Has developed an internal code of honest conduct.
Adolescence	Often violates societal rules. Unaware of own behavior and its impact on others.	Usually follows rules of society. Aware of own behavior and its impact on others.

Child Social Development: Bonding with others and learning social skills

Age	Struggling child	Successful child
Infant/toddler	Insecure attachment or bond with parent.	Secure attachment or bond with parent.
Preschool	Mostly negative interactions with parents and peers. Poor social skills.	Mostly positive interactions with parents and peers. Good social skills.
Elementary school	Mostly negative interactions or withdrawn with peers and teachers. Often affiliates with negative peers. Ineffective in solving social problems.	Mostly positive interactions with peers and teachers. Affiliates with positive peers. Solves social problems effectively.
Adolescence	Often engages in negative activities with peers or is withdrawn. Rejects family and has poor family relationships.	Engages in positive activities with peers. "Launches" from family but maintains strong family ties.

(cont.)

Child Emotional Development: Learning to understand/express feelings, think rational or helpful thoughts, and regulate stress-related emotions

Age	Struggling child	Successful child
Infant/toddler	Displays mostly negative basic emotions. Expresses negative emotions through play.	Displays all basic emotions. Expresses a wide range of emotions through play.
Preschool	Verbally unexpressive and keeps feelings inside.	Verbally expresses simple emotions.
Elementary school	Fears persist. Doesn't understand, express, and control intense emotions. Mostly negative and unhelpful thoughts about self and others.	Overcomes most fears. Understands, expresses, and controls intense emotions. Mostly positive and helpful thoughts about self and others.
Adolescence	Negative and unhealthy identity emerging. Often depressed, anxious, or angry.	Positive and healthy identity emerging. Often happy and satisfied.

Child Academic Development: Learning self-directed academic behaviors and pursuing educational opportunities

Age	Struggling child	Successful child
Infant/toddler	Apprehensive about environment. Avoids new situations.	Explores environment. Is curious and inquisitive.
Preschool	Engages in excessive television and video games versus looking at books. Poor adjustment to school setting. Indifferent about learning.	Enjoys looking at books. Good adjustment to school setting. Excited about learning.
Elementary school	Inattentive, off-task, doesn't complete tasks. Can't manage time, organize, and plan to get schoolwork done.	Concentrates, stays on task, gets tasks done. Can manage time, organize, and plan to get schoolwork done.
Adolescence	No particular special skills or interests. No viable vocational or career plans.	Consolidating special skills and interests. Engaging in vocational or career planning and preparation.

Parent and Family Well-Being

Parent Well-Being: Personal functioning of parent(s)

Stressed parent	Coping parent
Overwhelmed by everyday challenges and problems.	Managing everyday challenges and problems.
Marriage or intimate partner relationship problems.	Satisfactory marriage or intimate partner relationship.
Overwhelmed by parenting responsibilities.	Keeping up with parenting responsibilities.
Limited family or friend support system.	Supportive family and/or friends.

Family Well-Being: Functioning of family relationships

Stressed family	Coping family
Distant parent–child relationship.	Close parent–child relationship.
Lack of routines and/or rituals.	Predictable routines and rituals.
Mostly negative (coercive) parent–child interactions.	Mostly positive parent–child interactions.
Mostly negative family communication and inability to resolve conflict.	Mostly positive family communication and ability to resolve conflict.

Forms from Parent Book Chapter 2

Examining How Your Child and Family Are Doing

Name: _____ **Date:** _____

Read the descriptors from left to right that correspond to **areas of child functioning** and **areas of parent/family functioning**. Circle a number from 1 to 6 to reflect your best judgment. Underline specific words that best describe your child. *The first time you fill this out, think about your child/family in a general sense; other times you fill it out, think about your child/family over the past week or so to give you an idea of progress.* Any area rated as a 1, 2, or 3 indicates a concern, and any rating of 4, 5, or 6 indicates that things are moving in the right direction.

Areas of Child Functioning

Struggling ⟶ **In Progress** ⟶ **Successful**

Struggling		In Progress		Successful	
Defiant, doesn't follow rules, or lies, sneaks, or steals and can get upset when disciplined		*Child behavioral development*		Follows reasonable directions and rules from adults and is trustworthy and honest	
1	2	3	4	5	6
Aggressive, withdrawn, bothersome, or rejected (by peers and/or siblings)		*Child social development*		Bonded with others, has good social skills, and affiliates with peers who have a positive influence	
1	2	3	4	5	6
Keeps feelings inside, thinks unhelpful thoughts, or is stressed out, angry, or anxious		*Child emotional development*		Understands, expresses, and controls strong feelings	
1	2	3	4	5	6
Dislikes school, is achieving below potential, or has trouble completing school work		*Child academic development*		Satisfactorily completes schoolwork and is pursuing educational opportunities	
1	2	3	4	5	6

Areas of Parent/Family Functioning

Stressed ⟶ **In Progress** ⟶ **Coping**

Stressed		In Progress		Coping	
Feels overwhelmed, has adult relationship problems, has difficulty fulfilling parenting responsibilities, or has limited support of family/friends		*Parent well-being*		Managing personal, adult relationship and parenting challenges and has supportive family/friends	
1	2	3	4	5	6
Distant parent–child relationships, negative parent–child interactions, or problems with family communication and conflicts		*Family well-being*		Close and positive parent–child relationships, and family members get along with each other most of the time	
1	2	3	4	5	6

Selecting Skills-Building Strategies to Work On

Name: _____ Date: _____

Select child and parent/family skills-building chapters from this menu that are related to ratings of 3 or lower in the same areas on the ***Examining How Your Child and Family Are Doing*** form. Put a checkmark next to the selected chapters below. **Use your judgment and choose those chapters that seem to match your goals for your child and family.**

Enhancing Your Child's Behavioral Development

CHAPTER
____ 4. Doing What You're Told: Teaching Your Child to Comply with Parental Directives
____ 5. Doing What's Expected: Teaching Your Child to Follow Rules
____ 6. Doing the Right Thing: Teaching Your Child to Behave Honestly
____ 7. Staying Cool under Fire: Managing Your Child's Protesting of Discipline and Preventing Angry Outbursts

Enhancing Your Child's Social Development

CHAPTER
____ 8. Making Friends: Teaching Your Child Social Behavior Skills
____ 9. Keeping Friends: Teaching Your Child Social Problem-Solving Skills
____ 10. That Hurts!: Helping Your Child with Bullies
____ 11. Hanging with the "Right Crowd": Influencing Your Child's Peer Relationships

Enhancing Your Child's Emotional Development

CHAPTER
____ 12. Let It Out!: Teaching Your Child to Understand and Express Feelings
____ 13. You Are What You Think: Teaching Your Child to Think Helpful Thoughts
____ 14. Stress Busters: Teaching Your Child to Manage Stress

Enhancing Your Child's Academic Development

CHAPTER
____ 15. Surviving School: Teaching Your Child to Manage Time, Organize, Plan, Review, and Stay on Task
____ 16. Teaming Up: Collaborating and Advocating for Your Child at School

Enhancing Your Well-Being as a Parent

CHAPTER
____ 17. You Parent the Way You Think: Thinking Helpful Thoughts to Enhance Parenting
____ 18. Cool Parents: Managing Your Own Stress to Enhance Parenting

Enhancing Your Family's Well-Being

CHAPTER
____ 19. Let's Get Together: Strengthening Family Bonds and Organization
____ 20. We Can Work It Out: Strengthening Family Interaction Skills

Forms from Parent Book Chapter 3

Parent Checklist for Getting Going and Following Through

Name: _____ Date: _____

In the blanks below, check off whether you have accomplished any of the indicated ideas related to getting going and following through.

Determining the Stages of Change for Family Members

A. _____ Figuring out what stage each family member is at for making changes.

1. *Precontemplation:* Who in the family is not too aware of a problem or a need to change or work on goals?

2. *Contemplation:* Who in the family is beginning to think that it might be a good idea to make some changes or work on goals?

3. *Preparation:* Who in the family is coming up with a plan for change and has goals to work on?

4. *Action:* Who in the family is implementing a plan and actively working on achieving goals?

5. *Maintenance:* Who in the family has met their goals and is upholding changes with new behaviors that have become routine and long-lasting?

Note: Family members at the precontemplation or contemplation stages may need help with setting goals and getting motivated.

Parent's Use of Strategies to Get Going and Follow Through

B. _____ Setting and writing down specific parenting goals.

C. _____ Prioritizing what to work on and determining how important a parenting goal is in comparison to all other obligations and interests.

D. _____ Pledging how much effort will be put into working on parenting goals.

E. _____ Monitoring progress until parenting goals are reached.

Parent's Use of Strategies to Help Child Get Going and Follow Through

F. _____ Promoting parent–child or family teamwork approach to working on goals.

G. _____ Assisting child in declaring one or more personal goals to work on.

H. _____ Promoting child's *internal motivation* by calmly discussing personal goals, motivation to accomplish them, and steps to reach them.

I. _____ Promoting child's *external motivation* by providing rewards for working on personal goals.

J. _____ Monitoring progress until child's personal goals are reached.

From *The Practitioner Guide to Skills Training for Struggling Kids* by Michael L. Bloomquist. Copyright 2013 by The Guilford Press. Permission to photocopy this material is granted to purchasers of this book for personal use only (see copyright page for details).

Determining Stages of Change

Name of Person or Family: _____ **Date**: _____

Identify a problem or a challenge for the child, parent, or family that might be the focus of a plan for change. Then write down which stage of change different family members are at. It may be helpful for the family to discuss it until a consensus is achieved and everyone is at least at the **Preparation** stage.

The problem and/or skills-building strategy being considered is:

_____

_____

1. **Precontemplation:** Not too aware of a problem or a need to change. *Family member(s) at this stage*:

_____

_____

2. **Contemplation**: Beginning to think that it might be a good idea to make some changes.

Family member(s) at this stage:

_____

_____

3. **Preparation**: Coming up with a well thought-out plan for change and setting goals.

Family member(s) at this stage:

_____

_____

4. **Action:** Implementing the plan and working on goals, making changes in behavior for a few weeks to a few months. An occasional setback might occur, but you don't give up!

Family member(s) at this stage:

_____

_____

5. **Maintenance:** Sustaining changes with new behaviors that have become routine and long-lasting. Changes have been maintained with few setbacks for a few months or more.

Family member(s) at this stage:

_____

_____

Parenting Goals

Name: _____ **Date:** _____

Write down your parenting goal(s) and smaller steps to take to reach it (them). Every now and then, record a score in the circle or square to indicate how much progress you have made on each parenting goal and its steps.

Limited progress	**Some progress**	**A lot of progress**
1	**2**	**3**

Overall progress! ◯

Goal 1: _____

Progress on steps

Steps to achieve goal:

1. _____
2. _____
3. _____
4. _____

Overall progress! ◯

Goal 2: _____

Progress on steps

Steps to achieve goal:

1. _____
2. _____
3. _____
4. _____

Overall progress! ◯

Goal 3: _____

Progress on steps

Steps to achieve goal:

1. _____
2. _____
3. _____
4. _____

I commit to working on these goals.

Parent signature: _____

Personal Goals (Basic)

Name: _____ **Date:** _____

The time period when the chart will be used: _____

Indicate below which goal(s) will be worked on. At the end of the specified time period the child and parent can rate how much progress the child has made on goal(s).

Child Evaluation

I am working on the following goal(s):

How much progress have I made on goal(s)? (Circle one.)

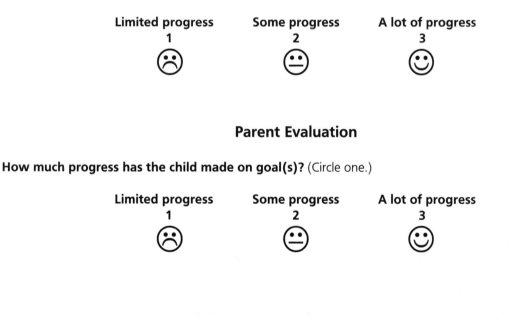

Limited progress	Some progress	A lot of progress
1	2	3
☹	😐	☺

Parent Evaluation

How much progress has the child made on goal(s)? (Circle one.)

Limited progress	Some progress	A lot of progress
1	2	3
☹	😐	☺

Signature: _____

Parent signature(s): _____

Personal Goals (Advanced)

Name: _____ Date: _____

Write down your personal goal(s) and smaller steps to take to reach it (them). Every now and then, record a score in the circle or square to indicate how much progress you have made on each personal goal and steps.

Limited progress	**Some progress**	**A lot of progress**
1	**2**	**3**

Overall progress!

○

Goal 1: _____

Progress on steps

Steps to achieve goal:
1. _____
2. _____
3. _____
4. _____

Overall progress!

○

Goal 2: _____

Progress on steps

Steps to achieve goal:
1. _____
2. _____
3. _____
4. _____

Overall progress!

○

Goal 3: _____

Progress on steps

Steps to achieve goal:
1. _____
2. _____
3. _____
4. _____

I commit to working on these goals and to working with my parent(s) to reach them.

Signature: _____

Parent signature(s): _____

Thinking about Personal Goals

Name: _____ Date: _____

It has been suggested that I work on a goal of: _____

_____

What are the "pros" or positives that might happen if I work on this goal? _____

_____

_____

What are the "cons" or negatives that might happen if I work on this goal?

_____

_____

_____

Which is greater—the *pros* or *cons* for working on this goal? (Circle one.)

How important is working on this goal compared to other activities in my life? (Circle one.)

1	2	3	4	5	6	7	8	9	10

Not important   Somewhat important   Very important

I agree to put in this amount of effort to work on this goal (circle one):

1	2	3	4	5	6	7	8	9	10

Little effort   Okay effort   Lots of effort

Rewards I might be able to earn for working on goal(s): _____

_____

I agree to work with my parent(s) on this goal.

Signature: _____

Parent signature(s): _____

From *The Practitioner Guide to Skills Training for Struggling Kids* by Michael L. Bloomquist. Copyright 2013 by The Guilford Press. Permission to photocopy this material is granted to purchasers of this book for personal use only (see copyright page for details).

5

Using the Child Behavioral Development Module

This practitioner book chapter corresponds to the parent book section "Enhancing Your Child's Behavioral Development" (Chapters 4–7). This module provides parents with strategies for dealing with defiant, rule-breaking, dishonest, and volatile/agitated behaviors. Behavioral training methods for parents are emphasized. The primary goal is to help parents get their child's problematic behavior under control to promote behavioral development. **The practitioner should read and fully understand the *content* in parent book Chapters 4–7 before using the related *procedures* described in this practitioner book chapter.**

An important procedural method is worth considering at the outset. It can be useful to begin training the parent in the child behavioral development module without the child present, typically for one to three parent-only sessions. This can help early on when the parent is beginning to learn the new skills related to managing the child, because it gives the parent and practitioner time to fully discuss, plan, model, role-play, etc., as described in this chapter. The child can be brought in later to be informed of, and discuss, the behavior management methods the parent will now be using. If the child is cooperative, some role playing can then be conducted with him or her. One example would be to first work with a parent to develop competency in doing time-out and then later bring a child in to be informed of the technique and to practice it. Another example would be to bring a teen into a session to discuss the new house rules the parent developed in an earlier session with the practitioner.

This sequence of meeting with the parent and then also with the child should be discussed in a collaborative fashion with the parent. If the parent prefers the child to be involved, and the child is not too disruptive, the training could occur with both parent and child together. If the parent prefers the child to be involved but the child is disruptive (e.g., arguing, refusing to cooperate), then it is important to discuss the issue further. In this instance, make sure the parent understands that the child is still the focus, but that it is useful to begin training without having to simultaneously manage the child in the session. Suggest that after a plan is in place and the parent has acquired some new skills, the uncooperative child can be brought in for some training. Perhaps "in-session rules" (discussed below) and other behavior management techniques could then be applied in the session. This in-session behavior management of the child will be much more successful, and can even be a training opportunity, if the early foundation has been laid by working with the parent alone.

Tailoring within the Child Behavioral Development Module

The *Overview of the Child Behavioral Development Module* chart at the end of this chapter summarizes the main concepts and strategies in this module. Reviewing this chart can help parents understand the nuts and bolts of the parenting skills-building strategies used to promote behavioral development in children. It's important for parents to understand that this module requires them to influence the child's behavior, which means that the focus in training is more on parents than on the child at this point. Inform the parents that although many of the basic ideas are the same for all children, there are differences in how the procedures are used with a younger child versus an older child or teen. For example, time-out can be used to help a younger child learn to comply and follow rules, whereas removal of privileges can be used to accomplish the same goals with an older child or teen. Also note that Chapter 7 in the parent book, which focuses on dealing with protesting and angry outbursts, is typically applied along with Chapters 4–6 in the parent book. The initial discussion should conclude in broadly stated options for pursuing skills training within the module.

Procedures for Applying the Overlapping Content in Parent Book Chapters 4–7

Each of the chapters in the child behavioral development module discusses the importance of increasing positive behavior (compliance, rule following, honesty, and staying calm when disciplined) and managing the child's protesting discipline. Although the specific type of targeted misbehavior differs across Chapters 4–7 in the parent book, the following methods are usually applied when a child's behavior is a problem. These ideas are tweaked to meet the unique goals of each chapter and are only briefly summarized here.

Training Parents to Build the Relationship and Increase Positive Behavior

Parent book Chapters 4–7 each begins by noting the importance of a positive approach when attempting to increase positive behaviors. Stress the importance of **building a relationship,** particularly the fact that this should not be contingent on the child's improved behavior. In other words the child gets to have bonding activities with the parent regardless of his or her behavior. This does not mean that parents cannot justifiably postpone a bonding activity if the child has just misbehaved, but it does mean that, overall, the child should get the message of goodwill and love from the parents just for who the child is, not for how the child behaves. Brainstorm specific ideas for activities the parent and child can do together and suggest that the parent schedule them on a personal calendar or planner so that they don't fall by the wayside in the crush of everyday responsibilities. It is often a good idea to involve the child in these discussions (see parent book Chapter 19 for more ideas on bonding activities). Make sure the parent understands that, when needed, discipline will go more smoothly if the parent and child have a good relationship and a strong bond.

Have the parent and child engage in some bonding-type activities—playing with toys for a younger child, playing cards or a board game with an older child or teen—during a session so that they get some practice. If the parents express disbelief that they need to practice playing with their child, suggest that when positive bonds have been compromised by behavioral–emotional problems, what may have come naturally in the past can be "unlearned." This in-session play also affords the opportunity for the practitioner to spot problems and gently coach the parents in ways to make the activity a positive experience. You can also ask the parents and child, during the activity, to plan how they can replicate this and other activities at home.

Another parent–child relationship factor commonly addressed in behavior management methods is the reduction of critical and negative statements that frustrated parents make to their misbehaving child. A section elaborating on this point in Chapter 4 of the parent book and brief mentions in Chapters 5–7 of the parent book provide psychoeducation on this topic. It is important to review this material with parents. Ask them if they ever get annoyed, upset, or discouraged and maybe engage in criticism, ask negative questions, blame, bring up old issues, and/or deliver put-downs on the spur of the moment. Ask what impact these types of statements might have on the child and on the parent–child bond. Discuss how these statements can actually increase, not decrease, challenging behavior in the child because they can give rise to mistrust and ill will on the child's side.

Then ask the parent if he or she would like to work on having a more constructive way to talk to the child and manage behavior. The goal is for the parent to increase awareness of negative verbalizations directed at the child and to utilize a more constructive, ongoing dialogue. Work with the parent on "catching 'em being good" and using the behavior management techniques in Chapters 4–7 as replacement methods for the critical and negative statements. A parent who is interested in reducing negative verbalizations toward his or her child might declare this as a goal to work on and keep track of his or her progress on the *Parenting Goals* form. Revisit this idea whenever you observe the parent making negative statements directly to the child in session or in reference to the child.

Emphasize the importance of "catching 'em being good" (praising compliance, following rules, honesty, and/or staying calm). Brainstorm ways that parents can remember to do this, such as posting reminders to themselves or to prompting each other (if applicable). Try to model catching the child being compliant, following rules, being honest, and/or staying calm in the session if the opportunity arises. For example, if the child sits down after the parent requests it, point this out and offer praise.

It is a good idea to ask the parent to practice giving praise for positive child behavior at home. For example, if the child is ready for school by 6:30 a.m., as stated on the ***Daily Privileges for Following House Rules*** form (in parent book Chapter 5 and also at the end of this chapter), then the parent could say, "I really appreciate your following the rule of being ready for school by 6:30." Another example: If the child admits to sneaking by playing video games during homework, the parent could say, "I appreciate your honesty in admitting that you were playing video games instead of doing homework." **To facilitate the learning of this behavior, ask the parent to write a list of praise-type statements to make when catching the child being compliant, following rules, being honest, and/or staying calm.** Then ask the parent to read and rehearse these statements privately on occasion so they are remembered in the moment. That way when the child is behaving positively, the parent will be prepared and know what to say.

Training Parents to Manage Child Protests of Discipline

The use of time-out or removal of privileges for noncompliance, rule breaking, and incidences of dishonesty is discussed in Chapters 4–6 of the parent book. Time-out or removal of privileges should be administered using a deferred method when children resist or protest the parent's attempts to discipline in this manner. This deferred method of time-out or removal of privileges is noted briefly in parent book Chapters 4–6 and discussed fully in Chapter 7. To summarize, the parent should be taught to deescalate and disengage from coercive power struggles with the child by ignoring the child's protesting and avoid interacting if the child whines, complains, or acts belligerent when the parent is trying to use time-out or removal of privileges. Instead the parent should (1) defer the time-out or privilege removal via a "patient standoff" until the child is calm, and (2) take safety precautions, if needed, for increasingly volatile child behavior (see "Specific Procedures for Applying Parent Book Chapter 7" later in this chapter for more information, examples, and role-play suggestions).

Specific Procedures for Applying Parent Book Chapter 4

This parent book chapter focuses on noncompliant behavior in a child. After encouraging the parent to build a positive parent–child bond and to notice and praise the child's compliance, as described above, this chapter offers strategies to get a noncompliant child to comply and to avoid power struggles that often typify parental interactions with such children. The parent accomplishes this by giving an effective command, giving an effective warning using an "if . . . then" statement, and following through with what was stated in the warning (i.e., putting child in time-out or taking away a privilege). For children who strongly resist this discipline, planned ignoring and a deferred time-out or privilege removal strategy is recommended (Patterson, 1975; Sanders, 1999; Warzak & Floress, 2009). This means ignoring verbal and physical power struggles and eventually following through with the time-out or privilege removal once the child has calmed down.

Note: *The forms and charts referred to in the discussion below are in parent book Chapter 4 and also at the end of this chapter unless otherwise noted.*

Discussing Child Compliance Problems with Parents

Noncompliant behavior should always be framed developmentally for parents. Explain that it is "normal" for children to be noncompliant to some extent (this includes being defiant, bargaining, and resisting), but that noncompliance above a normal level can be associated with future behavioral–emotional problems. Likewise, improvements in a child's compliance often lead to social and school-related success, thus placing the child on a more successful developmental track.

To help parents figure out what is "normal" compliance, say that typically developing children comply with reasonable parent requests about two-thirds of the time. **Make sure that parents understand that a fairly high rate of noncompliance (one-third) is normal.** Ask parents to estimate what percentage of the time their child complies with reasonable requests. If it is less than 67% (two-thirds) of the time, it should be addressed.

Note that noncompliance is also associated with irritability and moodiness. *Explain that it is therefore imperative for the parent to remain calm when dealing with this behavior in the child.* Parents need to understand that the way they interact with their child around this behavior can contribute to the problem, and it is important to reduce negative (coercive) parent–child interactions. Explain that reducing this type of interaction not only helps their relationship but promotes better emotional functioning in the child over the long term.

Getting Parents Started and Focused

Begin by reviewing the ***Parent Checklist for Child Compliance*** with the parent. The parent can rate and check off items that are going well and pinpoint areas needing some work. Inform the parent that this checklist summarizes the overall approach in this chapter. Answer any questions about the content conveyed on the checklist. The parent should be told that it is very important to fully understand the information summarized on this checklist and detailed in parent book Chapter 4.

It is also a good idea to elaborate on some of the commands that are mentioned in the text of parent book Chapter 4. Be sure to review **Ineffective Commands** (see the sidebar below) and ask if the parent uses any of them. This is often an "aha" moment as a parent realizes how ineffective the commands he or she typically uses are. Be sure to also review **Pre-Commands and "When . . . Then" Commands** (see the sidebar below). Note that these commands are particularly useful for rigid or inflexible children who need time to transition from an activity to complying with a parent command.

INEFFECTIVE COMMANDS

- Vague command (e.g., "Knock it off," "Shape up")
- Question command (e.g., "Do you want to pick up your clothes?")
- Rationale command (e.g., "You need to hurry or we will be late")
- Multiple commands (e.g., "Pick up your books, go wash your hands, and sit down at the table")
- Frequent commands (e.g., telling your child to do something again and again and again)

PRE-COMMANDS AND "WHEN . . . THEN" COMMANDS

Some children have a hard time transitioning from one task to another and benefit from **pre-commands**, which tell the child that compliance will soon be expected. For example, if a parent wants a child off a computer game at 4:00, it is a good idea to tell the child at 3:45, 3:50, and 3:55 that at 4:00 the computer must go off. Then at 4:00, the parent can give an effective command, such as "Okay, it is 4:00, and I expect you to turn off the computer now."

Another useful way to get a child to comply is by using a "when . . . then" command. A parent could tell a child that **when** he or she has completed a task, **then** he or she can have a privilege (e.g., "When you have finished with the dishes, then you can watch TV").

Training Parents to Use a Firm Approach to Reduce Child Noncompliance

Review the *Time Out* and/or *Removing Privileges for Noncompliance* charts with the parent and later with the child. These charts are very similar, with the exception of the third step, where either the child is placed in time-out or a privilege is removed. Make sure that the parent fully understands each of the three steps related to (1) command, (2) warning, and (3) follow-through with warning. Go through the precise definition of each of the steps as defined in parent book Chapter 4.

Have the parent also consider several other important factors. Suggest that time-out is usually preferred over removing a privilege for Step 3 with a younger child because it is more feasible and easier to follow through on than removing a privilege. Suggest further that removing a privilege for Step 3 is preferred if there is no time to do time-out (getting ready for school in the morning, going to bed at night, etc.) or with an older child or teen. Finally, if using time-out for Step 3, discuss where the time-out chair will be placed at home.

Ideally this would be somewhere that is free of distractions and fun activities and where the parent can visually monitor the child from a distance. This might be a corner of a room or a stairway, etc.

In-session practice with a parent of a **younger child** should focus on the time-out method. One can begin by modeling and role-playing the procedure with a child who does not protest (examples of enforcing time-out with a protesting child are discussed below in "Specific Procedures for Applying Parent Book Chapter 7") while referring to the ***Time Out*** chart. Ask if the parent can act like a child for a modeling demonstration in which the practitioner plays the part of the parent. Ask the "child" not to comply with a task (e.g., "Pick up those toys and put them in the basket") and then give a warning, followed by putting him or her in a time-out chair. Be sure to demonstrate each of the steps in a manner that is consistent with what is written in the text of Chapter 4. Then ask the parent if he or she would be comfortable playing the parent in a similar role play. Keep role-playing until the parent has mastered the procedure if he or she is comfortable doing so.

The same modeling and role-playing setup can be used to practice the strategy of removing a privilege with the parent of an **older child or teen**, first dealing with a nonprotesting child (examples of this strategy used with a protesting child are discussed below in "Specific Procedures for Applying Parent Book Chapter 7"). A similar series of modeling demonstrations and role playing could occur while referring to the ***Removing Privileges for Noncompliance*** chart. An older child or teen (the role-playing parent), for example, might be asked to comply with a command to "Get off the computer and begin your homework." The practitioner would demonstrate the skills consistent with the (1) command, (2) the warning, and (3) the follow-through with warning sequence. Step 3 would center on removing privileges for 24 hours, such as specific video games, Internet use, TV, cell phone use, sports equipment (e.g., bicycle, basketball, hockey skates), iPod, going out of the house, hanging out with friends, use of car (if older teen), and so on.

After the parent has practiced time-out or removing privileges for noncompliance, it is useful to bring the child in for a session so he or she can be informed of the consequence for noncompliance, and, if he or she is cooperative, could also participate in role playing. In these role plays the "child" role would be played by the actual child. The same scenarios already practiced by the parent could be replicated in these role plays (as described above).

Developing a Home Implementation Plan to Be Led by the Parent

The next step is to come up with a detailed plan to implement these strategies. Brainstorm about when to review this procedure with the child and when to do "practice" role plays with the child at home (if the child will cooperate). It is a good idea to discuss specific goals and ask the parent to write them on the ***Parenting Goals*** form. For example, the parent might write down a goal of using time-out when the child is noncompliant and also write steps for using effective warnings and disengaging from power struggles. Other goals might center on "catching 'em being compliant," and the parent's own personal stress management could be noted as a related goal (see parent book Chapter 18).

Specific Procedures for Applying Parent Book Chapter 5

This parent book chapter focuses on increasing rule-following behavior in a child. Again, parents begin by building a better parent–child relationship and noticing and praising child rule following when it occurs, as described above. Then the practitioner helps parents identify and write down house rules and learn to enforce them without power struggles by periodically reviewing the rules and imposing automatic time-out and/or privilege removal for violations. Parents learn to use a deferred time-out or privilege removal strategy with children who resist discipline. They also learn to establish and enforce situational rules for use away from home.

Note: *The forms and charts referred to in the discussion below are in parent book Chapter 5 and also at the end of this chapter unless otherwise noted.*

Discussing Child Rule-Following Problems with Parents

As with compliance, rule following should be explained to parents in developmental terms: House rules are behavioral expectations a child should follow without always having to be told. The goal is for children to eventually "internalize" standards of behavior, because children who frequently violate rules are at risk for future behavioral–emotional problems. Children who don't follow rules disrupt their own learning, both naturalistic learning that occurs during normal daily routines and interactions and formal learning at school and elsewhere. Tell parents that obeying the "rule" of sticking to a 30 m.p.h. speed limit on residential streets, without a reminder every time they get behind the wheel, helps keep them safe and frees their attention for traffic hazards, darting children, and safe navigating. In the same way that adults have to learn the "rules of the road," children need to be taught to follow rules so they can eventually internalize them. Doing so increases children's self-control, an essential developmental skill that makes significant parental effort highly worthwhile.

Getting Parents Started and Focused

Start by asking parents whether they have any house rules in place already. Often they will say yes, but when asked to state them, it becomes apparent that the house rules are vague, and sometimes the child has no idea of what they are (e.g., the child might say "I should be good"). Typically, this disparity shows parents how important it is that house rules be concrete and specific, and perhaps be written down to avoid confusion.

Next, review the *Parent Checklist for Child Rule Following* with the parent. The parent can rate and check off items that are going well and pinpoint areas needing some work. Indicate that the checklist summarizes the basic ideas in this chapter and answer all questions. Make sure that the parent understands it is necessary to really know the information on this checklist, and detailed in parent book Chapter 5, to do well.

Training Parents to State House Rules and Situational Rules Clearly

Ask the parent to generate a list of house rules. If the child is cooperative, he or she can also participate in generating house rules, but the parent has the final say. Guide the parent to select some easy rules to include with harder rules so that the child can experience some success. For example, an easier rule might be to "help with dishes after supper," and a harder rule might be "limit video games to 1 hour per day." Specific examples of house rules are in parent book Chapter 5. Discuss where the house rules will be posted in the family's home.

If there are siblings in the house, it is helpful to review the pros and cons for having one set of specific house rules for each child or one set of global house rules for all children at this juncture. The parent has to weigh the advantage of individualizing the house rules for each child versus the convenience of global house rules. Be sure to tell the parent that with either method, the parent still has to enforce the house rules on a child-by-child basis because each child will follow or violate house rules in his or her own unique way.

Parents should also consider whether they need situational rules for particular settings or activities where the child exhibits problematic behavior (e.g., shopping rules, rules at Grandma's house, rules for the Internet). Specific examples of situational rules can be found in parent book Chapter 5.

Training Parents to Take a Firm Approach to Enforcing House Rules

First ask the parents to choose among three options for use on a daily basis to improve the child's rule following: option 1, reviewing rules; option 2, automatic time-out; and option 3, removing privileges. Then review the *How Well Was I Following the House Rules Today?* worksheet if they select option 1, *Time-Out* if they select option 2, or *Daily Privileges for Following House Rules* if they select option 3. Tell the parent that just reviewing house rules each day for option 1 can be a powerful and relatively easier way to improve the child's rule following. Be sure to note, too, that it is sometimes useful to use option 1 for a few days or a week, followed by option 2 or 3, as an induction to get the child used to following rules. Suggest that removing a privilege for violating rules is preferred if there is no time to do time-out (getting ready for school in morning, going to bed at night, etc.) or with an older child or teen. It can also help to review parent book Chapter 4 on procedures related to time-out and removing privileges as part of this discussion.

To practice option 1, the child has to be present. Ask the parent to create some "in-session rules" (be quiet, listen to adults in the room, stay in the room, etc.) and encourage the parent to firmly inform the child that he or she is expected to follow them. Then after 15 minutes or so, review the ***How Well Was I Following the House Rules Today?*** worksheet (adapted for in-session rules) with the child to aid this practice. In accordance with the directions on this worksheet, ask the child to evaluate his or her own rule following and then ask the parent to give the child feedback. Discuss how the same procedure could be used at home but with house rules instead of in-session rules.

For option 2, inform the parent that when the **younger child** breaks a house rule, he or she is to be sent automatically to time-out. There is no warning because, in effect, the posted house rules are the warning. Ask the parent to participate in modeling and role-playing exercises related to putting a child in time-out for violating rules. For example, a young child broke a house rule stated as "Work out your disagreements in a respectful way with your brother" by hitting his brother. In this scenario he or she is sent automatically to time-out (see earlier examples of how to do time-out in "Specific Procedures for Applying Parent Book Chapter 4").

Option 3, usually best for an **older child or teen**, involves indicating specific privileges that can be earned for following house rules on the ***Daily Privileges for Following House Rules*** form. Help the parent generate a list of all privileges to which the child has access on a typical day. Parent book Chapter 5 has many examples of specific privileges, ranging from video games to cell phone access to the car (for older teen). An important concept to discuss is the idea that privileges earned should be wants, not needs. Some children may **need** to go outside to get exercise for relief of stress or to have social contact with peers on a social networking website to minimize social isolation. In these instances it would not be wise to require the child to have to earn the privilege of going outside or accessing the Internet by following house rules. The practitioner and parent should carefully **choose privileges that are clearly wants, not needs.**

Work with parents to figure out the daily time period for which house rules must be followed and when earned privileges will be accessed later (e.g., same day or next day, as described in parent book Chapter 5). Review the pros and cons for the same-day or next-day method that fits their child's age and their family circumstances. As a general rule the same-day method is best for a **younger child**, and the next-day method works best for an **older child or teen**.

Help the parent organize the privileges into three levels of decreasing value. A clear example of the three levels of privileges is depicted in parent book Chapter 5. Prompt the parent to tell the child that his or her access to the privileges depends on whether the house rules are followed. A clear example of this is also illustrated in parent book Chapter 5. Thereafter the child is told that access to privileges depends on whether house rules are followed.

Provide counsel to the parent on how to deal effectively with a child who sneaks a privilege that was removed for 24 hours. Rather than adding on more consequences, it is preferable to restart the clock for 24 hours. The parent should tell the child that the privilege will be withheld for a 24-hour time span before the child gets it back.

Developing a Home Implementation Plan to Be Led by the Parent

Guide the parent in articulating a detailed plan for how the rule-oriented strategies will be implemented. This could include specifying when rules will be discussed with the child and "practiced" at home using option 1. It is a good idea to set specific goals on the *Parenting Goals* form (see parent book Chapter 3 and the end of Chapter 4 in this book). For example, the parent might write down a goal to use the *Daily Privileges for Following House Rules* chart, with steps centering on providing reminders of the house rules to the child and catching 'em following those rules. Then the parent needs to execute the plan and monitor progress.

Specific Procedures for Applying Parent Book Chapter 6

This chapter provides strategies for parent use to quell dishonest behaviors such as lying, sneaking, cheating, or stealing and to promote a child's development of honesty. The parent is informed about different types of dishonesty and some of the common reasons for it. This parent book chapter also notes the utility of beginning with a positive parenting approach that strengthens the parent–child bond and noticing and praising a child's honesty, as described earlier. This positive method often needs to be augmented with a firm approach that includes the child's acknowledgment of incidences of dishonest behavior, the parent's provision of a mild or moderate consequence, the child's willingness to make restitution, and the parent and child together reviewing how the dishonest behavior impacted others. Time-out or privilege removal is often used as a consequence for dishonesty, and a deferred method of implementation is advocated for children who resist such discipline. Other methods to promote the development of honesty, such as the enforcement of house rules, parental monitoring, and parental redirection of the child to achieve goals through honest means are also covered.

> Note: *The forms and charts referred to in the discussion below are in parent book Chapter 6 and also at the end of this chapter unless otherwise noted.*

Discussing Child Honesty Problems with Parents

It is important to help parents fully understand the different types of dishonest behavior and the multiple reasons for them. Types of dishonest behavior include lying, sneaking, cheating, and stealing. Among the potential causes of these various behaviors are impulsivity, peer pressure, and valuing dishonesty. Spend some time considering types and causes of dishonesty for the child in question. Read through the descriptive information in parent book Chapter 6 and help parents pinpoint the information that applies to their child. Explain to the parents that the strategies described in parent book Chapter 6 attempt not only to reduce incidents of dishonesty but also to help the child "internalize" a moral code of honesty. Help the parent understand that a child who frequently engages in dishonest behavior is at risk for a variety of future behavioral–emotional problems. The parent should be advised to take immediate and thorough action to reduce these behaviors.

Getting Parents Started and Focused

Review the ***Parent Checklist for Child Honesty*** with the parent. The parent can rate and check off items that are going well and pinpoint areas needing some work. Inform the parent that the checklist summarizes the basic ideas in this chapter. Impress upon the parent the importance of understanding the content on this checklist and what is written in parent book Chapter 6.

Training Parents to Use a Firm Approach When Child Dishonesty Occurs

The firm approach described here is recommended when an incident of dishonest behavior has occurred. Since some children lie about their dishonest behavior, ask the parents how they feel about using a "gut reaction" to "prove" the child was dishonest. Sometimes the parent is uncomfortable with this idea and wants to give the child the benefit of the doubt. One way to frame this point and to make parents more comfortable is to remind them that we all guide our own behavior by using the past to predict the future. Judging a child's behavior should not be an exception; in fact, the child's knowing that this past behavior may expose him or her to false accusations could be an incentive for behaving honestly in the future. More than likely, if a child has lied in the past, a gut reaction about the possibility of current lying will be accurate.

Make sure the parent understands that if the child admits to the act of dishonesty, he or she should receive only a standard time-out (1 minute for each year of age, as described in parent book Chapter 4) for a younger child or loss of a privilege for 24 hours for an older child or teen. If the parent believes that the child is lying, a doubled time-out period or a 48-hour privilege removal should be imposed. Be sure to brainstorm with the parent to generate a list of examples of privileges that can be removed (as described in parent book Chapters 4 and 5). Then it is up to the parent to make sure that the child is held accountable by making restitution and reviewing how the dishonest behavior impacted others. For example, if a child steals something from another family member, he or she must return or replace it, apologize to the "victim," and discuss or write down how this act made the other person feel (e.g., feels sad and angry, thinks the child can't be trusted). After the parent fully comprehends this strategy, it is a good idea to review it with the child, noting what will occur in the future if the child exhibits lying, sneaking, cheating, or stealing.

Modeling and role-play exercises can be constructed based on a past event of the child's dishonesty. For example, say a child was recently caught after having stolen money from his mother's purse. The events surrounding this incident of stealing could be reviewed via modeling and role playing within the context of this new strategy. Someone acting as the child, or the child him- or herself, could act out the initial denial of stealing from the mother. A father could demonstrate the imposition of the consequence, saying, "I am sure that you stole from your mother's purse, and you are going to lose the privilege of screen time (computer, videogames, etc.) for 24 hours; this will be doubled to 48 hours if you do not own up to it." Then the modeling or role-play exercise could conclude with the child admitting to stealing from his mother and the father responding by enforcing a 24-hour loss of screen time as a consequence. Additional similar role plays can be constructed from any past example of the child's lying, sneaking, cheating, or stealing.

Training Parents to Promote the Development of Honesty in the Child

Review of this strategy is accomplished primarily through discussion and planning. It basically boils down to trying to prevent incidents of dishonesty by promoting alternative development of honest behavior. This can be accomplished by enforcing clearly defined house rules (see discussion in "Specific Procedures for Applying Parent Book Chapter 5") and by monitoring the whereabouts and activities of the child. The monitoring strategy entails the parent's knowing the "four W's": what the child is doing, whom the child is with, where the child is going, and when the child will be home each time the child goes out. This particular strategy can be very useful in addressing the problems of a child who has a habit of sneaking and doing dishonest things behind the parent's back.

Tell the parent that another useful technique is to provide opportunities for the child to earn what he or she wants rather than obtaining it via dishonest means. The practitioner can guide the parent to set up a deal so that the child could earn something by working for it around the house or actually assist the older child or teen in getting a job. This concept can also include telling the child that instead of sneaking, trust will be earned, leading to more privileges, if he or she follows house rules for a few weeks. Brainstorm with the parent about other options for redirecting the child toward achieving his or her goals via honest versus dishonest means.

Developing a Home Implementation Plan to Be Led by the Parent

The manifestation of dishonest behavior can take many forms; many strategies for ameliorating these behaviors are discussed in parent book Chapter 6. It is essential that the practitioner guide the parent to focus on specific target behaviors of dishonesty and the corresponding strategies. Then a plan for how the chosen strategies will be used should be developed. It is helpful to identify specific goals on the **Parenting Goals** form (see parent book Chapter 3 and also the end of Chapter 4 in this book). For example, the parent might write down a goal to take a firm approach when the child sneaks and lies, to notice and praise the child for telling the truth, and to provide opportunities for the child to earn what he or she wants instead of getting it by sneaking and lying. Encourage the parent to execute the plan and monitor progress.

Specific Procedures for Applying Parent Book Chapter 7

Some of the firm strategies in parent book Chapters 4–6 can elicit reactive protests and anger outbursts from the child that can derail the parent's effort and resolve to correct the child's misbehavior. Chapter 7 of the parent book focuses on strategies and techniques that the parent can use to deal with the child's reactive and volatile behavior. As in the rest of this module, this parent book chapter notes the importance of beginning with a positive parenting approach. Then one section focuses on methods for managing child protests when a parent is disciplining for misbehavior (defiance, rule breaking, or dishonesty). Another section describes methods for preventing angry child outbursts through structure, predictability, and stopping the nagging that can trigger parent–child conflict. It is important to inform the parent that this chapter is not about teaching a child to internally calm him- or herself down. Rather it provides information and techniques for the parent to *externally* manage the child's emotional agitation.

Note: *The forms and charts referred to in the discussion below are in parent book Chapter 7 and also at the end of this chapter unless otherwise noted.*

Discussing Child Protesting/Outbursts with Parents

In earlier chapters it was noted that a child sometimes protests when a parent tries to get the child to behave or attempts to discipline him or her for misbehavior. The most important point to convey to parents here is that **protesting should be distinguished from misbehavior.** Misbehavior includes the noncompliance, rule breaking, and dishonesty targeted in this module. Protesting is a reaction to the parent's attempts to get the child to behave. Yet many parents confuse the two. For example, sometimes parents complain that their child is defiant and describe it as not listening, talking back, and "being disrespectful." A parent might say something like "He won't do what I say, and I'm not going to let him talk to me that way." This statement reflects a type of thinking that often leads to nonproductive and coercive power struggles. The practitioner needs to educate the parent about protesting and advise him or her to think of noncompliant, rule-breaking, and dishonest behaviors as separate from protesting. **Make sure the parent knows that the targeted misbehavior and the protesting each requires its own unique strategy.**

The practitioner should also inform the parent about the emotional component of protesting and suggest that the parent can help the child with "emotion regulation" (discussed in Chapter 7 of this book and covered in the emotional development module, Chapters 12–14, of the parent book) by effectively managing protesting. Frame the child's protesting as difficulties learning to regulate frustration and staying calm when challenges come up. In this case the challenge for the child is that he or she is being held accountable for misbehavior and has to deal with a consequence (i.e., time-out or removal of a privilege). Tell the parent that child protesting is an indication of immature emotion regulation. Encourage the parent not to personalize protesting (e.g., "I'm not going to stand for that disrespect") and instead reframe it so the parent can view it as a delay in emotional development. Suggest that the parent can help the child learn to cope with frustration-based emotions by responding to the child's emotional outbursts in a calm manner while still following through with discipline.

Tell the parent that gradually, over time, if he or she is consistent in responding to the child's protesting calmly, the length of the child's protesting behavior should get briefer and less intense. Shorter and moderated outbursts are evidence that the child is learning to cope with intense emotions and making progress. Explain that, conversely, responding to the child's protesting by engaging in power struggles can have an unintended effect of actually strengthening emotion dysregulation through the back-and-forth escalation. Explain that this can paradoxically make the child's protesting worse over time. It can also be useful to tell the parent that emotion dysregulation is a significant precursor for future behavioral–emotional problems. It therefore behooves the parent to respond to it in an effective manner, thus preventing future problems from emerging.

It is not too surprising that many children with emotion dysregulation difficulties also have a parent with similar problems. Parent book Chapters 17 and 18, which focus on helping a parent develop personal coping skills related to parenting, can also be a useful adjunct to parent book Chapter 7.

Chapter 7 in the parent book also discusses that many children with volatile behavior will need much more than better parental management of their protesting and outbursts. Other modules in the book may also be useful to work on, including the child-focused emotional development module, the parent-focused well-being module, and the family-focused well-being module. Other non-skill-related interventions may be needed (including possible medications) as well. It is a good idea to brainstorm with the parent about whether other skills or interventions would be useful with the volatile child in question.

Getting Parents Started and Focused

Review the ***Parent Checklist for Child Protests and Angry Outbursts*** with the parent. The parent can rate and check off items that are going well and pinpoint areas needing some work. Inform the parent that the checklist summarizes the basic ideas in this chapter. Highly recommend that the parent fully comprehend the content on this checklist and what is written in Chapter 7.

Training Parents to Manage Child Protesting and to Disengage/Deescalate

Educate the parent that protesting typically occurs when the parent attempts to get the child to behave or when using time-out (with a younger child) or removing privileges (with any age child) to discipline him or her. It is important at the outset for the parent to distinguish between different levels of protesting behavior in the child. Typically, mild protesting takes the form of grunting, complaining, talking under the breath, etc. Moderate protesting may manifest as refusing to be disciplined, stomping off, slamming doors, and the like. Severe protesting could entail destruction of property, threats to self or others, violence, dangerous behaviors, and so on. Thoroughly discuss and review mild, moderate, and severe forms of child protesting, as defined in parent book Chapter 7. It can help to discuss past events when the child protested and ask the parent to categorize those protests as mild, moderate, or severe. To promote awareness, discuss typical ways in which the child exhibits protesting behaviors at the different levels.

Next ask the parent to imagine putting the child in time-out (for the parent of younger children) or removing a privilege (for the parent of children at all ages) and then being confronted with the child's protesting. Talk to the parent about ways he or she can respond to different levels of protesting. The three levels of protesting can be presented as steps upon which the parent will add strategies to manage the child's emotional reactions. **Tell the parent that the strategy for dealing with mild protesting is to ignore it.** Lead the parent to identify different ways to ignore the child's mild protesting behavior. For example, the parent could stop talking, avoid eye contact, and walk away.

When moderate protesting occurs, the parents should continue to ignore the behavior and add a "patient standoff" strategy. Inform the parent that the goal of the patient standoff is to remain calm, avoid power struggles, and eventually "win," with the child doing what he or she has been told. For example, when using time-out, the parent could take away the TV viewing privilege until the child completes it. Another example is when a parent takes away TV for 24 hours and the child keeps watching it anyway, to which the parent informs the child that as soon as he or she stops watching television, the 24-hour restriction will begin. If need be, tell parents they can **"go on strike"** until the child cooperates with relinquishing the privilege. When on strike, the parent does not do favors for the child, such as chauffeuring, ironing, making meals for friends, getting the child's favorite snack at the store, etc. Make sure parents understand that the "favors" they identify are indeed extras and that going on strike does not mean denying the child the fundamental care that parents owe their children (feeding them, keeping them safe, maintaining a positive and loving bond, etc.). Inform the parent that a patient standoff can sometimes last for several days!

For example, one mother took away TV until her protesting 10-year-old son completed his time-out 2 days later.

When severe protesting occurs, advise the parent that the ignoring and patient stand-off strategy should remain in effect, and safety procedures should be added. This means isolating/removing the child from others (or others from the child), deescalating/disengaging, and still keeping track of what the child is doing. One idea to review is the notion of sending the child to his or her room to "cool down," and then once calm, the child can go to time-out or surrender the stated privilege(s). Suggest that the parent may need to get help from other adults. **Advise the parent that restraining the child or calling the police is the very last resort and should be avoided except when the child is "out of control."**

The parent must understand that it typically does not help to add more consequences for protesting because that can escalate the situation. Tell the parent that the preferred strategy is to keep restarting the time interval for time-out or privilege removal with each new infraction or incident of misbehavior. With time-out, for example, each time the child gets out of the chair and/or misbehaves, the timer is restarted. With privilege removal, if the child will not relinquish the privilege, calm down, or stop misbehaving, the 24-hour privilege loss cannot begin until all problem behaviors desist.

It is imperative to instruct the parent on how to disengage/deescalate emotionally, verbally, and physically in accordance with the techniques outlined in parent book Chapter 7. The basic idea is to stay calm, minimize talking, and physically separate from the severely protesting child. Make sure the parent knows that "I understand" statements **can** be used to acknowledge a child's feelings ("I see that you are frustrated," "I know how important this is to you," etc.). In addition, the parent can use the broken record technique to remind the child to calm down in order to have a discussion (e.g., "As soon as you calm down, we can discuss it"). The parent should be counseled, however, not to engage in dialogue with a child about the **content** of the protests or complaints (e.g., "You are so unfair," "That's not what you said before," "You never told me") as this will escalate matters.

The use of modeling and role playing to teach the parent how to handle the protesting child is strongly advised. It might be best to model and role-play the strategy without the child at first and then later consider involving the child in the exercises if he or she has a positive attitude and demeanor. Modeling and role-play scenarios can be constructed from the parent's recounting of past incidences of the child's protests in response to time-out and/or removal of privileges. For example, consider a role play for a **younger child** who broke the house rule of "Work out disagreements in a respectful way with your siblings" by hitting her brother, and she angrily protested an automatic time-out by refusing to go. The practitioner could model stating to the child "You broke the 'respect your sibling' rule, so you must go to the time-out chair and you can't watch TV until you do it," or something similar. Then the practitioner could demonstrate deescalating/disengaging from the child by using self-talk to stay calm, looking away, providing an occasional "I understand" statement, or using the broken record technique and attempting to walk away. As soon as the child calms down, the practitioner could prompt her to go to the time-out chair. After the modeling demonstration, ask the parent to practice with the same scenario in a similar manner via role playing.

Imagining an **older child or teen** breaking the same house rule, the modeling or role-play practice with the protesting behavior might center on the child's getting angry and refusing to relinquish his cell phone for 24 hours. In this case the parent might say "You violated the 'respecting your sibling' rule, and now you will lose your cell phone for 24 hours. The time begins only after you hand it over." Then the parent could also practice deescalating and disengaging from the older child or teen by staying calm, not talking to him or her, and attempting to walk away. It is particularly useful for the practitioner to model for the parent the use of coping self-talk when dealing with a protesting child, such as "Stay cool," "I can handle it," etc.

Another series of modeling and role-playing exercises could center on putting a child in time-out or removing privileges while he or she is protesting severely. The same modeling and role-play scenarios could be used, with the addition of more severe protesting. Ask whoever is playing the younger child to refuse, yell, maybe tip a chair over, etc. Make sure everyone understands that this behavior is "just pretend" and not real. If someone is getting upset with this modeling or role play, it should be halted. This exercise provides an opportunity to practice isolating/removing the child from others (or others from the child), getting help from other adults (restraining or calling the police as a last resort), and deescalating/disengaging while still keeping track of what the child is doing. It is useful for the practitioner who models and the parent who later practices this strategy to talk out loud about what they are doing to illustrate the importance of self-talk. The most productive self-talk when dealing with a severely protesting child is to say things to oneself such as "Stay cool," "I can handle it," etc.

Training Parents to Prevent Angry Child Outbursts

This strategy is accomplished primarily through discussion and planning. It emphasizes trying to prevent angry outbursts by strategically using many of the methods and procedures described in this behavioral development module in a **proactive fashion.** Educate the parent about the four stages that a child will go through in the angry outburst process as described in parent book Chapter 7. The parent should be told that it is preferable to focus his or her efforts on preventing angry outbursts (Stages 1 and 2) rather than reactively dealing with them (Stage 3) and dealing with the aftermath (Stage 4).

The proactive strategy for Stage 1 centers on maintaining a state of calm in the child by providing predictable household routines, enforcing clearly stated house rules, and attending to positive behaviors in the child. Brainstorm with parents on how they might implement a schedule or routine in their home (see parent book Chapter 19 for more ideas) so that the child's environment is predictable. Tell the parent that this predictability can be particularly useful for a child who is inflexible and has a hard time with transitions. Also tell the parent that setting up and following through with house rules, as discussed in parent book

Chapter 5, can serve as a preventive strategy because children will understand exactly what is expected and have less to react to. Parent book Chapters 4–7 all emphasize different variations of "catching 'em being good." Inform the parent that it is useful to promote positive behavior and prevent emotional outbursts from the child by attending to the child's positive behavior.

The proactive strategy for Stage 2 pertains to redirecting an increasingly agitated child by guiding him or her in the use of stress management and/or family cool-down. Tell the parent that this is useful only if the foundation has been laid by teaching the child these coping-related skills. The practitioner and parent will need to do some background work of teaching the child to use stress management techniques (see parent book Chapter 14) and family conflict management methods (see parent book Chapter 20). If the child has been taught these skills, the parent can prompt the child to engage in them in the early stages of agitation. Help the parent plan how he or she might go about teaching the child personal stress management skills and/or teaching family members the family conflict management procedures. In addition, the techniques for handling mild and moderate protesting can also be useful at Stage 2.

Inform parents that at Stages 3 and 4 they are basically in a "crisis management" mode. The emphasis at Stage 3 is on maintaining safety for the child and other family members. Procedures reviewed earlier, pertaining to severe protesting and disengaging/deescalating while maintaining safety, are useful at this point. In addition, at Stage 4, after calming down, the child is held accountable for his or her actions during the outburst. This accountability might involve the parent requiring the child to clean up, possibly make restitution, and process or discuss what happened (if the child is cooperative).

Developing a Home Implementation Plan to Be Led by Parents

Protesting behaviors and angry acting out on the part of the child are stressful and complicated to manage. The practitioner must help parents focus on specific ways of responding to their child's volatile reactions using techniques in parent book Chapter 7. The *Parenting Goals* form (see parent book Chapter 3 and also the end of Chapter 4 in this book) can be used to identify and track progress with specific goals. For example, the parent might choose the patient standoff procedure as a goal to work on, with steps related to staying calm and using coping self-talk. Another goal might be to work at deescalating/disengaging with an emphasis on using "I understand" statements and the broken record technique. Encourage parents to execute their plan and monitor progress.

Modifications for Implementing the Child Behavioral Development Module in Parent Groups

The *Overview of Child Behavioral Development Module* chart can be used to orient parent group members to the primary methods for enhancing children's behavior. Ask group members to discuss behavioral challenges they have with their children and what parenting methods they have tried in the past. Often a parent will say something like "I tried that and it didn't work." Chances are that such a parent did try something like the strategies depicted but did not implement them very well and did not PERCON. Tell parents these techniques work most of the time with the caveat that they have to be implemented well.

Facilitate a discussion to help group members reach a consensus regarding which areas could be emphasized for that meeting or over several meetings. The topics can be introduced over one meeting, but if a parent group chooses to emphasize this module, it could take three or more meetings to review the topics of using a positive approach; teaching a child to comply, follow rules, and behave honestly; as well as teaching the parent to manage a child's protesting and preventing angry outbursts. All of the charts and forms found in parent book Chapters 4–7 (and at the end of this chapter) can be used, as needed, to impart information and strategies for improving a child's behavior. The role plays in the training sections above for parent book Chapters 4–7 could be replicated in parent groups. It can be useful to have parents take turns in role plays if they are comfortable. It helps to do role plays first without managing a child who is protesting and then later with managing a child who is protesting. Help each parent individually pinpoint specific behavioral management goals and strategies to work on using the ***Parenting Goals*** form.

Overview of the Child Behavioral Development Module

Beginning with a Positive Approach in Chapters 4–7

- *Building a relationship*—make an extra effort to establish rapport and "bond" with child

- *Avoiding critical or negative comments*—be aware and try not to engage in criticism, asking negative questions, blaming, bringing up old issues, and/or delivering put-downs, etc.

- *Catching 'em being good*—make three positive comments or praise for one correction or reprimand

Chapter 4. Doing What You're Told: Teaching Your Child to Comply with Parental Directives

Avoiding Ineffective or Unclear Commands When Giving Directives

- Vague command (e.g., "Knock it off," "Shape up")

- Question command (e.g., "Do you want to pick up your clothes?")

- Rationale command (e.g., "You need to hurry or we will be late")

- Multiple commands (e.g., "Pick up your books, go wash your hands, and sit down at the table")

- Frequent commands (e.g., Telling your child to do something again and again and again . . .)

Using Three Steps for Increasing Compliance

- *Stating effective command*—make it clear, specific, one-step, with eye contact and voice *slightly* raised (e.g., "Turn off the TV and come to dinner now")

- *Stating warning as "If . . . then"*—warning with time-out or privilege removal until there is compliance or for 24 hours (e.g., "*If* you don't . . ., *then* . . . [time-out or privilege removal]")

- *Following through with warning*—put child in time-out or take away privilege (see Chapter 7 for when child does not cooperate with time-out or privilege removal)

See the **Time-Out** and **Removing Privileges for Noncompliance** charts.

Chapter 5. Doing What's Expected: Teaching Your Child to Follow Rules

Writing Down and Posting House Rules

- Worded as *dos*, not as *don'ts* (e.g., "Be ready for the bus at 7:00 A.M. on school days," instead of "Don't be late for the bus")

Following Through to Enforce Rules (Three Options)

- Regular monitoring of rule following and providing verbal feedback

- Automatic time-out for rule violations (for a younger child)

(cont.)

- Privileges earned or lost according to how well house rules were followed

  - *Same-day method*—privileges for the evening are based on how well house rules were followed that same day (e.g., privileges allowed after homework until bedtime depend on how well house rules were followed to that point on a Tuesday)

  - *Next-day method*—privileges for the next day are based on how well house rules were followed the previous day (e.g., privileges on a Wednesday depend on how well house rules were followed on a Tuesday)

See **How Well Was I Following the House Rules Today?** and **Daily Privileges for Following House Rules** forms.

Chapter 6. Doing the Right Thing: Teaching Your Child to Behave Honestly

Using Four Steps to Reduce Dishonesty (e.g., Lying, Sneaking, Cheating, or Stealing)

- *Noting that dishonest behavior has occurred*—use "gut reaction" as "proof" if child denies it but parent is certain it occurred

- Providing a consequence—to teach a lesson, not to punish

  - Enforce mild consequence if infraction admitted (e.g., remove privileges for 24 hours)

  - Enforce moderate consequence if infraction denied (e.g., remove privileges for 48 hours)

  - Avoid severe consequences

- *Arranging apology and restitution*—apologize and do "extras" for "victim." If stealing is involved, stolen item is returned or replaced

- *Helping child understand impact on others*—communicate disappointment in the dishonest behavior and its impact on others

Promoting Development of Honesty

- Enforcing house rules and monitoring child's activities

- Providing opportunities for child to earn things or privileges

Chapter 7. Staying Cool under Fire:
Managing Your Child's Protesting of Discipline and Preventing Angry Outbursts

Managing "Protesting" of Disciplining (When Using Time-Out or Removing a Privilege)

- *Mild protesting: Ignore*—do not pay attention to grunting/groaning, huffing/puffing, talking under breath, etc., as long as child is cooperating with time-out or privilege removal

(cont.)

- *Moderate protesting: Ignore + patient standoff*—patiently follow through when child is banging things, yelling loudly, getting out of time-out chair, and/or will not give up a privilege that has been removed

  - *When using time-out*—take away a privilege until child goes to and stays in time-out (e.g., no TV until time-out is completed)

    - *When using privilege removal*—go "on strike" (e.g., do not provide extra favors) until a privilege is surrendered or turned over

- *Severe protesting: Ignore + patient standoff + safety procedures*—isolate or remove others from a child who is harming self, others, or property (get help, if needed). Once calm, consider asking child to clean up and make restitution (e.g., apologize, pay damages)

Disengaging and Deescalating When Child Is Highly Agitated

- *Emotional level*—stay calm

- *Verbal level*—minimize talking

- *Physical level*—minimize eye contact and try to walk away

Don't Add on Consequences for Protesting or Other Incidences of Noncompliance

- If using time-out, the child returns there and time is restarted

- If using privilege removal, the time is restarted with each incident

Emphasizing the Prevention of Angry Outbursts

- *Maintaining a state of calm*—have predictable household routines and clearly stated rules and expectations and pay attention to positive behaviors

- *Redirecting an increasingly agitated child*—use calming strategies such as recognizing child's feelings (e.g., "I see you look upset") and/or guiding child to use stress management and/or to participate in a family cool-down

- *Dealing with the angry outburst*—disengage/deescalate and maintain safety

- *Recovery from the angry outburst*—consider having child clean up, and/or make restitution, and/or discuss what happened (only if child is calm)

Training Parent in Behavior Development Skills (Chapters 4–7)

- Identify parenting skills and goals related to promoting child's behavioral development

- Learn, practice, and monitor progress with behavioral development skills and goals

See **Parent Checklist** for each chapter and **Parenting Goals** form (in Chapter 3 and at the end of Chapter 4 in this book).

Forms from Parent Book Chapter 4

Parent Checklist for Child Compliance

Name: _____ Date: _____

In the blanks below, indicate a score for **how well** you make use of that parenting behavior at this time.

	Not too well	Okay	Very well
	1	2	3

Parent's Use of a Positive Approach to Increase Child's Compliance

A. ____ Building a relationship and bond

B. ____ Avoiding use of critical or negative comments

C. ____ Catching 'em being compliant by using three positive comments or praise about the child's compliance for every one correction or reprimand about child's noncompliance

Parent's Use of a Firm Approach to Reduce Child's Noncompliance

D. ____ Giving *effective commands* by making them clear, specific, one-step, and while having eye contact with the child and with voice slightly raised

E. ____ Giving *effective warnings* that *if* the command isn't followed, *then* the child will go to time-out *or* lose a privilege

F. ____ *Following through* by putting the child in time-out *or* taking away a privilege at that moment or in a delayed and patient manner if the child protests (acts up) significantly

Parent's Use of Strategies to Manage Child's Protesting of Discipline for Noncompliance

G. ____ Ignoring and not getting caught up in the child's talking back, acting up, complaining, and so on, when trying to get the child to comply (see Chapter 7 for more information)

H. ____ Disengaging from power struggles and avoiding yelling, threatening, forcing, and so on, to get the child to comply (see Chapter 7 for more information)

I. ____ Following through with D–F above in a calm manner (see Chapter 7 for more information)

Time-Out

1. **Command**—"I want you to. . . . "

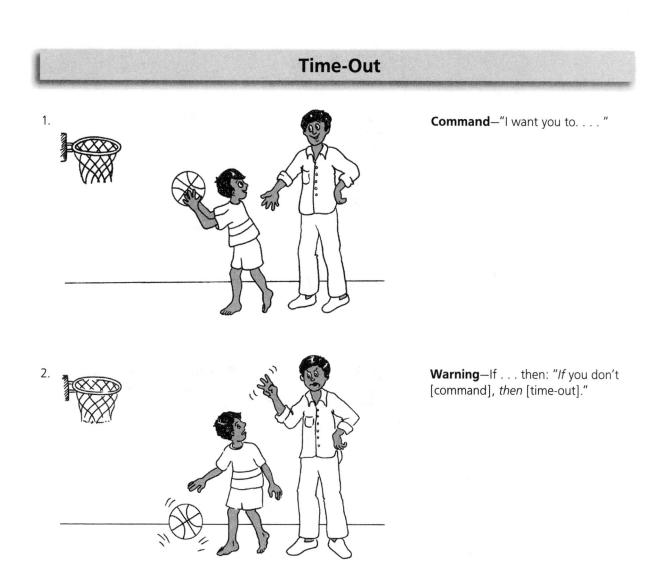

2. **Warning**—If . . . then: "*If* you don't [command], *then* [time-out]."

3. **Time-out**—Have the child sit and then set a timer.

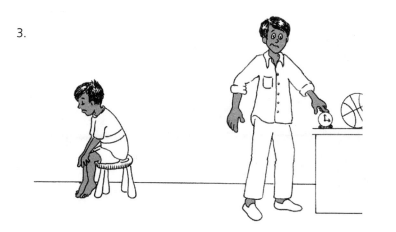

Time-Out

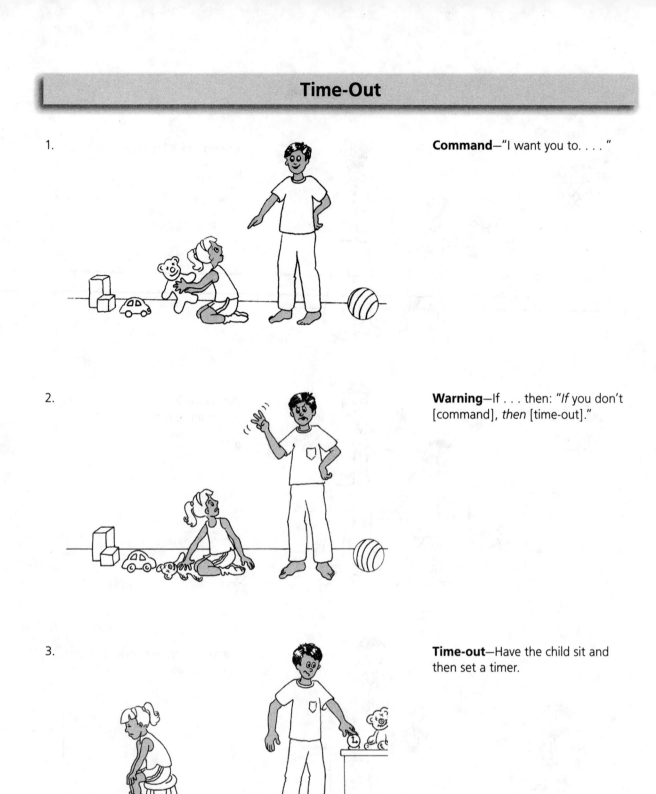

1.

Command—"I want you to. . . . "

2.

Warning—If . . . then: "*If* you don't [command], *then* [time-out]."

3.

Time-out—Have the child sit and then set a timer.

Time-Out

1.

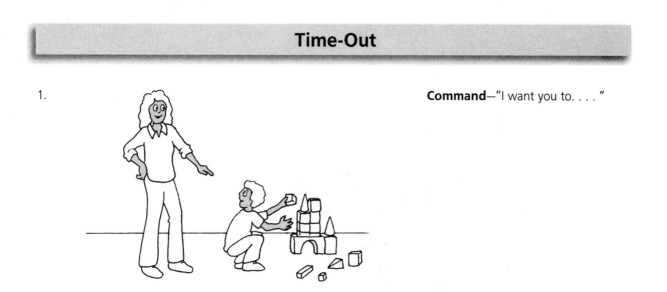

Command—"I want you to. . . . "

2.

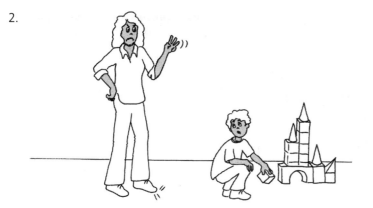

Warning—If . . . then: "*If* you don't [command], *then* [time-out]."

3.

Time-out—Have the child sit and then set a timer.

1.

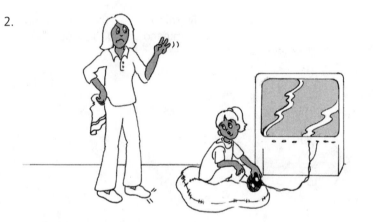

Command—"I want you to. . . . "

2.

Warning—If . . . then: "*If* you don't [command], *then* [time-out]."

3.

Time-out—Have the child sit and then set a timer.

Removing Privileges for Noncompliance

1. **Parent states a brief, clear, and specific command to child or teen.**

2. **Give a warning:** "If . . . then" statement.

   - **Option 1:** The child or teen is told *if* he or she doesn't follow command, *then* a privilege will be lost until he or she complies with the command.

   - **Option 2:** The child or teen is told *if* he or she doesn't follow command, *then* a privilege will be lost for a specified period of time (e.g., 24 hours), and he or she is still expected to comply with command.

3. **Loss of privilege.** Follow through with option 1 or 2 above.

4. Privilege return. **The lost privilege is restored in accordance with the specification of option 1 or 2 above.**

Forms from Parent Book Chapter 5

Parent Checklist for Child Rule Following

Name: _____ Date: _____

In the blanks below, indicate a score for **how well** you make use of each parenting behavior at this time.

Not too well	Okay	Very well
1	2	3

Parent's Use of a Positive Approach to Increase Child's Rule Following

A. _____ Building a relationship and bond

B. _____ Avoiding the use of critical or negative comments

C. _____ Catching 'em following the rules by using three positive comments or praise for the child's rule following for every one correction/reprimand for not following them

Parent's Use of Clearly Stated House Rules for Child

D. _____ Discussing house rules so that the child definitely knows them

E. _____ Writing down house rules in clear terms and posting them

Parent's Use of a Firm Approach to Reduce Child's Rule Violations

F. _____ Periodically reviewing the house rules

G. _____ Putting a younger child in automatic time-out for house rules violations

H. _____ Providing access to privileges according to how well the child or teen has followed house rules

Parent's Use of Strategies to Manage Child's Protesting of Discipline for Breaking Rules

I. _____ Ignoring and not getting caught up in the child's talking back, acting up, complaining, and so on, when trying to get the child to follow house rules (see Chapter 7 for more information)

J. _____ Disengaging from power struggles and avoiding yelling, threatening, forcing, and so on, to get the child to follow house rules (see Chapter 7 for more information)

K. _____ Following through with D–H above in a calm manner (see Chapter 7 for more information)

How Well Was I Following the House Rules Today?

1. I think I was following the rules . . .

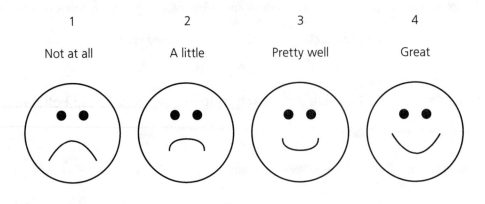

2. You think I was following the rules . . .

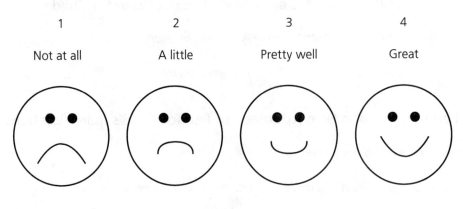

Daily Privileges for Following House Rules

Name: _____

Write down daily time period for which house rules must be followed and when earned privileges can be accessed (e.g., same day or next day): _____

Write down four house rules to be followed each day. Put a *Y* (Yes) in the box if the rule was followed or an *N* (No) in the box if the rule was not followed. At the end of the day, tally up the *Y*'s and then provide privileges that were earned that day or the next day.

House rules	Mon.	Tues.	Wed.	Thurs.	Fri.	Sat.	Sun.
1.							
2.							
3.							
4.							
Total Y's (Yes) for the day							

Daily Privileges Earned

4 *Y*'s (Yes) for Level A Privileges = _____ privileges

2–3 *Y*'s (Yes) for Level B Privileges = _____ privileges

0–1 *Y* (Yes) for Level C Privileges = _____ privileges

Forms from Parent Book Chapter 6

Parent Checklist for Child Honesty

Name: _____ Date: _____

In the blanks below, indicate a score for **how well** you make use of that parenting behavior at this time.

Not too well	**Okay**	**Very well**
1	**2**	**3**

Parent's Use of a Positive Approach to Increase Child's Honesty

A. _____ Building a relationship and bond

B. _____ Avoiding the use of critical or negative comments

C. _____ Catching 'em being honest by using three positive comments or praise related to the child's honest behavior for every one correction/reprimand for dishonest behavior

Parent's Use of a Firm Approach When Child's Dishonesty Occurs

D. _____ Publicly acknowledging the specific incidence of dishonesty either by the child's admitting it or by your saying it occurred based on a "gut reaction"

E. _____ Providing a mild consequence (e.g., remove privileges for 24 hours) if dishonesty is admitted or a moderate consequence (e.g., remove privileges for 48 hours) if dishonesty is denied

F. _____ Making sure that the child apologizes and makes restitution to the "victim" of dishonesty

G. _____ Communicating disappointment and reviewing how the dishonest behavior impacted others

Parent's Use of Strategies to Promote Development of Child's Honesty

H. _____ Enforcing clearly defined house rules

I. _____ Keeping close tabs on the child through monitoring, including when out of house

J. _____ Promoting the child's earning what is wanted instead of getting it dishonestly

Parent's Use of Strategies to Manage Child's Protesting of Discipline for Dishonesty

K. _____ Ignoring and not getting caught up in the child's talking back, acting up, complaining, and so on, when trying to teach the child to behave honestly (see Chapter 7 for more information)

L. _____ Disengaging from power struggles and avoiding yelling, threatening, forcing, and so on to teach the child to behave honestly (see Chapter 7 for more information)

M. _____ Following through with D–J above in a calm manner (see Chapter 7 for more information)

Forms from Parent Book Chapter 7

Parent Checklist for Child Protests and Angry Outbursts

Name: _____ Date: _____

In the blanks below, indicate a score for **how well** you make use of that parenting behavior at this time.

Not too well	Okay	Very well
1	2	3

Parent's Use of a Positive Approach to Increase Child's Calmness

A. ____ Building a relationship and bond

B. ____ Avoiding the use of critical or negative comments

C. ____ Catching 'em staying calm by using three positive comments or praise related to staying calm for every one correction or reprimand for getting angry or having an outburst

Parent's Use of a Patient Approach to Manage Child's Protesting

D. ____ Managing *mild* child protesting (grunting, complaining, etc.) by ignoring it

E. ____ Managing *moderate* child protesting (refusing to be disciplined, stomping off, slamming the door, etc.) with ignoring, remaining calm, avoiding power struggles, and patiently getting the child to eventually do what he or she was told (i.e., a "patient standoff")

F. ____ Managing *severe* protesting with ignoring, patiently prevailing, and taking safety precautions as needed (isolating and removing others; calling police as last resort)

Parent's Use of Disengaging and Deescalating Techniques with an Agitated Child

G. ____ Reducing unproductive discussions when the child is agitated; making occasional *"I understand"* *statements* ("I see that you are upset") and using the *"broken record technique"* (repeating "As soon as you calm down, we can discuss it" and so on)

H. ____ Minimizing eye contact and trying to walk away

I. ____ Staying calm!

Parent's Use of Prevention to Avoid or Reduce Child's Angry Outbursts

J. ____ Maintaining a state of calm in the child by using predictable household routines, clearly stated rules, and attending to positive behaviors in the child

K. ____ Redirecting an increasingly agitated child by guiding in the use of stress management and/or family cool-down at first signs of child agitation

L. ____ Dealing with the child's angry outburst by disengaging/deescalating while maintaining safety

M. ____ Helping the child recover by prompting him or her to clean up, possibly make restitution, and process what happened if the child is cooperative

6

Using the Child Social Development Module

This practitioner book chapter corresponds to the parent book section "Enhancing Your Child's Social Development" (Chapters 8–11). In this module the parent is given ideas and strategies for enhancing the child's social behavior and social problem-solving competencies, as well as focused strategies for dealing with bullies and negative peer influence. **The practitioner should read and fully understand the *content* in parent book Chapters 8–11 before using the related *procedures* described here.**

It is important for the practitioner to consider who should be involved and when during training of the social development module. With a **younger child** it is often best to train the child and parent simultaneously. This allows the parent to learn all social-type skills and then be actively involved in helping the child use those skills at home. Alternatively, since this module is focused on the child's acquiring skills, it can be productive to train the child first and then bring the parent in to learn, support, and encourage skill development in the child. This approach—train the child and then train the parent—is particularly useful when an **older child or teen** might benefit from private discussion of social concerns; it also assists in garnering the child or teen's buy-in and motivation. It is a good idea to collaborate with the child and parent about when to involve the parents, although it is imperative to involve the parent in the process at some point.

Tailoring within the Child Social Development Module

The *Overview of the Child Social Development Module* chart at the end of this chapter provides a concise review of the ideas and methods contained in this module. This chart can be used to guide a psychoeducation-focused discussion with a parent regarding broad goals and skills-building strategies used to promote competency in children who are struggling in the social development area. Tell the parent that each chapter deals with increasingly more sophisticated social skills and that work with a younger child should focus on basic skills (e.g., taking turns), whereas work with an older child or teen can work on advanced skills (e.g., being assertive in peer pressure situations). Sometimes it is best to begin with earlier chapters and proceed to later chapters as a child's skills become increasingly advanced. The initial discussion should culminate in talking through skills-building options for improving the child's social development and beginning to formulate an individualized plan.

Specific Procedures for Applying Parent Book Chapter 8

This chapter targets rudimentary social skills and emphasizes behavioral rehearsal as a primary training method. **It is most useful for younger children, but the older child or teen with social delays can often benefit too.** The chapter explains how parents can teach and coach the child in positive social behavior skills: identifying social behaviors to work on (basic or advanced); explaining, demonstrating, and role-playing/practicing specified social behavior(s) with the child; and periodically reviewing to create more awareness and/or using charts to promote use of social behavior skills. The parent is also encouraged to arrange social activities to give the child social opportunities and a venue in which to practice social behavior goals.

Note: *The forms and charts referred to in the discussion below are in parent book Chapter 8 and also at the end of this chapter unless otherwise noted.*

Discussing Child Social Interaction Problems with Parents

Parents who already know that their child is having difficulty in the social arena can often relate incidents illustrating the child's problems that typically center on aggressive, withdrawn, and/or bothersome social behaviors with peers and/or siblings. Explain that the best way to deal with negative social behaviors is to promote the child's use of positive replacement social behaviors. For parents who describe social problems in their child but do not seem to take them as seriously as problems in other arenas, it may be important to emphasize how difficulties making friends can impact the child's longer-term development. Describe how children who have social interaction difficulties sometimes end up being rejected or neglected by positive-influence peers and occasionally end up affiliating or hanging out with the "wrong crowd." Helping a child acquire social behavior skills now is an important first step to enhance social development and reduce the likelihood of later problems. Once the child has built good social behavior skills, the parent can help him or her with more complex social skills such as problem solving, coping with bullies, and handling peer pressure, presented in later chapters of the parent book.

Getting Parents Started and Focused

Parents can use the *Parent Checklist for Child Social Behaviors* to see what is working and what needs to be worked on to make progress. This checklist summarizes the overall approach in the chapter; be prepared to answer any content questions so that the parents understand all the information summarized on the list and described in parent book Chapter 8.

Training the Parent and Child to Promote Child Social Behavior Skills

Parent book Chapter 8 provides examples of negative child social behaviors, and it makes sense to spend a little time discussing them and the similar behaviors that parents are seeing in their child to clarify where their problems lie. But then you would be wise to move quickly to identifying specific positive social behaviors for the child to work on to *replace* those negative social behaviors. Ask the parent to examine the *Identifying Social Behaviors to Work On* form and identify basic or advanced social behaviors for the child to work on. The goal is to identify the best social behavior to work on by first examining the problem behavior and then finding the opposite adaptive behavior and to get the parent oriented to that way of thinking (i.e., replacing problem behaviors with adaptive behaviors). Because there are many other social behaviors that are not on the form, you will need to prompt the parent to identify all of the problematic ones observed in the child and then help the parent funnel them down to one or two that seem to be the most important.

To teach the child the targeted social behavior(s), you can first use modeling and role plays in the training context and then ask the parent to duplicate the role plays at home. Either train the child alone and then invite the parent in for a demonstration or train the child and parent together.

For example, with a **younger child** who tends to dominate playtime with other children, the role play might center on the two social behaviors of cooperating during play and inquiring about others' interests. The practitioner could act as the child and physically model the give-and-take of cooperatively playing with another "child" (perhaps the parent acting as the other child) during a game while asking questions about what he or she likes to do (e.g., "What do you like to do for fun?" or "Do you have a favorite game?"). The same role-play scenario could be repeated with the child assuming his or her true role.

Another example could apply to an **older child or teen** who tends to argue too much by role-playing how to disagree respectfully and compromise. The practitioner could act as the older child or teen and verbally model staying calm while disagreeing with someone about what TV show to watch and then strike some kind of compromise (e.g., "This is one of my favorite shows, so how about if I choose the show now and you can choose the next one?"). The same role-play scenario could be repeated with the older child or teen assuming his or her true role.

With problems in verbally oriented social behaviors, such as starting conversations, inquiring about others' interests, asserting self, etc., ask the child and/or parent for examples of one- or two-sentence statements the child could make and then suggest that the child review and rehearse this script periodically.

Explain that coaching involves prompting or reminding the child to be aware of and to physically perform positive social behaviors. Use the ***Personal Goals (Basic*** or ***Advanced)*** form (see parent book Chapter 3 and the end of Chapter 4 in this book) in the session to practice using the form and prompting the targeted social behaviors with parents and siblings (if they are in attendance). For example, the child could work on "waiting your turn to talk" as a replacement for interrupting others during the session. At the end of the session the parent could be guided to go through the steps on the ***Personal Goals (Basic*** or ***Advanced)*** form. This approach enables both the parent and child to practice using a new skill in the training context before using it at home.

Helping Parents Create Opportunities for the Child to Use Social Behavior Skills

Brainstorm with the parent about ways to provide opportunities for the child to practice social behavior skills. Perhaps the parent could arrange play dates for a **younger child** or organize outings (e.g., to a baseball game or movie) with an **older child or teen** and one or more peers. It may be helpful to enroll the child in ongoing structured and routine activities (e.g., Scouting, sports teams, orchestra). The parent could guide the child in planning specific social behavior goals to work on during the upcoming activity and afterward process how well it went.

Developing a Home Implementation Plan to Be Led by Parents

Brainstorm with the parent about when and how often to review social behaviors with the child at home. Discuss ways in which the parent will coach the child to practice the new targeted social behavior in everyday interactions with friends, siblings, and/or parents. Discuss specific goals that the parent can enter on the ***Parenting Goals*** form (see parent book Chapter 3 and the end of Chapter 4 in this book). For example, the parent might write down a goal of using the ***Personal Goals (Basic*** or ***Advanced)*** form to guide the child to work on the social behaviors of **sharing** (younger child) or **negotiating in a calm manner** (older child or teen). Another related goal for the ***Parenting Goals*** form might be to create two social opportunities per week for the child to practice using social behavior skills. Establishing when (evenings, weekends, etc.), where (home, school, in the neighborhood, etc.), and how often (once per day or week, several times per day or week, etc.) social behaviors will be worked on will help parents follow through.

Suggest that another way to monitor progress and refine methods is for the parent to conduct occasional *10-minute family meetings* (see parent book Chapter 2) at home to review social behavior skills. During these meetings the parent should focus on the child's use of specified social behaviors and note the child's efforts toward reaching social behavior goals. The parent should encourage the child to "keep it going."

Typical problems for parents that affect home implementation of the material in this chapter are the parents' lack of direct opportunity to guide the child in using social behavior skills and the child's discontinued use of social behavior skills as they fall by the wayside. Brainstorm with the parents about taking advantage of situations that do arise in which it **is** possible to guide the child, such as a visit to a cousin's house, a neighbor's birthday party, sports practice, etc. Also remind parents that the parent–child relationship is a social one at its core, so there may be opportunities to guide the child in that ever-present context.

Delivery Procedures for Applying Parent Book Chapter 9

This chapter uses behavioral training methods to promote adaptive social–cognitive skills. Children of all ages can benefit as long as work with younger children focuses on basic social problem-solving skills and advanced skills are reserved for older children. Because it may be difficult for a child under the age of 8–10 to independently apply social problem solving, children of that age typically require more guidance.

Parent book Chapter 9 explains how parents can teach the child to recognize when a social problem exists and to use a step-by-step process to solve it. The parents will discuss and practice social problem-solving skills (basic or advanced) with the child, periodically discuss and/or use charts to guide social problem solving, and use social problem solving to mediate sibling conflict (if applicable). The parents are also encouraged to arrange social activities to give the child social opportunities and a venue in which to practice social problem-solving skills.

Note: *The forms and charts referred to in the discussion below are in parent book Chapter 9 and also at the end of this chapter unless otherwise noted.*

Discussing Child Social Problem-Solving Difficulties with Parents

Discuss with parents that a child who has frequent and/or varied problems getting along with peers or siblings might benefit from working on social problem-solving skills. **Of particular importance to note is that a child who is upset usually has difficulty solving social problems.** Therefore, the parents might want to teach the child to calm down and manage stress (see parent book Chapter 14) and/or use a family cool-down method (see parent book Chapter 20) along with or before prompting the use of social problem solving.

Getting Parents Started and Focused

Parents should begin by using the ***Parent Checklist for Child Social Problem Solving,*** which summarizes the basic ideas in this chapter, to examine what is going well and to identify areas needing some work. Be sure to answer all the questions the parents raise so that they thoroughly understand these basic ideas and the material in parent book Chapter 9.

Training the Parent and Child to Promote Child Social Problem-Solving Skills

Begin by explaining social problem solving to the parent and child using either the ***Basic Social Problem Solving*** or the ***Advanced Social Problem Solving*** chart, depending on the child's age and developmental capacity. Generally, children ages 5–8 do better with basic social problem solving, and children ages 10 and up can profit from advanced social problem solving. Children between ages 8 and 10 are in the gray area and need to be considered for their capabilities on a case-by-case basis. **It can be very helpful to read out loud the scripts provided in "Step 1: Discussing and Practicing Social Problem-Solving Skills"** of parent book Chapter 9. These scripts provide verbal examples of basic or advanced social problem solving.

The next step is to do some modeling and role playing to teach basic or advanced social problem-solving steps (using the corresponding charts). Role-play exercises could focus on using the new social problem-solving skills to replay episodes of social difficulties or conflicts from the child's past with a positive spin. These role plays can be done in a training session and then repeated by parents at home. Prompt the parent to use the **"parental instruction"** methods for basic problem solving and **"parental guidance"** methods for advanced problem solving (as discussed in Step 1 in parent book Chapter 9) during the role plays.

For example, with a **younger child** the ***Basic Social Problem Solving*** steps can be used to resolve a role-played dispute with a sibling about which television show to watch. The practitioner could first act out the part of the child, and perhaps the parent or the child could take on the role of the sibling. Then go through the five problem-solving steps to solve the television show dilemma. In subsequent role plays the child could assume his or her natural role to practice using social problem-solving with the same problem.

The **older child or teen** can benefit from conducting role plays to practice ***Advanced Social Problem Solving.*** An example of a problem to solve could be two siblings trying to figure out who gets to use the bathroom at what times on school-day mornings. Another problem might be how to cope with someone spreading rumors about a teen at school. In each of these examples the practitioner could first model the skills, acting as the child to go through the advanced social problem-solving steps, with the older child or teen stepping in and doing the same role play afterward. In addition, the older child or teen can be guided to complete the ***Advanced Social Problem-Solving Worksheet*** during the role play.

If there is a sibling, the sibling mediation option is a good way to practice social problem solving at home. Role plays similar to those just described, especially including the sibling, can be used with the basic or advanced problem-solving steps.

To emphasize the importance of calming down to facilitate good problem solving, construct at least one role play in which a parent figure deescalates a highly charged situation. For example, a parent could send a younger child to a cool-down area (e.g., bedroom) for a few minutes, attempting social problem solving only once the child is calmer. For an older child or teen, a reminder to calm down before trying to solve the problem may be sufficient. With conflicted siblings it is good to redirect both of them to cool down and then try to work out their differences. Brainstorm specific ways to get the child to calm down with the ideas in parent book Chapters 14 and 20.

Helping Parents Create Opportunities for the Child to Use Social Problem-Solving Skills

There are many ways to provide opportunities for a child to practice social problem-solving skills. Brainstorming is the best way to identify good opportunities for a particular child. Two that often work well are (1) sibling mediation procedures, with the parent prompting and guiding the siblings to cool down and then use the basic or advanced social problem-solving steps, and (2) play dates for a younger child or outings with an older child or teen and one or more peers in which the parent prompts the child to use social problem solving and then reviews with the child later how the problem solving went.

Developing a Home Implementation Plan to Be Led by the Parent

Be sure to spend some time helping the parent make specific plans to implement the social problem-solving methods. Discuss how the parent could guide the use of "practice" role plays at home. Ask the parent to set specific goals and designate them on the *Parenting Goals* form (see parent book Chapter 3 and the end of Chapter 4 in this book). For example, the parent might write down a goal of rewarding an older child or teen for using the *Advanced Social Problem-Solving Worksheet* when social problems come up. Another related goal might be to focus on sibling mediation at home for the next 2 weeks.

As with building positive social behaviors, it's important to designate when (e.g., Tuesday evenings, weekends), where (e.g., home, school, in the neighborhood), and how often (e.g., once per day or week, several times per day or week) the parent will use role-play practicing and reviewing of progress. The parent should also be prodded to use a strategy to monitor a child's progress with social problem solving. This could involve using the *Personal Goals (Basic* or *Advanced)* form (see parent book Chapter 3 and also the end of Chapter 4 in this book) or the *Advanced Social Problem-Solving Worksheet* form with an older child or teen. Assist the family in figuring out how often they might want to use a chosen monitoring form.

Specific Procedures for Applying Parent Book Chapter 10

This chapter deals with the difficult and often emotionally charged issue of bullying. An important intervention is to get the parent and other adults involved and organized in monitoring and setting limits on the bully. The parent identifies adults who are regularly involved with the child and attempts to get them to intervene when bullying occurs.

Once adult monitoring is in place, it is helpful to teach the child to use the coping skills of ignoring and assertiveness. The parent is taught how to explain, demonstrate, and role-play/practice ignoring and assertiveness skills with the child. Using ignoring and assertiveness skills is difficult for most children when dealing with bullies, so the parent has to be heavily involved.

Note: *The forms and charts referred to in the discussion below are in parent book Chapter 10 and also at the end of this chapter unless otherwise noted.*

Discussing Child Bullying with Parents

Bullying includes physical aggression, verbal abuse, intimidation, and social exclusion (see parent book Chapter 10 for definitions). Ask the parents which of these behaviors have been directed toward their child and then review who does this, how often it occurs, and where it happens. If the parents have sought professional help because they know their child is being bullied, they do not need to be told that bullying is harmful, but sometimes they are not fully aware of the insidious and devastating consequences, so it is wise to explain how bullying can affect a child's behavioral and emotional development. Some bullied children are prone to anxiety and depression. What many parents don't want to face is that some children who are bullied are also bullies. To stop the cycle of intimidation, it is very important for parents to address the bullying of their child in an effective way.

It can't be stressed enough that parents, teachers, and other adults must get involved to assist a child who is bullied by monitoring and setting limits on the bully or bullies. Some parents make the mistake of thinking a child can handle the situation alone by "standing up to" the bully. Yet through intimidation the bully has more power than the victim. A child who is being bullied must have the help and support of adults, though the child might also benefit from learning bully-coping skills.

Getting Parents Started and Focused

Parents can start by checking off items on the *Parent Checklist for Bullying* that are already being used and pinpointing what needs to be worked on. Make sure that the parents understand everything on the form (and in the parent book chapter) since the checklist summarizes the main ideas. Spend whatever time is needed to answer questions.

Training Parents in Adult Monitoring/Intervention

Explain to the parents that their primary role is to organize adults to minimize the bullying incidents. Brainstorm with the parents to generate a list of the key adult allies in the child's life—people who might be involved with the child and have knowledge of the bullying, such as teachers, coaches, and neighbors. Suggest that the parents arrange informal or formal contact with these key adults to organize a **"no bullying tolerated"** policy. The goal is to take whatever steps are necessary to help the adults' observe, coordinate with each other, and convey no tolerance of bullying behavior toward the child.

Parents should be encouraged to tell their child that, although the child cannot be responsible for halting the bullying, the adults in the child's life cannot help him or her unless they are informed about the bullying.

Training Parents to Promote and the Child to Learn Ignoring of Bullies

Describe, model, and role-play the Turtle Technique for a child or an ignoring strategy for an older child or teen. As parent book Chapter 10 explains, reviewing past episodes of bullying might provide an example the parent and child can use to practice ignoring. With a **younger child,** the role play might center on being teased on the playground. The child or parent could act as the bully. The practitioner could act as the "child" and physically model the Turtle Technique, including avoiding eye contact, turning away, keeping quiet, and verbally stating coping thoughts such as "Don't let him [her] bug me," "I'm going to be okay," "I'll try to ignore her [him]." The same role-play scenario could be repeated with the child assuming his or her own role. Encourage the parent to ask guiding questions to elicit the child's ideas for ignoring the teasing. For an **older child or teen,** the same procedure could be followed to build coping skills in someone who is, for example, frequently ridiculed by a teammate on a sports team.

Training the Parent and Child to Promote Assertiveness with Bullies

The practitioner should again describe, model, and do role playing, but this time focus on the Courageous Lion Technique (for younger children), or the assertiveness strategy (for older children or teens). The role plays described above could be recycled to practice this alternative coping strategy, which focuses on sticking up for oneself when bullied. First act out specific **"say and do"** behaviors and then trade with the child, who can do the same. For example, in response to being teased on the playground, a **younger child** might say, "Stop bothering me or I will tell the teacher," and walk into the school building. For an **older child or teen** being ridiculed on a sports team, the child could say, "Knock it off," and walk toward the coach. Here, too, the parent can be coached to ask guiding questions to elicit the child's ideas for being assertive when teased or ridiculed. This is another place where coming up with a list of one- or two-sentence statements to rehearse and use in responding assertively will be a fruitful exercise for parent and child.

Developing a Home Implementation Plan to Be Led by the Parent

A concrete plan is critical to dealing with bullying in a child's life. Ask the parent to identify specific goals on the *Parenting Goals* form (see parent book Chapter 3 and the end of Chapter 4 in this book) that are designed to help the child cope with bullying. For example, the parent might write down a goal of organizing a meeting at school to come up with an adult monitoring plan to deal with the bullying. Perhaps another goal would be for the parent to do role plays each night for a week to help the child practice ignoring the bully and making assertive responses to him or her. Encourage the parent to execute the plan and monitor progress.

The parent should also be advised to use a strategy to monitor the child's progress with bullies. This could involve using the *Personal Goals (Basic* or *Advanced)* form (see parent book Chapter 3 and the end of Chapter 4 in this book). On this form the child, with the help of the parent, could indicate personalized goals related to dealing with bullies. Aid the family in determining how often they might want to review this goal and monitoring form to assess progress.

Specific Procedures for Applying Parent Book Chapter 11

This chapter deals with the sometimes thorny issue, especially for teens, of with whom the child hangs out and whom he or she identifies as friends. One important intervention involves the parent's setting of parameters with the child to guard against negative peer influences while directing him or her to more positive peers. The parent is taught specific techniques to monitor and supervise the child's peer-related activities. The focus is not typically on restricting a child from associating with peers, but more on *how* the child associates with those peers. In other words the parent sets parameters on the child's social network. There may be exceptions, however, when prohibition of certain very-high-risk peers might be warranted (e.g., a 6-year-old boy who is influenced by a highly aggressive peer in the neighborhood, or a 13-year-old girl who is hanging out with a 19-year-old boy). It is important to discuss potentially very-high-risk peers with the parent and brainstorm all possible responses the parent has available, including possibly calling the police.

After the adult is involved in setting up social boundaries the cooperating child can be taught to use peer pressure coping skills, based on avoiding and/or assertively responding to peer pressure situations. The parent is taught how to help the child make good decisions about peer pressure and then learn to apply the skills as needed. This chapter is useful for children of all ages but has to be calibrated according to the age-related examples provided in the chapter.

Note: *The forms and charts referred to in the discussion below are in parent book Chapter 11 and also at the end of this chapter unless otherwise noted.*

Discussing Peer Influence Problems with Parents

The parent may already know this, but it is worth emphasizing that it's not easy being a child or teen these days. This is especially true due to an increase in peer pressure. Discuss the fact that children are dealing with peers almost all the time, by interacting with them in person or via Internet social networking and/or cell phones. Point out that peer pressure can be direct, such as one peer or a group of peers actively persuading a child to do something wrong, or indirect, such as when the child is present in a group that is doing something wrong at the moment.

Getting Parents Started and Focused

Have the parent check off the items from the ***Parent Checklist for Peer Relationships*** that are going well and identify areas needing some work. Because the checklist summarizes the ideas in this chapter, parents should understand all the items as well as the text in the chapter. Be sure to solicit questions and answer them thoroughly.

Training Parents to Monitor and Supervise Peer Contacts

Depending on the age of the child, parents are often concerned about with whom their child affiliates but uncertain about how much to intervene, especially if the child has had difficulty making and keeping friends. Practitioners should guide concerned parents to strongly consider monitoring and setting limits on the child regarding those peers. One relatively easy way to stay on top of peer relationships is to get to know the child's friends and, if possible, their parents. Brainstorm ways that the parents can connect with the child's friends, such as talking to them in public settings like school events, inviting them over for dinner, and/or going to a sports event or movie with the child and his or her friend. Also think about ways the parents can get to know other parents, such as introducing themselves in public settings, making a phone call, or sending an e-mail.

Monitoring children's friendships and their activities with friends is a tough balancing act as children get older. Older children, and especially teens, often object to having their activities monitored closely. Practitioners need to emphasize the importance of parents knowing the **four W's** for events or activities that the child attends or participates in. Facilitate a discussion between parent and child on this important topic so that the child at least understands the rationale for parental monitoring. Emphasize that the child and parent can work out together where the child may go, with whom, to do what, and when the child will return home, but that the parent has the final say. It can be helpful for the parent to indicate the four W's as a house rule (see parent book Chapter 5).

Discuss how the parent currently monitors the child's Internet social networking and cell phone usage and suggest that the four W's apply here too. Brainstorm about how the monitoring of these activities could be tightened up. Perhaps the parent could set up house rules about how much and when the child can use Internet social networking and his or her cell phone. The parent should also be asked to consider setting parental controls on these devices.

Discuss the potential for drug/alcohol use and how the parent can better monitor the child if this is a concern. Chapter 11 in the parent book contains suggestions for how the parent can "dial up" the monitoring and supervision process to be more intensive. In addition to the four W's, brainstorm with the parent about how to best check up on the child to prevent drug/alcohol use. For example, if the child says that he or she is going to a friend's house and that a parent will be home, one way to verify this is by calling the friend's home to speak to a parent.

Brainstorm with the parent and the child about specific adult-supervised organizations that the child could get involved in where a positive peer culture exists. As mentioned in parent book Chapter 11, this might include settings such as churches, community centers, schools, park and recreation boards, and activities such as Scouts, sports, after-school programs, art classes, youth theater groups, dance and music programming, volunteer work, cultural activities, and religious activities. Make a list and help the parent plan how to get the child involved.

There are several potential pitfalls in using variations of monitoring and supervising that may need to be discussed. Sometimes a parent is more like a "friend" than a "parent" to the child. In other words the parent may have a history of being too permissive, which makes tightening up the reins a challenge. It may help to discuss how it will take effort to move from permissiveness to monitoring and supervising. Be sure to encourage and support that parent to follow through. Another outcome to be alert for: When the parent ratchets up his or her monitoring and supervising efforts, the child may protest the new limits. This protesting could derail the parent's efforts and resolve to follow through. It may be necessary to work with the parent on how to handle protesting from the child (see parent book Chapter 7).

Training the Parent and Child to Promote Coping Skills in Response to Peer Pressure

Coping skills for peer pressure involve teaching the child to avoid peer pressure and/or to be assertive in response to it. Not surprisingly, some children are not immediately on board with the need to develop and use these skills. When this initial resistance from the child occurs, the parent's work may need to begin with motivating the child. Facilitating a discussion between the parent and child with the goal of getting the child to acknowledge peer pressure and to be open to suggestions on how to make it better can be the best entry point for practitioners. It will be useful to guide the child and possibly the parent to apply the decision-making ideas for peer pressure described in the "Guiding Your Child in Making Decisions about Peer Pressure" section of parent book Chapter 11 and broader motivational methods found in parent book Chapter 3. The goal of such a discussion is to get the child primed and ready to learn coping skills for peer pressure.

The **peer pressure avoidance skills** are a good place to begin. The practitioner should facilitate a brainstorming meeting or two with the parent and child. First guide them to write down a list of peer pressure situations that are unique to the child. Parent book Chapter 11 provides some examples, but this is by no means an exhaustive list. Peer pressure situations will vary greatly from one child to the next, so carefully pinpointing the specific situations can be very valuable. Then guide the parent and child to write a list of peer pressure avoidance techniques that can be used in those peer pressure situations. Again, parent book Chapter 11 provides several examples but only a beginning. Help the parent and child think of as many peer pressure avoidance techniques as possible. In subsequent meetings, ask how well the child has been using the peer pressure avoidance methods and whether the parent has been coaching the child to use them.

Describe, model, and role-play the **peer pressure assertiveness strategies** that can be used when moments of peer pressure arise. First identify specific situations in which the child has been, or expects to be, negatively influenced by peers. The answers could be similar to the examples provided in parent book Chapter 11. Explain to the parent and child that a good coping strategy is to be assertive—to stick up for oneself—when feeling peer pressure. Engage the parent and child in discussion of specific "**say and do**" assertiveness behaviors. It can be helpful to generate a "script" for a role play involving peer pressure and the use of specific "**say and do**" assertiveness behaviors.

The practitioner could first model the use of assertiveness skills for peer pressure and then trade with the child, who can do the same. For example, when peers pressure him or her to make fun of or tease another child on the playground, a **younger child** could say, "I don't want to do that," and walk into the school building. An **older child or teen** could say, "No thanks, I have to go home," and then walk away when peers pressure him or her to go to a party. The parent can be coached to ask guiding questions to elicit ideas for how the child could be assertive when pressured directly or indirectly by peers. As in the other social skills chapters, encourage parent and child to generate a list of one- or two-sentence statements that can be practiced and called into play when peer pressure arises.

Developing a Home Implementation Plan to Be Led by the Parent

Encourage the parent to identify specific goals on the **Parenting Goals** form (see parent book Chapter 3 and the end of Chapter 4 in this book). The parent might, for example, write down a goal of sitting down with the child to review the four W's for going out with friends and specific rules for Internet and cell phone usage. Another goal could be for the parent to reach out and connect with the parent of the child's best friend. The parent might set a goal about discussing and writing down ways for the child to avoid peer pressure situations. Encourage the parent to execute the plan and monitor progress.

Suggest to the parent that it is best to use a strategy to monitor the child's progress with peer pressure. Again, the **Personal Goals (Basic** or **Advanced)** form (see parent book Chapter 3 and the end of Chapter 4 in this book) can be used for this purpose. On this form the child, with the assistance of the parent, could indicate personalized goals related to dealing with peer pressure. Help the family decide how often they might want to review this goal and monitoring form to assess progress.

Modifications for Using the Child Social Development Module in Parent Groups

Discuss the **Overview of the Child Social Development Module** chart with parent group members to introduce the primary methods for enhancing children's social competency. Prompt parents to reveal social challenges they have observed with their children and what they have tried in the past. Parents typically have a lot of empathy for their children because they have seen them struggle socially. Allowing parents to discuss their feelings about their children's social struggles can be a very potent way to introduce and motivate them to work on this developmental area. Inform parents that the main goal of this module is to train children in social skills and for parents to guide them to use the skills.

Help parents reach a consensus about which areas could be emphasized for that meeting or over several meetings. This module can be introduced over one meeting, but three or more meetings will be needed to cover the topics of facilitating child motivation/commitment, making friends using social behavior skills, keeping friends using social problem-solving skills, dealing with bullies, and promoting positive peer affiliations. The charts and forms found in parent book Chapters 8–11 can be used, as needed, to convey information and approaches for improving a child's social functioning. The role plays described in the training sections above for parent book Chapters 8–11 can be used in parent groups by having parents take turns if they are comfortable doing so. Help each parent individually pinpoint specific child social goals and strategies to work on and designate them on the **Parenting Goals** form.

Overview of the Child Social Development Module

Chapter 8. Making Friends: Teaching Your Child Social Behavior Skills

Selecting and Training Basic Social Behaviors for Younger Child

- Taking turns
- Sharing
- Expressing feelings
- Cooperating
- Making eye contact
- Conversing
- Listening to others
- Complimenting others
- Accepting compliments
- Following rules of play
- Apologizing to others
- Asking questions
- Telling others about oneself

- Playing fair
- Inquiring about others' interests
- Talking in a brief manner
- Asking for what one wants/needs
- Helping others
- Inviting others to do something
- Greeting others
- Introducing oneself
- Entering a group
- Getting someone's attention
- Being a good winner/loser
- Using a quieter "inside voice"
- Other basic social behaviors

Selecting and Training Advanced Social Behaviors for Older Children or Teens

- Respectfully disagreeing with someone
- Compromising with someone
- Ignoring when appropriate
- Being assertive or sticking up for oneself when appropriate
- Displaying social confidence

- Resisting peer pressure
- Negotiating
- Resolving conflicts
- Being aware of how one's behavior affects others
- Being aware of behaviors that irritate others
- Staying calm with others

Chapter 9. Keeping Friends: Teaching Your Child Social Problem-Solving Skills

Selecting and Training Basic Social Problem Solving for Younger Children

1. Stop! What is the problem?
2. What are some plans?
3. What is the best plan?
4. Follow the plan.
5. Did the plan work?

See **Basic Social Problem Solving** form.

(cont.)

Selecting and Training Advanced Social Problem Solving for Older Children or Teens

1. Stop! What is the problem?

2. Who or what caused the problem?

3. What does each person think and feel?

4. What are some plans?

5. Which plan is the most likely to work?

6. Follow the plan.

7. Did the plan work?

See ***Advanced Social Problem-Solving*** chart and ***Advanced Social Problem-Solving Worksheet.***

Chapter 10. That Hurts!: Helping Your Child with Bullies

Using Adult Monitoring and Intervention

- Coordinate with adults between home and school if bullying occurs at school

- Adults are vigilant in watching for and intervening with instances of bullying

- The victim of bullying is encouraged to tell adults about bullying incidents

- Adults communicate via phone, e-mail, or notes about child and bullying incidents

- Adults provide consequences for bullying behavior

- It may be a good idea for authority figures (e.g., school administrators) to have "serious talks" with the bully and/or the parents of the bully

Training "Turtle Technique" (Younger Child) or Ignoring Behavior (Older Child or Teen)

- Teach child to avoid eye contact and turn away

- Teach child to keep quiet

- Teach child to think "coping thoughts" (e.g., "Don't let him [her] bug me," "I'm going to be okay," "I'll try to ignore her [him]")

Training "Courageous Lion Technique" (Younger Child)
or Assertiveness Behavior (Older Child or Teen)

- Explain difference between passive, assertive, and aggressive responses to bullying

- Help child understand that the assertive response is best

- Teach child to deal with bullying with assertive **"say and do"** behaviors

(cont.)

Chapter 11. Hanging with the "Right Crowd": Influencing Your Child's Peer Relationships

Monitoring and Directing Activities

- *Getting to know 'em*—reach out to child's friends and their parents

- *Monitoring and supervising activities, Internet, cell phone via four W's*—knowing **w**here, **w**ho, **w**hat, and **w**hen to keep track of child

- *Creating and posting house rules*—emphasize rules that set guidelines for peer relationships

- *Getting your child involved in positive organizations*—make sure there is structure and adult monitoring in outside organizations

Teaching Coping Skills for Peer Pressure

- Discuss and encourage child to make decision to work on peer pressure

- Brainstorm strategies to avoid peer pressure situations

- Encourage assertive **"say and do"** behaviors to deal with peer pressure situations

Training Child in Social Development Skills (Chapters 8–11)

- Focus on the family "team" working together

- Guide child to choose and then work on social development skills and goals

- Identify parenting goals related to promoting child's social development at home

- Learn, practice, and monitor progress with social development skills and goals

See **Parent Checklist** for each chapter, as well as **Personal Goals (Basic** or **Advanced)** form for child and **Parenting Goals** form for parent (both in Chapter 3 and also at the end of Chapter 4 in this book).

Forms from Parent Book Chapter 8

Parent Checklist for Child Social Behaviors

Name: _____ Date: _____

In the blanks below, indicate a score for **how well** you make use of that parenting behavior at this time.

	Not too well	Okay	Very well
	1	2	3

Parent's Efforts in Teaching Child Social Behavior Skills

A. _____ Identifying specific social behavior(s) to work on that match the child's age, such as sharing or taking turns or assertiveness or negotiating

B. _____ Teaching specific social behaviors by explaining, demonstrating, and role-playing/practicing of specified social behavior(s) with the child

C. _____ Coaching specific social behavior(s) by periodically reviewing to create more awareness and/or using a chart to promote use of social behavior skill(s)

Parent's Efforts in Creating Social Opportunities for Child

D. _____ Arranging and orchestrating social activities to give the child social opportunities

E. _____ Planning social behavior goals prior to the activity and processing how well it went afterward

Identifying Social Behaviors to Work On

Name: _____ **Date:** _____

Below are lists of basic and advanced positive social behaviors. Circle one or two social behaviors that your child can work on at this time. Put a square around any social behaviors that could be worked on later.

Examples of Basic Social Behaviors

- Taking turns
- Sharing
- Expressing feelings
- Cooperating
- Making eye contact
- Conversing with others
- Listening to others
- Complimenting others
- Accepting compliments
- Following rules of play
- Apologizing to others
- Asking questions
- Using a quieter "inside voice"

- Telling others about self
- Playing fairly
- Inquiring about others' interests
- Talking in a brief manner
- Asking for what one wants/needs
- Helping others
- Inviting others to do something
- Greeting others
- Introducing oneself
- Entering a group
- Getting someone's attention
- Being a good winner/loser
- Other basic social behaviors

Examples of Advanced Social Behaviors

- Respectfully disagreeing with someone
- Compromising with someone
- Ignoring when appropriate
- Being assertive or sticking up for oneself when appropriate
- Displaying social confidence
- Resisting peer pressure
- Negotiating

- Resolving conflicts
- Being aware of how one's behavior affects others
- Being aware of behaviors that irritate others
- Staying calm with others
- Stopping, thinking, and planning to resolve a conflict or disagreement
- Other advanced social behaviors

Write down other social behaviors not listed that might be good to work on:

_____

_____

_____

_____

Forms from Parent Book Chapter 9

Parent Checklist for Child Social Problem Solving

Name: _____ **Date:** _____

In the blanks below, indicate a score for **how well** you make use of that parenting behavior at this time.

Not too well	Okay	Very well
1	2	3

Parent's Efforts in Teaching Child Social Problem-Solving Skills

A. ____ Discussing and practicing social problem-solving skills by reviewing and role-play practicing of social problem-solving steps

B. ____ Coaching social problem solving in "real life" by using questions and dialoguing and/or social problem-solving charts to periodically guide the process

C. ____ Using social problem solving to resolve sibling conflict (if applicable) by acting as a mediator to guide siblings to use this process to work it out

Parent's Efforts in Creating Social Opportunities for the Child

D. ____ Arranging and orchestrating social activities to give the child social opportunities

E. ____ Planning social problem-solving goals prior to the activity and processing how well it went afterward

Basic Social Problem Solving

1. **Stop! What is the social problem?**

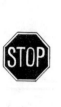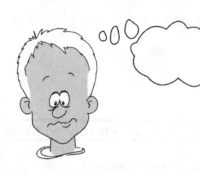

2. **What are some plans?**

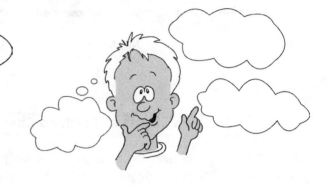

3. **What is the best plan?**

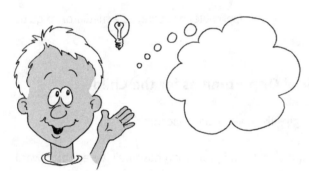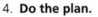

4. **Do the plan.**

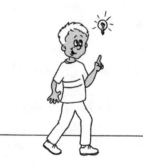

5. **Did the plan work?**

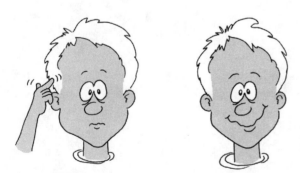

Basic Social Problem Solving

1. **Stop! What is the social problem?**

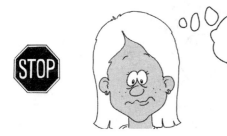

2. **What are some plans?**

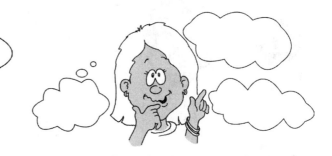

3. **What is the best plan?**

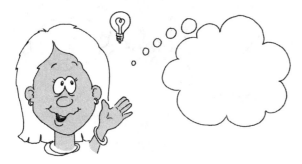

4. **Do the plan.**

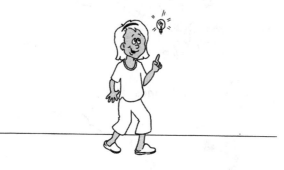

5. **Did the plan work?**

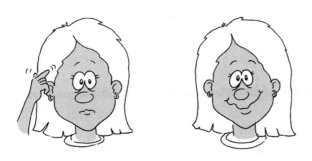

Advanced Social Problem Solving

1. **Stop! What is the social problem?**

 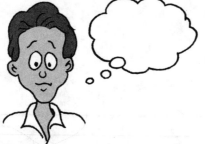

2. **Who or what caused the social problem?**

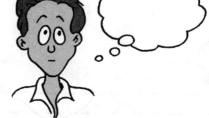

3. **What does each person think and feel?**

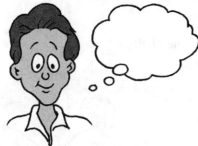

4. **What are some plans?**

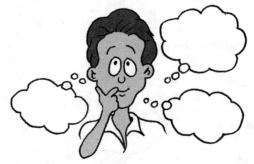

5. **Which plan is the most likely to work?**

6. **Do the plan.**

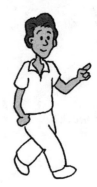

7. **Did the plan work?**

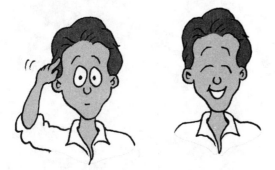

Advanced Social Problem Solving

1. **Stop! What is the social problem?**

 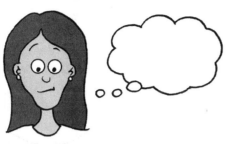

2. **Who or what caused the social problem?**

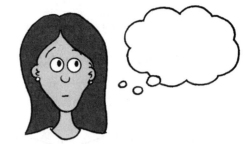

3. **What does each person think and feel?**

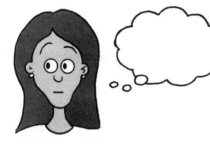

4. **What are some plans?**

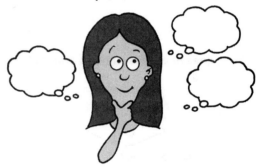

5. **Which plan is the most likely to work?**

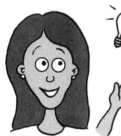

6. **Do the plan.**

7. **Did the plan work?**

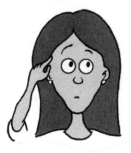

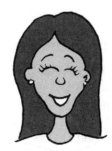

Advanced Social Problem-Solving Worksheet

Name: _____ **Date:** _____

A child/teen and/or parent can complete this worksheet. It's best to fill out the worksheet while you are having a social problem, but it's also okay to fill it out afterward.

1. **Stop! What is the social problem?**

2. **Who or what caused the social problem?** Try to figure out your role and other people's roles in causing the social problem.

3. **What does each person think and feel?** Put yourself in the "other guy's shoes" to see how that person thinks and feels.

4. **What are some plans?** List as many plans or solutions as possible that could be used to solve the social problem.

5. **Which plan is the most likely to work?** Think ahead about what would happen if you used the plans above. Then decide which one will work best.

6. **Do the plan.** How will I do the plan? What will I do to make the plan work?

7. **Did the plan work?**

How Well Did It Work?
(Circle *1, 2, 3,* or *4.*)

1. I didn't really try too hard.
2. I sort of tried, but it didn't really work.
3. I tried hard, and it kind of worked.
4. I tried really hard, and it really worked.

Forms from Parent Book Chapter 10

Parent Checklist for Bullying

Name: _____ **Date:** _____

In the blanks below, indicate a score for **how well** you make use of that parenting behavior at this time.

	Not too well	Okay	Very well
	1	2	3

Parent's Efforts in Adult Monitoring/Intervention Plan

A. _____ Taking steps to help adults be observant, coordinate with each other, and not tolerate bullying behavior toward the child

Parent's Efforts in Teaching the Child to Ignore Bullies

B. _____ Explaining, demonstrating, and role-playing/practicing how to ignore bullies

C. _____ Coaching the child and periodically reviewing how it's going

Parent's Efforts in Teaching the Child to Be Assertive with Bullies

D. _____ Explaining, demonstrating, and role-playing/practicing with the child how to be assertive with bullies

E. _____ Coaching the child and periodically reviewing how it's going

Forms from Parent Book Chapter 11

Parent Checklist for Peer Relationships

Name: _____ Date: _____

In the blanks below, indicate a score for how well you make use of that parenting behavior at this time.

Not too well	Okay	Very well
1	2	3

Parent's Efforts in Monitoring and Directing Peer Contacts

A. _____ Making an extra effort to establish a rapport and bond with the child to enhance the child's willingness to work on positive peer relationships

B. _____ Getting to know the child's friends and their parents

C. _____ Knowing the four W's when child is out and monitoring Internet and cell phone use

D. _____ Checking up on the child to prevent drug use

E. _____ Getting the child involved in programs and places that provide positive structured activities with adult supervision

Parent's Efforts in Teaching the Child Peer Pressure Coping Skills

F. _____ Discussing peer pressure with the child

G. _____ Helping the child make decisions to work on dealing with peer pressure

H. _____ Discussing and brainstorming ideas and techniques that the child can use to avoid peer pressure situations

I. _____ Explaining, demonstrating, and role-playing/practicing methods that the child can use to respond assertively to peer pressure situations

J. _____ Coaching the child and periodically reviewing how well he or she is dealing with peer pressure

7

Using the Child Emotional Development Module

This practitioner book chapter corresponds to the parent book section "Enhancing Your Child's Emotional Development" (Chapters 12–14). This module provides the parent with ideas and strategies for enhancing the child's awareness and expression of emotions, ability to recognize and change unhelpful thinking, and capacity to cope with stress. **The practitioner should read and fully understand the *content* in parent book Chapters 12–14 before using the related *procedures* described here.**

This module is based on cognitive-behavioral therapy methods. The goal is to change maladaptive feelings, thoughts, and behaviors that underlie behavioral–emotional problems. Techniques include affective education, self-instruction, cognitive restructuring, and stress-inoculation-based skills training. Parent book Chapter 12 incorporates affective methods that increase a child's "feelings vocabulary" and teaches him or her how to express feelings. Parent book Chapter 13 focuses on cognitive methods aimed at helping a child identify and alter beliefs and automatic thoughts. Finally, Chapter 14 is based on behavioral activation methods designed to teach stress management via activity scheduling, routine regulation, and replacing avoidant behaviors with action coping, as well as acute stress-coping skills derived from relaxation, self-talk, and effective action strategies. The classic cognitive-behavioral triangle depicting the interacting relationship between feelings, thoughts, and behaviors is introduced in parent book Chapter 12 and serves to orient the parent and child to the methods. Ideas for tailoring the strategies for younger versus older children and teens are offered throughout.

The practitioner should be aware that many parents also lack emotion-related skills. In some instances, the practitioner may well be teaching both the parent and child these methods at the same time. Although child-focused practitioners typically have not formally assessed parents, it is important to gauge parents' comprehension of the skills and calibrate training to them as well as the child. More general support, explanation, role playing, and repetition will be needed for less sophisticated parents and their children.

During a given session within the child skills-focused emotional development module, it is important for the practitioner to consider whom to work with and when. With a **younger child** it is usually most productive to train the child and parent together, so the parent can fully learn all emotion-related skills and then be actively involved in facilitating the child's use of those skills at home. With an **older child or teen**, however, it can be fruitful to train the child first and then the parent. This way the child learns important skills in a one-on-one private context and the parent is brought in to learn, support, and encourage skill development in the child. It is important to decide with the child and parent together about when to involve the parents. It is highly recommended that the parent be involved in the process at some point.

Tailoring within the Child Emotional Development Module

The *Overview of the Child Emotional Development Module* chart at the end of this chapter summarizes the main ideas and techniques in this module. Reviewing this chart can give the parent an overview of the skills-building strategies used to promote emotional competency in children. Because the chapters deal with increasingly sophisticated skills, the parent of a **younger child** should focus on basic skills (e.g., identifying and expressing feelings), whereas the parent of an **older child or teen** can work on advanced skills (e.g., advanced helpful thinking). Likewise a young child may not have the capacity to profit from some of the more complicated skills of stress management described in Chapter 14, whereas an older child may balk at the "childish" nature of the material on feelings in Chapter 12. These developmental considerations need to be weighed by the practitioner and the parent. The objective is to carefully determine which skills-building strategies best fit the child in question.

Specific Procedures for Applying Parent Book Chapter 12

This chapter helps parents teach their child to identify and express feelings in a healthy way. Understanding something about the nature of emotion is the first step toward emotional competency, but many children (and some parents) do not comprehend how feelings, thoughts, and behavior are connected, and therefore practitioners might need to spend some extra time explaining this interconnection and giving examples to illustrate. To build the child's emotional vocabulary, parents can review feelings-oriented charts (basic or advanced) with the child. To enhance the child's growing fluency, parents should be encouraged to model identifying and expressing feelings, as well as to prompt and reinforce the child for using newly acquired skills.

Note: *The forms and charts referred to in the discussion below are in parent book Chapter 12 and also at the end of this chapter unless otherwise noted.*

Discussing Child Emotion Identification and Expression Problems with Parents

Explain that some children with behavioral–emotional concerns do not have the words in their vocabulary to express their feelings outright. To find out how fluent the child is in describing his or her emotional experience, ask the parent how often the child currently uses feelings words such as "I feel **sad**" or "That makes me **mad.**" Ask the parent for a global impression of how well the child expresses feelings verbally.

If the child seems to have very little vocabulary for emotions, impart to the parents how important it is to give the child that language. Children who don't understand what they are feeling may misinterpret and express their emotions in ways that confuse or alienate others (e.g., acting angry when sad) and that interfere with their own problem solving. If they don't understand that what they are feeling is sadness, they may not be able to soothe themselves or solve the problem that is making them feel sad. Obviously, then, a lack of emotional fluency can have far-reaching developmental ramifications, hampering children's social and cognitive development along with their emotional maturation. Suggest that parents spend plenty of time on Chapter 12 before moving on to more complex emotion-coping skills such as helpful thinking and stress management.

Getting Parents Started and Focused

Start by asking the parent to rate and check off items on the *Parent Checklist for Child Feelings* that are going well and identify areas that need to be strengthened. Because this checklist is a synopsis of the approach described in the chapter, it's important to answer any questions parents have about the checklist. Parents should also be told that is very important to fully understand the text in Chapter 12.

Training the Parent and Child to Promote Emotion Identification and Expression Skills

Discuss the child's age and maturity with the parent to collaboratively determine whether the basic or advanced feelings vocabulary would be best for the child. Then go through each feeling-related word on the appropriate chart and ask the child to define the word. Provide the definition for a child who is stumped, giving examples of when someone might feel a particular feeling.

When children are having trouble understanding their feelings, it's particularly important to help them build vocabulary in a way that acknowledges their age and relative sophistication, or they are likely to feel patronized and possibly humiliated, which will halt learning.

For a **younger child** a visual image can be helpful when words are tougher to grasp. The analogy of a balloon is one effective possibility. Explain that keeping feelings inside is similar to continuously blowing up a balloon, which will eventually pop if you keep blowing in air without letting any out (the balloon analogy is also in parent book Chapter 12). A child who keeps too many feelings inside can feel like "popping," such as when a child keeps sad and angry feelings inside and then yells at someone. If the child had expressed those sad and angry feelings in words, he or she might not have yelled. Such explanations can be followed up in the session or at home through the practice exercises of matching facial expressions and "Simon says" feelings games. These activities can be used to get a younger child interested in, and familiar with, feelings on the ***Basic Feelings Vocabulary Chart.***

With an **older child or teen,** it is fruitful to discuss each feeling-related word on the ***Advanced Feelings Vocabulary Chart.*** Help the child decipher and think about the more advanced feelings (e.g., disapproving, exasperated) and discuss how these various feelings relate to his or her experiences in life. The parent might also be able to give the older child or teen some feedback or examples. An older child or teen may not need a lot of work on identifying the feelings themselves but might not understand how feelings can be influenced by thoughts and behaviors. Review the ***Feelings, Thoughts, and Behaviors Go Together*** chart. The goal is for the older child or teen to understand the relationship between feelings, thoughts, and behaviors in the manner depicted on this chart. Review the examples on the chart, and ask the child (and parent) for other examples he or she can think of, to illustrate how feelings are related to thoughts and behavior. Make sure the child (and parent) understands that to cope with feelings, it is advantageous to express them (the topic of Chapter 12) or change thinking and behaving (the topics of Chapters 13 and 14, respectively). Explain that the goal here is to focus on expressing feelings and that those thoughts and behaviors can be addressed later with other methods.

Familiarity with basic or advanced feelings can be cemented for any-age child by discussing the child's actual emotional experiences. Review events that occurred that day in the child's life and how they made him or her feel. Have the child write down positive and negative events and the accompanying feelings on the ***Feelings Diary***. For example:

- *Positive event for a young child*: "I got a star on my math worksheet."
  My feeling: happy and joyful.
- *Positive event for an older child or teen*: "I made some good comments in class discussion at school today."
  My feeling: confident and proud.
- *Negative event for a young child:* "Some kids called me names on the bus."
  My feeling: lonely and scared.

- *Negative event for an older child or teen:* "One of my friends did not answer my text message today."
  My feeling: hurt, nervous, and disappointed.

Throughout this discussion of feelings, encourage the parents to participate so that the child understands what a natural and normal part of human experience it is to have and express emotions. Parents can assist their child in discussing feelings, and they can also talk about their own feelings. Advise parents to stick to feelings related to everyday experiences (e.g., frustration at having to wait in traffic, joy at seeing their child achieve something special) and avoid personal, intimate stories.

Assisting Parents in Creating Opportunities for the Child to Use Emotion Identification and Expression Skills

Parents play a crucial role in coaching the children to continue the work done in training at home. Discuss ways in which the parent will coach the child to practice identifying and verbally expressing feelings in everyday interactions with friends, siblings, and/or parents. Explain that coaching involves prompting or reminding the child to be aware of, and go through the process of, talking about feelings.

Discuss with the child and parent how they might use one of the feelings charts and the *Feelings Diary* at home. Perhaps the child and parent could develop a routine in which the child completes the *Feelings Diary* and discusses it with the parent. The parent can ask questions to encourage the child to expand on events and feelings. The parent can also fill out a *Feelings Diary* to share with the child, again as long as the parent does not disclose personal feelings about an intimate relationship that might upset the child. This mutual use of the *Feelings Diary* allows the parent to be a role model for identifying and expressing feelings at home.

It is also a good idea to brainstorm with the parent about ways to guide the expression of feelings in real-life moments. If the parent observes the child exhibiting either positive or negative feelings, for example, the parent could guide and/or dialogue with the child to help

WHEN TALKING ABOUT FEELINGS UPSETS THE CHILD

If a child resists the parent's prompt to label a feeling, the parent can try labeling the feeling for the child, saying "You look sad and hurt" to a child who has just slammed a door, for example. Or the parent can simply ask the child to talk about his or her feelings. But if the child gets too defensive or upset, the parent should be counseled to discontinue talking about or labeling feelings until the child calms down.

him or her label and verbally express the feelings. Review the section in parent book Chapter 12 that suggests the parent ask limited-choice questions such as "Are you sad or hurt or both?" or open-ended questions such as "What are you feeling right now?" For parents who are not comfortable doing this kind of prompting or seem likely to forget to do it, role playing can help, with the practitioner demonstrating the technique to the parent who is acting the part of the child and then the two switching roles.

Developing a Home Implementation Plan to Be Led by the Parent

Discuss ways in which the parent can review feelings with the child at home. This plan might include details pertaining to when (evenings, weekends, etc.), where (home, school, in the neighborhood, etc.), and how often (once per day or week, several times per day or week, etc.) to use the chosen feelings-related techniques. Suggest that the parent consider writing down specific ideas to accomplish this plan on the *Parenting Goals* form (see parent book Chapter 3 and also the end of Chapter 4 in this book). For example, the parent might declare a goal of completing a *Feelings Diary* form with the child every day for several weeks. Another goal might be to motivate the child by providing a tangible reward for completing a certain number of *Feelings Diary* forms (see parent book Chapter 3 for more details on motivating the child). Still another goal might be for the parent to be more aware of his or her feelings and model how to express them during everyday family activities.

Suggest to the parent that it is best to use a strategy to monitor the child's progress with identifying and expressing feelings. The *Personal Goals (Basic* or *Advanced)* form (see parent book Chapter 3 and also the end of Chapter 4 in this book) can be used by the child, with the assistance of the parent, to set goals related to feelings. Help the family decide how often they will review this goal and monitoring form to assess progress.

Specific Procedures for Applying Parent Book Chapter 13

This chapter focuses on teaching the child how to change thoughts commonly associated with anxious, depressed, and/or angry emotional states. Parents can help children understand the difference between helpful and unhelpful thoughts, as introduced in Chapter 12. Methods for instructing and guiding the helpful thought strategies for different ages are discussed in parent book Chapter 13 and later in this section of the practitioner book.

Note: *The forms and charts referred to in the discussion below are in parent book Chapter 13 and also at the end of this chapter unless otherwise noted.*

Discussing Unhelpful Child Thoughts with Parents

"I'm so stupid!" "This is too hard!" "You are so unfair!" "I hate you!"—these are all examples of unhelpful statements that children tend to make and with which parents are undoubtedly familiar. To find out how the child tends to use unhelpful thoughts, ask the parents what statements like these they have heard from their child. Then ask them what the child generally does after making such a statement. Parents are likely to say "He bursts into tears" or "She slams her workbook shut and storms out of the room" or "He stamps his feet and glares at me." These observations can lead into a discussion of how unhelpful thoughts negatively affect the child's emotions and behavior. Explain how habitual unhelpful thinking can perpetuate anxiety, depression, and/or anger. This is why it's important for the child who has those negative feelings to form the habit of trying to think helpful thoughts. To illustrate this point to parents and children, you could ask the parent to pick any problematic behavior of the child's and talk about the kinds of unhelpful thoughts that might produce it. Then the child and parent could come up with some preliminary ideas for a helpful thought to replace the negative thought and lead to some more productive behavior.

Getting Parents Started and Focused

Ask parents to rate how well they are helping their child use helpful thoughts by rating the items on the *Parent Checklist for Child Helpful Thoughts* on a 1–3 scale. They should plan on working on the 1's and possibly the 2's. Before they get started, however, be sure that they thoroughly understand the items on the list, since this is an overview of the chapter contents, and answer any questions they have.

Training the Parent and Child to Promote Child Helpful Thoughts Skills

Before going too far, discuss the child's age and maturity with the parent to determine whether basic or advanced helpful thinking would be best for the child. It can be hard for the youngest children addressed in this program to **think about thinking** because they lack abstract thinking capacity. The basic helpful thoughts procedures can be of benefit to a younger child, however, if the presentation is geared to his or her developmental level. It should be based more on self-instruction and the parent's provision of direct instruction (i.e., telling the child how to think). The older child or teen can comprehend abstract thoughts, so the procedure is rooted more in cognitive restructuring, with parental guidance emphasized (i.e., guiding the older child how to think).

The first goal is to promote awareness of thinking and how it can affect someone. Begin by asking the **younger child** to consider different situations and how thoughts can affect what happens with a child. For example, ask what might happen if a child attempts a piano recital, is up to bat in a baseball game, or is about to give a dance performance and thinks something like "I can't do it," or "I bet I'll goof it up." Younger children are usually able to explain that they will feel nervous and might indeed goof it up in this situation when thinking those thoughts. Ask the child if he or she has ever had any "unhelpful thoughts" like this. Ask the parent to give the child some specific examples.

With an **older child or teen** it is useful to promote awareness of how thoughts affect someone by reviewing the *Feelings, Thoughts, and Behaviors Go Together* chart back in parent book Chapter 12. Discuss the examples depicted on this chart. Then ask the older child or teen and parent if they comprehend the connection between feelings, thoughts, and behaviors. Make sure that the older child or teen understands that this connection can go in a negative or positive direction, depending on whether the thoughts are unhelpful or helpful. Ask the child for examples from his or her life that might be similar to those shown on the chart. **If the older child or teen was already exposed to this chart in Chapter 12, and seemed to grasp the ideas, it can be skipped or just briefly reviewed again if needed.**

To facilitate a personal understanding in the **older child or teen,** review the *Unhelpful Thoughts List,* ask the child if he or she typically has such thoughts, and if so, whether or not the child would characterize them as worrying, downer, and/or unfriendly thoughts. Prompt the parent to give the older child or teen some empathic feedback about what the child has said out loud that is unhelpful or helpful. Ask for specific examples of which thoughts the child thinks on the unhelpful list and then ask him or her to ponder the questions at the bottom of the *Unhelpful Thoughts List*. Keep discussing specific thoughts of the older child or teen and how they make him or her feel and act. Ask whether or not the older child or teen might want to think more helpful thoughts.

Next review the *Helpful Thoughts List* with the **older child or teen.** Ask the child to "counter" previously identified unhelpful thoughts with the corresponding helpful thought on this list. Again ask the older child or teen to consider the questions at the bottom of the *Helpful Thoughts List*. Keep discussing this topic until the older child or teen understands that these helpful thoughts are associated with more positive emotions and actions. Ask the older child or teen if he or she would like to cultivate helpful thoughts. Ask the parent if he or she would like that too.

The next stage involves assisting the child in using helpful thoughts skills on a regular basis. Discuss the *Basic Helpful Thoughts* chart (which is like self-instruction) or the *Advanced Helpful Thoughts* chart (which is like cognitive restructuring) with the younger child or older child/teen, respectively. Explain that these charts can be used to guide the child in using helpful thoughts. Then conduct role-play practice while using the chart or form. Generate made-up or real-life past scenarios (perhaps with parent input) and process using helpful thoughts.

For example, with a **younger child**, it would be useful to role-play a playground situation such as standing there not knowing which group of children with which to play. The younger child might think something like "Nobody likes me" or "They are so mean because they won't let me play." Go through the steps of the **Basic Helpful Thoughts** chart to change these unhelpful thoughts into more helpful ones. As stated in parent book Chapter 13, the younger child will need direct instruction and prompting to think something like "These thoughts are not going to help me, and I should ask someone to play with me," or "Maybe they don't see me and I should ask if I can play." Keep reviewing similar scenarios and get the parent to provide some input. Explain that the parent can use a similar instructional strategy at home whenever the child exhibits unhelpful thinking.

With an **older child or teen**, role-play a situation in which he or she thinks something like "I hate my mother because she is trying to run my life." Guide the older child or teen to use the **Advanced Helpful Thoughts Worksheet** in this situation to consider whether this is an unhelpful thought and to go through the steps of making it more helpful. Be sure to note that the objective is not to determine whether a thought is correct (the parent may indeed sometimes be "trying to run" the child's life); rather, the objective is to consider whether the thought is helpful in how it affects feelings and actions. Prompt the parent to give the child some constructive feedback and encouragement in this endeavor.

CHILL BEFORE THINKING!

Make sure the child and parent understand how emotions can derail helpful thinking. Tell them that when someone is upset, it is really hard to think helpful thoughts. Discuss the "chill before thinking" idea: One must calm down to think helpful thoughts. This can be accomplished by stepping away, taking deep breaths, etc. (see parent book Chapter 14 for more ideas on calming down).

After explaining the "chill before thinking" principle, repeat the role plays, adding a brief cooling-down period before using helpful thoughts. In other words, have the child practice first calming down and then using the helpful thinking strategies during the role plays.

Helping Parents Create Opportunities for the Child to Use Helpful Thoughts Skills

Suggest that the parent assist the child in using helpful thinking skills in real-life situations. Discuss ways in which the parent will coach the child to practice the basic or advanced helpful thinking steps using the **Basic Helpful Thoughts** chart or the **Advanced Helpful Thoughts** chart (depending on developmental age) at home during everyday interactions with friends, siblings, and/or parents. Explain that coaching involves prompting or reminding the child to be aware of and go through the steps. Suggest that parents facilitate this process by asking limited-choice questions such as "Is that an unhelpful or helpful way to think?" or "Are those worry thoughts?" or open-ended questions such as "Are you thinking unhelpful thoughts?" and "What is a more helpful way to think?"

As with the discussion of feelings in Chapter 12, parents could model helpful thoughts by talking about events that occurred in their day and related unhelpful or helpful thoughts (again, without getting into intimate/personal subjects). They should also guide and/or dialogue with the child when they observe the child having unhelpful thoughts to help him or her move to more helpful thoughts. They can ask limited-choice or open-ended questions, as described above, but should discontinue questioning if the child becomes upset. Brief role playing with the parents can help them internalize the practice of prompting the child to examine unhelpful thoughts.

Developing a Home Implementation Plan to Be Led by the Parent

Collaborate with the parent to come up with a plan for reviewing helpful thoughts at home—when (evenings, weekends, etc.), where (home, school, in the neighborhood, etc.), and how often (once per day or week, several times per day or week, etc.) to use the chosen techniques. Refer to parent book Chapter 13 for examples of limited-choice and open-ended questions the parent can use to guide the child in using helpful thinking skills at home.

Note that it helps the parent to write goals on the *Parenting Goals* form (see parent book Chapter 3 and the end of Chapter 4 in this book) to ensure follow-through. The parent might, for example, write down a goal of reviewing the *Basic (or Advanced) Helpful Thoughts* chart each evening for 2 weeks to remind the child. The parent and child could also discuss examples of unhelpful and helpful thinking each day at dinner. Another related goal for the *Parenting Goals* form might be for the parent to be more aware of opportunities to guide the child using limited-choice and open-ended questions.

Tell the parent it is important to monitor the older child or teen's progress using the *Personal Goals (Basic* or *Advanced)* form (see parent book Chapter 3 and the end of Chapter 4 in this book). On this form the child, with the assistance of the parent, can declare personalized goals related to helpful thinking. Assist the family in determining how often they will review this goal and monitoring form to assess progress.

Specific Procedures for Applying Parent Book Chapter 14

This chapter focuses on stress (including anxiety and anger), using a **stress-reduction** framework (e.g., good daily health habits) and training the child in **stress-coping skills** to use in the moment when stress is acute. The focus is on teaching the child behaviors or actions that can be taken to reduce stress—like developing good health habits and behavior acti-vation as well as learning to manage high-stress episodes, including recognizing "stress signals" and calming down using various relaxation techniques, coping self-talk, and taking effective action. Parents are given ideas for coaching the child's stress management skills in real life.

Parents and practitioners will have to collaborate on determining whether the child is mature enough to learn to use stress-coping skills. The stress-reduction skills are good for all ages, and even young children can use the stress-coping skills in a basic manner. Make sure that parents understand that a child under age 8–10 may not have the abilities required to learn how to cope with stress on his or her own and therefore will need considerable instruc-tion on how to use the skills at home.

Note: *The forms and charts referred to in the discussion below are in parent book Chapter 14 and also at the end of this chapter unless otherwise noted.*

Discussing Child Stress Problems with Child and Parents

This chapter is aimed at helping children who seem emotionally stressed. Here the term *stress* connotes distress, tension, frustration, upset, anxiety, and/or anger responses to life's challenges that can be overwhelming. This term is intentionally broad to encompass a host of negative emotions associated with overarousal. It's noteworthy that many children who display one of the forms of overarousal often also display some of the others. It follows, then, that stress-coping skills can help the child decrease arousal, which improves daily function-ing.

Explain stress to the child and parent. For a **younger child** it may be best to say that stress is getting upset sometimes, whereas an **older child or teen** can understand the more nuanced definition given above. Ask the child and parent if the child gets "stressed out," and if so, in what ways. If the child has stress responses across situations and settings, then the ideas in parent book Chapter 14 will be helpful.

Be alert for answers that indicate a problem that is much narrower than stress as defined above. If the child has an "anger problem" only when told to do something, explain that this may be more indicative of **noncompliance,** and therefore the skills in this chapter may not be the first-line approach (in which case the initial focus should be on parent book Chapter 4). Or if the child "gets too angry," but so do the parent and other family members, this may be more related to **family conflict,** and therefore the skills in this chapter may not be the best place to start (in which case the beginning focus should be on parent book Chapter 20). Nonetheless tell the parent that stress is often associated with behavior problems and fam-ily quarrels, so helping a child with stress may help as long as the other strategies are also emphasized.

Getting Parents Started and Focused

Start by asking the parent to rate and check off items on the *Parent Checklist for Child Stress Management* that are going well and identify areas needing continued parenting effort. Tell the parent that this checklist summarizes the overall approach in this chapter and answer any questions about the content conveyed. Inform the parent that it is important to understand the information summarized on this checklist and detailed in parent book Chapter 14.

Promoting the Child's Awareness of Stress

Practitioners and parents must take into account the child's developmental age in explaining stress. For **younger children,** just talk about the importance of staying calm when dealing with a stressful or difficult situation. Ask the child to report times when he or she felt nervous, upset, or angry and how it affected him or her. Get the parent involved in providing examples. A child might remember feeling nervous when called on at school and not knowing what to say. Or maybe someone called the child a name, and the child responded by hitting the other child and getting in trouble with the teacher. In both cases the practitioner can then ask the child to think back about how it might have gone if he or she could have stayed calm.

With an **older child or teen,** review the *Feelings, Thoughts, and Behaviors Go Together* chart from parent book Chapter 12 to promote awareness of how "unhelpful" behaviors are related to higher stress and how "helpful" behaviors are connected to lower stress. Solicit similar examples from the child that may be illustrative for him or her. Practitioners may be able to get a child to open up by using humor and by giving examples of behaviors of their own that cause them stress. Parents should also be encouraged to chime in with examples, but the practitioner will have to be alert for overly critical, unconstructive contributions that will only derail the discussion and steer it back to the constructive. Ending this discussion on a positive, optimistic note is essential if children are to be open to learning strategies for managing stress.

Training the Child and Parent in Stress-Reduction Skills

A thorough discussion of stress-reduction habits with the child and parent is indicated no matter the child's age. **Tell the parent that stress-reduction habits can be worked on to reduce global stress in the child.** Emphasize that this prevents stress, which is better than dealing with it as it occurs. Likewise, tell the child that these preventive-type methods "fill up the gas tank to keep going" (younger child) or provide the "staying power" (older child or teen) needed to face everyday challenges and to avoid being overwhelmed by them.

Brainstorm how the child and parent can work together to reduce the child's overall stress level. This could include, but is not limited to, making an intentional effort to improve diet, exercise regularly, improve sleep routines (see parent book Chapter 19 for more ideas on sleep routines), avoid procrastination with homework, etc. It is also beneficial to plan occasional pleasant events to combat general stress. Help the child and parent consider options such as having friends over for an evening, playing a game with a parent, attending a concert, taking the dog for a walk, or engaging in a favorite hobby.

Assist the child and parent in selecting one or two stress-reduction habits to work on and in setting up a plan to follow through. Note that most people succeed in developing stress-reduction habits if they work on goals and schedule when to tackle them (see parent book Chapter 3 for ideas on how the child and parent can set and monitor progress on goals). Suggest that the parent and child both work on stress-prevention habits as a team.

Training the Child and Parent in Behavior Activation Skills

Discuss the child's age, maturity, and openness to change with the parent to determine collaboratively whether the child can benefit from a targeted behavioral activation strategy. The targeted behaviors—avoiding, withdrawing, and/or overthinking—can be difficult to change, and success depends on the child's motivation. Additionally, some children (and parents) may believe mistakenly that feeling better is a prerequisite to taking action, not understanding that taking action (through behavioral activation) can lead to feeling better. Some psychoeducation about how behavioral activation is proven to reduce stress (and improve mood and lower anxiety) might be useful.

It is obvious that targeted behavioral activation requires buy-in on the child's part, so much effort to promote motivation is required before implementing this intervention. With a **younger child** it can be useful to discuss the plan of "having more fun when feeling down" or something similar. It can help to ask an **older child or teen** to fill out the ***Thinking about Personal Goals*** worksheet (at the end of Chapter 3 in the parent book and Chapter 4 in this volume) to further consider the value of working on behavioral activation. External rewards for children of any age can be helpful in getting them to try this method (also see Chapter 3 in the parent book and Chapter 4 in this volume for more ideas on motivating a child).

Once the child and parent are on board, it is a matter of educating and brainstorming about how the child will apply behavioral activation methods and how the parent can support this effort. This usually entails writing down personal examples and "signals" that tell the child that he or she is avoiding, withdrawing, and/or overthinking. It also helps to generate a list of specific coping behaviors that the child can use to take action, such as exercising, relaxing with a favorite activity, socializing with friends/family, or engaging in some kind of helpful goal-directed behavior, such as cleaning one's bedroom, homework, etc. For example, a child may recognize that he or she is watching too much TV, and when this occurs will go for a bike ride. The ***Personal Goals (Basic*** or ***Advanced)*** form (at the end of Chapter 3 in the parent book and Chapter 4 of this book) can be used to work on behavioral activation. A goal might be to "Stop thinking and go for a walk," "Stop withdrawing and talk to Mom," etc. Parents can encourage or reward follow-through to increase the child's motivation to use behavioral activation (also see Chapter 3 in the parent book and Chapter 4 in this volume).

Training the Child and Parent to Use In-the-Moment Stress-Coping Skills

Remind the parent that stress-coping skills can be used to help a child deal with moments of high stress, but that the skills need to be adjusted to the child's age.

Review the *Staying Calm* chart with the child and parent to present the big picture of what it takes to handle high-stress episodes. There are *Staying Calm* charts with younger or older kids depicted, so be sure to use the one that best fits the child. These charts present the steps of recognizing stress, relaxing the body, using calming self-talk, and taking effective action. Tell the parent that these are forms of coping behavior that the child can use to better manage high-stress episodes. You will teach each individual subskill first, as detailed below, and then how to use them all together. You can train the child and then invite the parent in for a demonstration or train both together. Collaborate with the child and parent about how they would like to proceed. Perhaps the parent of a less-motivated child could be prompted to provide a reward to the child for practicing and using these new skills at home between sessions (see parent book Chapter 3 for ideas on motivating the child).

Elicit specific past incidences of the child being stressed out to educate the child and parent about how the child can **recognize stress signals** related to the body, thoughts, and actions. Typical incidents include not being able to find something needed for school, being called a name, or having a sibling suddenly grab the TV remote from the child without asking. Use the examples of stress signals in the parent book Chapter 14 to enrich the discussion of the body, thought, and action signals present during the child's discussion of past stressful episodes. Also use the "Practice Exercises" described in the parent book to help the child learn about stress signals.

One or more sessions can be devoted to teaching the child **relaxation** methods. Model and then have the child and parent practice the belly breathing, muscle tension–release, and visualizing techniques described in the parent book, and then assign homework practice of one or more of the relaxation strategies for a specified time each day.

Another session or two can be used to teach the child to use **calming self-talk**. Although the focus is on thoughts, this is more like self-talk than the thought-changing techniques discussed in Chapter 13. Model, and then have the child and parent practice, using calming self-talk in stressful situations such as having too much homework or dealing with a name-calling sister. **Ask the child and parent to generate a personalized list of calming self-statements that the child could think during stressful situations (e.g., "Don't let her get to you," "Take some deep breaths," "Chill out").** Do some role playing with the child and parent in which these situations are acted out and the child recites the generated self-statements to stay calm. Encourage the child to review the calming self-statements at home and to use them whenever stressed out.

Still another meeting or two could be allocated to teaching the child to take **effective action** when stressful events arise. These effective actions could include going to a cool-down spot in the house, expressing feelings verbally, asking for a hug, going for a walk, relaxing, or being assertive with someone. Prompt the child and parent to create a personalized written list of effective actions the child can take when stressed out. This list could be referred to at home when stressful events occur.

Be sure to model and role-play the specific effective action methods that the child and parent have thought of and written down. For example, do a role play of getting tense over having too much homework and then taking effective action via a 5-minute break. Another example for a role play could be dealing with a name-calling sister by assertively saying "Stop it, I don't like that" and walking away.

Once the child is good at recognizing stress, taking steps to create relaxation and calming self-talk, and taking effective action, teach him or her to use all of the skills together. Describe, model, and do role playing for the entire staying-calm procedure. The *Staying Calm* chart or *Staying Calm Worksheet* (usually best for an older child or teen) can be used to facilitate this training. For example, the stressed-out homework scenario and/or name-calling sister episode could be reenacted with all of the subskills together. Be sure to go through each step of the *Staying Calm* chart or *Staying Calm Worksheet* as the child practices all of the steps. Ask the parent to practice guiding the child during the role plays (e.g., "Take some deep breaths," "What are some calming thoughts you can think?"). Repeat this procedure several times until it goes smoothly. Then ask the child to practice using the skills at home, with the parent guiding this effort, for a specified amount of time every day via role play.

Helping Parents Create Opportunities for the Child to Use Stress Management Skills

The parent can provide opportunities for the child to incorporate stress-reduction strategies into routine family life by providing, for example, access to exercise equipment to increase exercise or taking the child to the grocery store to buy healthier food. Another route would be to brainstorm with the child about how to improve the nightly routine so that he or she can get to bed on time to get enough sleep.

It is also important to help the parent come up with ways to guide the child in using stress-coping skills at home. Talk about ways in which the parent will coach the child to use the *Staying Calm* chart or *Staying Calm Worksheet* whenever a high-stress episode comes up. Note that coaching involves prompting or reminding the child to go through the staying-calm steps as stress is being dealt with in the moment. Sometimes it is helpful to review retroactively how a child could have stayed calm by using the *Staying Calm* chart or *Staying Calm Worksheet* after the fact.

It can be very helpful to conduct brief role plays with the parent about how to guide the child in using staying-calm methods. Model how to assist the child (played by the parent), who gets frustrated with a difficult homework assignment. Demonstrate how to use guiding questions: "It looks like you are upset"; "Is there anything you can do to calm down?"; "Let's look at the *Staying Calm* chart for ideas"; "Are you aware of any stress signals at this time?"; "Can you do anything to relax your body?" Then the parent could try to do the same role play, this time with the practitioner acting out the child's role.

Encourage the parent to model skills by using the steps delineated on the *Staying Calm* chart or *Staying Calm Worksheet* (depending on which one the child is using). Propose that when the parent is stressed out around the house, he or she could pause and use the same methods. For example, say, the parent burns something on the stove while preparing dinner, gets upset, pauses, and then models using the items on the *Staying Calm Worksheet*. During this demonstration the parent could fill out the worksheet and talk out loud while going through the steps.

Developing a Home Implementation Plan to Be Led by the Parent

It is not too difficult to plan with the parent how to incorporate stress-prevention methods into daily life. For example, the family could schedule going on bike rides on Monday, Wednesday, and Sunday evenings. Another example might involve the parent's incorporating the child's input into how to improve diet and what to buy at the grocery store.

Help the parent articulate concrete plans for when (evenings, weekends, etc.), where (home, school, in the neighborhood, etc.), and how often (once per day or week, several times per day or week, etc.) to use the chosen stress management skills. Recommend that the parent write goals on the *Parenting Goals* form (see parent book Chapter 3 and the end of Chapter 4 in this book) that pertain to the plan. For example, the parent might write down a goal of going to the gym with the child at least four times per week for some exercise, setting a firm bedtime to make sure that the child gets enough sleep, and rewarding an older child or teen for using the *Staying Calm Worksheet* when stressful situations arise.

Make sure that the parent understands the importance of monitoring the child's progress with stress management skills. The *Personal Goals (Basic* or *Advanced)* form (see parent book Chapter 3 and the end of Chapter 4 in this book) can be used by the child to facilitate accountability. On this form the child, with the assistance of the parent, can declare personalized goals related to stress management. Assist the child and parent in determining how often they will review the child's progress with personal goals.

Modifications for Using the Child Emotional Development Module in Parent Groups

Encourage parents to discuss concerns for their child's emotional well-being and what they have tried in the past to help the child. Listening to one another's trials and tribulations can be a catalyst to work with their child in this developmental area. In addition, their children's emotional distress distresses parents, and allowing parents to discuss this with other parents can be cathartic.

The *Overview of the Child Emotional Development Module* chart can be employed with parent group members to review strategies for enhancing children's emotional capabilities. Inform parents that the main goal of this module is to train children in emotion skills and for parents to guide them in using these skills. Then brainstorm with parents about specific chapters and/or techniques within this module that they would like to learn more about in upcoming weeks.

The emotional development module can be introduced over one meeting, but three or more meetings will be needed to cover all of the topics. The charts found in parent book Chapters 12–14 can be used as needed to convey information and approaches for improving a child's emotional well-being. The role plays described in the preceding training sections for parent book Chapters 12–14 can be used in parent groups by having parents take turns if they are comfortable doing so. Help each parent individually pinpoint specific emotional development goals and strategies to work on with their child and designate them on the *Parenting Goals* form.

Overview of the Child Emotional Development Module

Facilitating the Child's Emotional Awareness

- Discuss **Feelings, Thoughts, and Behaviors Go Together** chart to promote awareness

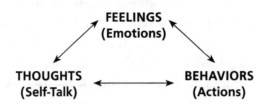

- Explain that each part influences the other two parts

- Explain further that expressing feelings, thinking helpful thoughts, and using stress management behaviors can make someone feel better

Chapter 12. Let It Out!: Teaching Your Child to Understand and Express Feelings

Increasing Awareness of Feelings

- Review and discuss basic feelings with a younger child or advanced feelings with an older child or teen

Training Feelings Expression Skills

- Informally review and dialogue about feelings (can refer to a feelings chart)

- Formally review and dialogue about feelings and consider using a diary

See **Basic Feelings Vocabulary Chart**, **Advanced Feelings Vocabulary Chart**, and **Feelings Diary** form.

Chapter 13. You Are What You Think: Teaching Your Child to Think Helpful Thoughts

Increasing Awareness of Unhelpful and Helpful Thinking

- Review types of **unhelpful** thoughts with child (usually best for older child or teen):

  - *Worry thoughts*—thinking that something terrible is going to happen, which is related to nervousness and avoidance behavior

  - *Downer thoughts*—thinking that life is going badly and nothing can make it better, which is related to sadness and withdrawn behavior

  - *Unfriendly thoughts*—thinking that people are unfair or doing mean things on purpose, which is related to anger and aggressive or defiant behavior

- Ask child if he or she has any unhelpful thoughts and how those thoughts make him or her feel and act

(cont.)

- Review types of **helpful** thoughts with child (usually best for older child or teen):

  - *Confidence thoughts*—thinking you can try your best, which is related to calmness and facing-your-fears behavior

  - *Upper thoughts*—thinking that life has good in it and that one can make it better, which is related to happiness and getting-involved behavior

  - *Friendly thoughts*—thinking that people are okay and fair most of the time, which is related to calm and cooperative behavior

- Ask child if he or she would like to think more helpful thoughts and how those thoughts would make him or her feel and act

See **Unhelpful Thoughts List** and **Helpful Thoughts List** forms.

Selecting and Training Basic Helpful Thinking with a Younger Child

1. Am I thinking unhelpful thoughts?

2. Are these thoughts going to help me?

3. What is a different and more helpful way I can think?

See **Basic Helpful Thoughts** chart.

Selecting and Training Advanced Helpful Thinking with an Older Child or Teen

1. Am I thinking unhelpful thoughts?

2. What kind of unhelpful thoughts am I having?

3. How are these unhelpful thoughts going to make me feel and act?

4. What is a different and more helpful way I can think?

5. What kind of helpful thoughts am I having?

6. How are these helpful thoughts going to make me feel and act?

See **Advanced Helpful Thoughts** chart and **Advanced Helpful Thoughts Worksheet** form.

Chapter 14. Stress Busters: Teaching Your Child to Manage Stress

Promoting General Stress-Reduction Activities

- Eat a healthy diet
- Get regular exercise
- Relax periodically
- Play a game with a parent
- Spend time with a friend
- Get enough sleep
- Follow routines and schedules
- Engage in a favorite hobby or interest
- Take the dog for a walk
- Avoid homework procrastination

(cont.)

- Promoting behavior activation

  - Raise awareness in the child that avoiding behavior, withdrawing behavior, and overthinking are signs of stress

  - Help the child learn to recognize avoiding, withdrawing, and overthinking and to respond to it by taking action

Training to Handle In-the-Moment High-Stress Episodes

- *Recognizing stress*—be aware of "signals" from body, thoughts, and actions related to stress

- *Belly breathing*—slow, low, and through-the-nose technique

- *Muscle tension and release*—relax muscles via "robot/rag doll" (younger child) or step-by-step muscle progression methods (older child or teen)

- *Visualization*—"see" self as calm; imagine being at favorite personal space or place

- *Helpful self-talk*—make statements such as "Take it easy," "Stay cool," "Don't let him bug me," "I'll be okay"

- *Effective action*—express feelings, ask for a hug, go for a walk, be assertive (instead of aggressive or passive), try to solve the problem, etc.

See **Staying Calm** chart (usually best for younger child) and **Staying Calm Worksheet** form (usually best for older child or teen).

Training Child in Emotional Development Skills (Chapters 12–14)

- Focus on the family "team" working together

- Guide child to choose and then work on emotional development skills and goals

- Identify parenting goals related to promoting child's emotional development at home

- Learn, practice, and monitor progress with child's emotional development skills and goals

See **Parent Checklist** for each chapter, as well as **Personal Goals (Basic** or **Advanced)** form for child and **Parenting Goals** form for parent (both in Chapter 3 of the parent book and at the end of Chapter 4 in this book)

Forms from Parent Book Chapter 12

Parent Checklist for Child Feelings

Name: _____ Date: _____

In the blanks below, indicate a score for **how well** you make use of that parenting behavior at this time.

	Not too well	Okay	Very well
	1	2	3

Parent's Efforts in Teaching Child Feelings Skills

A. _____ Reviewing feelings-oriented chart(s) to educate the child about different feelings and words to describe them

B. _____ Teaching the child about how feelings are related to thoughts and behaviors

C. _____ Using informal discussion and/or feelings charts to periodically guide feelings expression

D. _____ Being a good role model about how to express feelings

Basic Feelings Vocabulary Chart

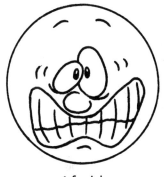

Afraid

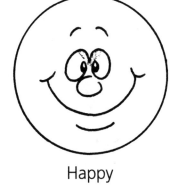

Happy

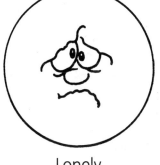

Lonely

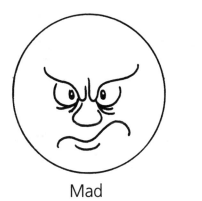

Mad

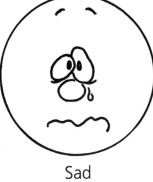

Sad

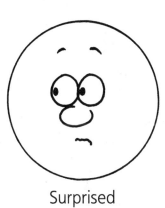

Surprised

Advanced Feelings Vocabulary Chart

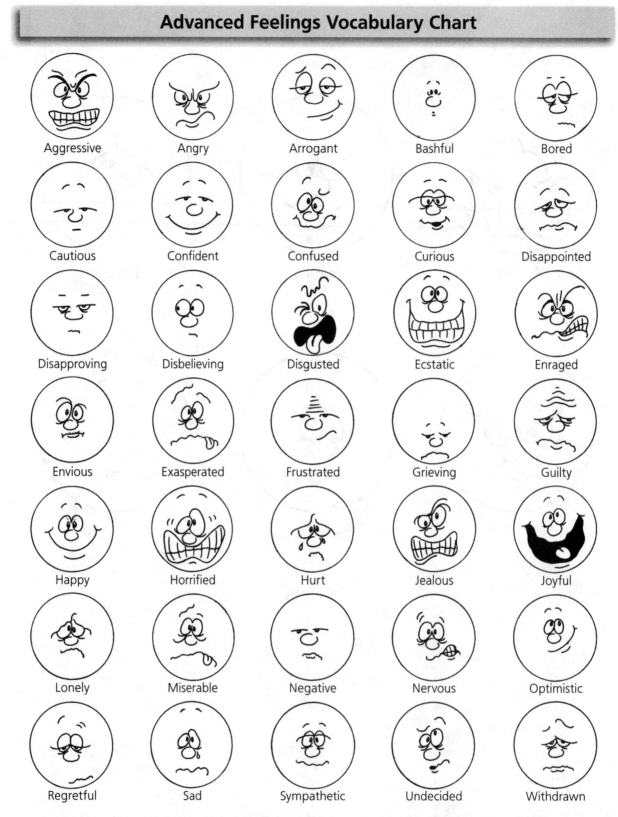

Aggressive	Angry	Arrogant	Bashful	Bored
Cautious	Confident	Confused	Curious	Disappointed
Disapproving	Disbelieving	Disgusted	Ecstatic	Enraged
Envious	Exasperated	Frustrated	Grieving	Guilty
Happy	Horrified	Hurt	Jealous	Joyful
Lonely	Miserable	Negative	Nervous	Optimistic
Regretful	Sad	Sympathetic	Undecided	Withdrawn

Feelings, Thoughts, and Behaviors Go Together

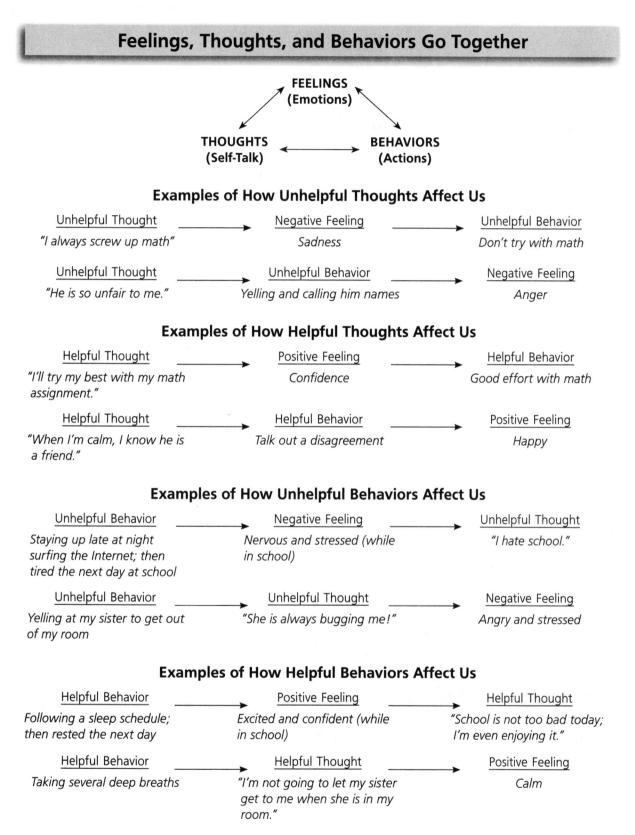

FEELINGS
(Emotions)

THOUGHTS
(Self-Talk)

BEHAVIORS
(Actions)

Examples of How Unhelpful Thoughts Affect Us

Unhelpful Thought → Negative Feeling → Unhelpful Behavior

"I always screw up math"   *Sadness*   *Don't try with math*

Unhelpful Thought → Unhelpful Behavior → Negative Feeling

"He is so unfair to me."   *Yelling and calling him names*   *Anger*

Examples of How Helpful Thoughts Affect Us

Helpful Thought → Positive Feeling → Helpful Behavior

"I'll try my best with my math assignment."   *Confidence*   *Good effort with math*

Helpful Thought → Helpful Behavior → Positive Feeling

"When I'm calm, I know he is a friend."   *Talk out a disagreement*   *Happy*

Examples of How Unhelpful Behaviors Affect Us

Unhelpful Behavior → Negative Feeling → Unhelpful Thought

Staying up late at night surfing the Internet; then tired the next day at school   *Nervous and stressed (while in school)*   *"I hate school."*

Unhelpful Behavior → Unhelpful Thought → Negative Feeling

Yelling at my sister to get out of my room   *"She is always bugging me!"*   *Angry and stressed*

Examples of How Helpful Behaviors Affect Us

Helpful Behavior → Positive Feeling → Helpful Thought

Following a sleep schedule; then rested the next day   *Excited and confident (while in school)*   *"School is not too bad today; I'm even enjoying it."*

Helpful Behavior → Helpful Thought → Positive Feeling

Taking several deep breaths   *"I'm not going to let my sister get to me when she is in my room."*   *Calm*

Feelings Diary

Name: _____ **Date:** _____

Write down positive and negative events that happened and how you felt. Use the (**Basic** or **Advanced**) **Feelings Vocabulary Chart** to help label your feelings. You can fill the diary out when an event occurs or afterward. You can share this **Feelings Diary** with others or keep it private.

Positive Events   **My Feelings**

1.   1.

2.   2.

3.   3.

4.   4.

Negative Events   **My Feelings**

1.   1.

2.   2.

3.   3.

4.   4.

Forms from Parent Book Chapter 13

Parent Checklist for Child Helpful Thoughts

Name: _____ Date: _____

In the blanks below, indicate a score for **how well** you make use of that parenting behavior at this time.

Not too well	Okay	Very well
1	2	3

Parent's Efforts in Promoting Child's Awareness of Unhelpful and Helpful Thoughts

A. _____ Explaining how unhelpful and helpful thoughts relate to how one feels and behaves so that the child is more aware

Parent's Efforts in Teaching a Child Helpful Thoughts Skills

B. _____ Reviewing and role-playing/practicing of helpful thoughts steps

C. _____ Using informal discussion and/or helpful thoughts charts to periodically guide helpful thoughts skills

D. _____ Modeling helpful thinking

E. _____ Coaching the child to calm down so that thoughts can be more helpful (i.e., "chill before thinking")

Unhelpful Thoughts List

Listed below is a variety of thoughts children may have about themselves. Read each thought and indicate how frequently that thought (or a similar thought) typically occurs for you over an average week. There is no right or wrong answer to these questions. Use the 3-point rating scale to answer how often you have these thoughts:

7

1	**2**	**3**
Rarely	**Sometimes**	**Often**

Worry Thoughts

1. ____ Something bad will happen to me (family member, friend, teachers, etc.).
2. ____ It will be terrible (horrible, scary, etc.).
3. ____ Everyone will be looking at me, and I won't know what to say.
4. ____ I don't fit in with the crowd.
5. ____ I won't be able to do it.
6. ____ My future doesn't look good. Nothing will work out for me.
7. ____ *My usual worry thoughts are (write in):* _____

_____

Downer Thoughts

8. ____ I'm no good (stupid, ugly, weak, etc.).
9. ____ I can't do anything right (I'm a failure).
10. ____ I have to do well in school, sports, and so forth, or people will look down on me.
11. ____ I give up. I've tried everything. There's nothing more I can do.
12. ____ It's my fault.
13. ____ No one likes me.
14. ____ *My usual downer thoughts are (write in):* _____

_____

Unfriendly Thoughts

15. ____ Lots of peers (siblings) are mean to me on purpose.
16. ____ Lots of peers (siblings) are unfair to me.
17. ____ My parent (teacher) is unfair to me.
18. ____ Lots of peers (siblings) mess with me (tease me, pick on me).
19. ____ My parent (teacher) is to blame.
20. ____ My parent wants to run my life.
21. ____ *My usual unfriendly thoughts are (write in):* _____

_____

For each thought you rated a 3, ask yourself the following questions:

1. How am I going to **feel** if I have this thought?
2. How am I going to **act or behave** if I have this thought?
3. Is this an unhelpful thought that I should be more aware of and try to change?

Helpful Thoughts List

Listed below are helpful counterthoughts that children can use instead of unhelpful thoughts. Unhelpful (Worry) Thought #1 corresponds to Helpful (Confidence) Thought #1, and so on. Compare the unhelpful thoughts to the helpful thoughts.

Confidence Thoughts

1. It's not likely that something bad will happen to me (family member, friend, teachers, etc.).
2. It will be all right (just fine, etc.) if I do my best.
3. I am imagining that everyone will be looking at me. I'll know what to say once I get there.
4. I fit in with some people. I do have friends.
5. I can do my best if I try.
6. My future will be fine as long as I do my best.
7. *Other confident thoughts I could think are (write in):* _____

_____

Upper Thoughts

8. I know I have lots of good points. I'm just fine the way I am.
9. I do lots of things quite well, actually.
10. I'll just try my best. People respect others who try.
11. It doesn't help to give up. I need to keep trying.
12. It doesn't help to find fault. I need to think of how to make it better.
13. I have some friends. If I want more, I can do something about that if I try.
14. *Other upper thoughts I could think are (write in):* _____

_____

Friendly Thoughts

15. When I'm calm, I realize that most peers (my siblings) treat me okay.
16. When I'm calm, I realize that most peers (my siblings) are fair to me.
17. When I'm calm, I realize that my parent (teacher) is usually fair to me.
18. Most of the time I get treated okay by peers (siblings).
19. It doesn't help to blame my parent (teacher). I need to think about solutions.
20. My parent is just trying to make sure I am safe and that I do well.
21. *Other friendly thoughts I could think are (write in):* _____

_____

For each counterthought you choose, ask yourself the following questions:

1. How am I going to **feel** if I have this thought?
2. How am I going to **act or behave** if I have this thought?
3. Is this a helpful thought that I should be more aware of and try to keep?

Basic Helpful Thoughts

1. Am I thinking unhelpful thoughts?

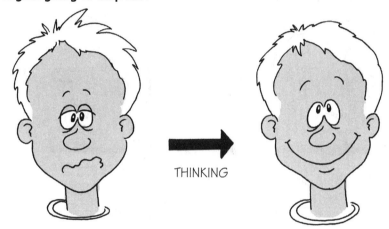

I'M NO GOOD. I GIVE UP. NO ONE LIKES ME. IT'S MY FAULT. THEY ARE SO UNFAIR. I ALWAYS . . . I HATE . . . I CAN'T DO IT. I SHOULD HAVE . . .

2. Are these thoughts going to help me?

THINKING

3. What is a different and more helpful way I can think?

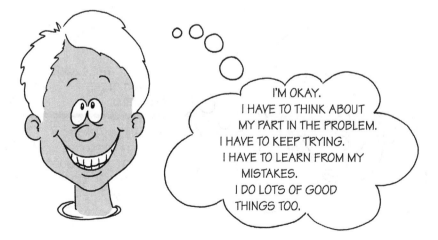

I'M OKAY.
I HAVE TO THINK ABOUT
MY PART IN THE PROBLEM.
I HAVE TO KEEP TRYING.
I HAVE TO LEARN FROM MY
MISTAKES.
I DO LOTS OF GOOD
THINGS TOO.

Basic Helpful Thoughts

1. Am I thinking unhelpful thoughts?

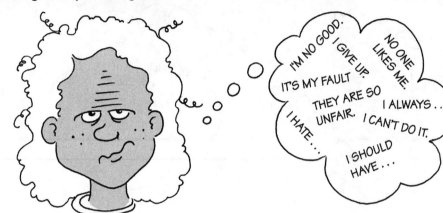

2. Are these thoughts going to help me?

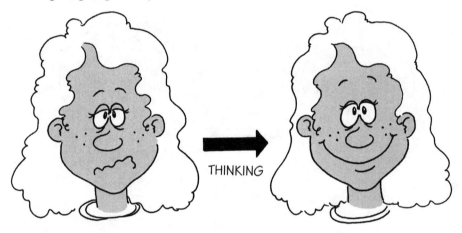

3. What is a different and more helpful way I can think?

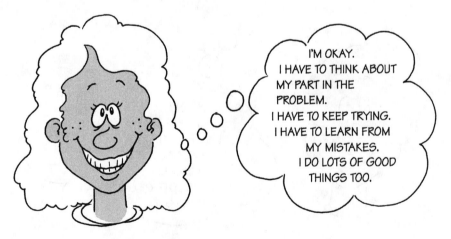

Advanced Helpful Thoughts

1. Am I thinking unhelpful thoughts?

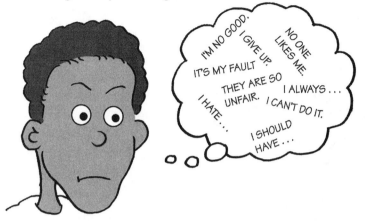

2. What kind of unhelpful thoughts am I having? Are they . . .

- **Worry Thoughts**—like thinking the worst or that something bad will happen?
- **Downer Thoughts**—like things are bad and nothing can make them better?
- **Unfriendly Thoughts**—like people are unfair and doing mean things on purpose?

3. How are these unhelpful thoughts going to make me feel and act?

4. What is a different and more helpful way I can think?

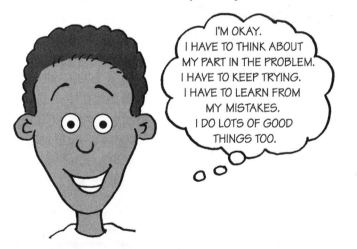

5. What kind of helpful thoughts am I now having? Are they . . .

- **Confidence Thoughts**—like I can handle it if I try?
- **Upper Thoughts**—like I can make them better if I try?
- **Friendly Thoughts**—like most people treat me okay most of the time?

6. How are these helpful thoughts going to make me feel and act?

Advanced Helpful Thoughts

1. Am I thinking unhelpful thoughts?

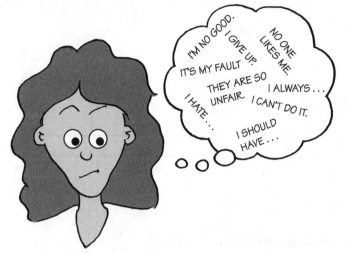

2. What kind of unhelpful thoughts am I having? Are they . . .

- **Worry Thoughts**—like thinking the worst or that something bad will happen?
- **Downer Thoughts**—like things are bad and nothing can make them better?
- **Unfriendly Thoughts**—like people are unfair and doing mean things on purpose?

3. How are these unhelpful thoughts going to make me feel and act?

4. What is a different and more helpful way I can think?

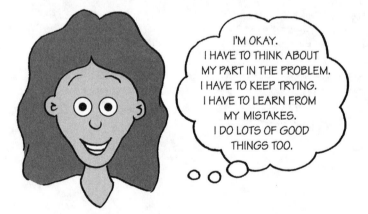

5. What kind of helpful thoughts am I now having? Are they . . .

- **Confidence Thoughts**—like I can handle it if I try?
- **Upper Thoughts**—like I can make them better if I try?
- **Friendly Thoughts**—like most people treat me okay most of the time?

6. How are these helpful thoughts going to make me feel and act?

Advanced Helpful Thoughts Worksheet

Name: _____ Date: _____

Fill out the worksheet during or after you have experienced an unhelpful thought.

1. What are my thoughts? Am I thinking unhelpful thoughts?

2. What kind of unhelpful thoughts am I having? Are they (circle those that apply) **..** .
- **Worry Thoughts**—like thinking the worst or that something bad will happen?

- **Downer Thoughts**—like things are bad and nothing can make them better?

- **Unfriendly Thoughts**—like people are unfair and doing mean things on purpose?

3. How are these unhelpful thoughts going to make me feel and act?

4. What is a different and more helpful way I can think?

5. What kind of helpful thoughts am I now having? Are they (circle those that apply) **..** .
- **Confidence Thoughts**—like I can handle it if I try?

- **Upper Thoughts**—like I can make them better if I try?

- **Friendly Thoughts**—like most people treat me okay most of the time?

6. How are these helpful thoughts going to make me feel and act?

How Well Did It Work?
(Circle *1, 2, 3,* or *4.*)

1. I didn't really try too hard.
2. I sort of tried, but it didn't really work.
3. I tried hard, and it kind of worked.
4. I tried really hard, and it really worked.

Forms from Parent Book Chapter 14

Parent Checklist for Child Stress Management

Name: _____ **Date:** _____

In the blanks below, indicate a score for **how well** you make use of that parenting behavior at this time.

Not too well	Okay	Very well
1	2	3

Parent's Efforts in Promoting Child's Awareness of Stress

A. _____ Explaining what stress is so that the child is more aware

Parent's Efforts in Teaching a Child Stress-Reduction Skills

B. _____ Helping the child develop good habits related to diet, exercising, relaxing, sleeping, etc.

C. _____ Incorporating routines and schedules into everyday life

D. _____ Taking action to follow through with healthy habits

E. _____ Guiding behavioral activation as needed by helping the child recognize ineffective coping and taking action as planned to enhance coping

Parent's Efforts in Teaching a Child In-the-Moment Stress-Coping Skills

F. _____ Educating the child about stress and body, thought, and action "stress signals"

G. _____ Guiding use of breathing, muscle tension–release relaxation, and visualization techniques to relax

H. _____ Guiding use of coping self-talk when stressed out

I. _____ Guiding taking action, like expressing feelings, asking for a hug, going for a walk, relaxing, asserting, etc.

J. _____ Asking guiding questions and/or using charts to prompt the child to use stress management in real life

K. _____ Being a good model for managing stress

Staying Calm

1. What am I stressed, angry, or nervous about?

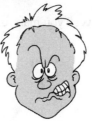

2. How stressed, or angry, or nervous am I?

1	2	3	4	5
Not at all	A little	Somewhat	A lot	Very much

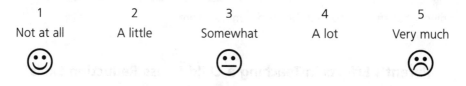

3. Calm down my body with slow breathing, muscle relaxation, and visualization.

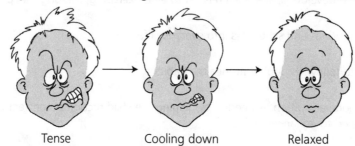

Tense   Cooling down   Relaxed

4. Use calming self-talk.

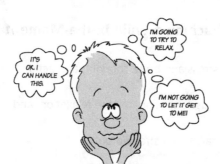

IT'S OK. I CAN HANDLE THIS.

I'M GOING TO TRY TO RELAX.

I'M NOT GOING TO LET IT GET TO ME!

5. Take some action to solve the problem.

Staying Calm

1. What am I stressed, angry, or nervous about?

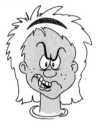

2. How stressed, or angry, or nervous am I?

1	2	3	4	5
Not at all	A little	Somewhat	A lot	Very much

3. Calm down my body with slow breathing, muscle relaxation, and visualization.

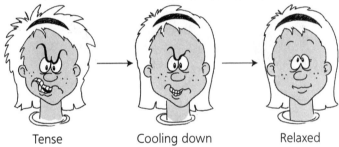

Tense   Cooling down   Relaxed

4. Use calming self-talk.

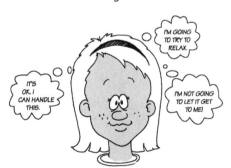

5. Take some action to solve the problem.

Staying Calm

1. **What am I stressed, angry, or nervous about?**

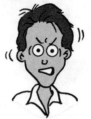

2. **How stressed, or angry, or nervous am I?**

1	2	3	4	5
Not at all	A little	Somewhat	A lot	Very much

3. **Calm down my body with slow breathing, muscle relaxation, and visualization.**

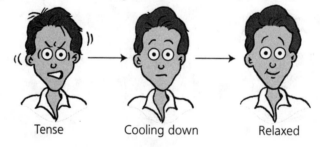

Tense   Cooling down   Relaxed

4. **Use calming self-talk.**

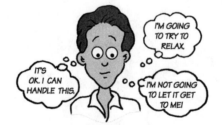

IT'S OK. I CAN HANDLE THIS.

I'M GOING TO TRY TO RELAX.

I'M NOT GOING TO LET IT GET TO ME!

5. **Take some action to solve the problem.**

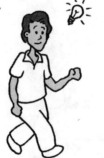

Staying Calm

1. What am I stressed, angry, or nervous about?

2. How stressed, or angry, or nervous am I?

1	2	3	4	5
Not at all	A little	Somewhat	A lot	Very much

3. Calm down my body with slow breathing, muscle relaxation, and visualization.

Tense → Cooling down → Relaxed

4. Use calming self-talk.

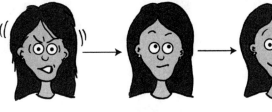

IT'S OK. I CAN HANDLE THIS.

I'M GOING TO TRY TO RELAX.

I'M NOT GOING TO LET IT GET TO ME!

5. Take some action to solve the problem.

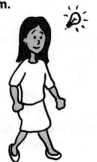

Staying Calm Worksheet

Name: _____ Date: _____

A child/teen and/or parent can complete this worksheet. It's best to fill out the worksheet while you are upset, but it's also okay to fill it out afterward.

1. **What am I stressed, angry, or nervous about?** _____

2. **How stressed, angry, or nervous am I? (Circle one.)**

1	2	3	4	5
Not at all	A little	Somewhat	A lot	Very much

3. **What are the signals that tell me I am stressed out?**

   a. **Body signals:**

   b. **Thought signals:**

   c. **Behavior signals:**

4. **What can I do to slow my breathing and relax my body?**

5. **What calming self-talk can I use to cope?**

6. **What action can I take to deal with the situation or solve the problem?**

   How Well Did It Work?
   (Circle *1, 2, 3,* or *4.*)

   1. **I didn't really try too hard.**
   2. **I sort of tried, but it didn't really work.**
   3. **I tried hard, and it kind of worked.**
   4. **I tried really hard, and it really worked.**

Using the Child Academic Development Module

This practitioner book chapter corresponds to the parent book section "Enhancing Your Child's Academic Development" (Chapters 15 & 16). The chapters in this section are designed to help the child do better academically and succeed at school. The parent is given (1) ideas and strategies for enhancing the child's self-directed academic behaviors and (2) methods to collaborate with school officials on the child's behalf. **The practitioner should read and fully understand the *content* in parent book Chapters 15 and 16 before using the related *procedures* described here.**

Within the child-focused academic development module, the practitioner has to carefully weigh considerations about whom to work with and when. This module is in many ways a very practical one; its primary goal is to help the child with schoolwork, and the parent's active involvement is crucial throughout. With school survival skills (parent book Chapter 15), it usually works best to train the child and parent together no matter the age of the child. This allows the practitioner to concurrently teach skills and also facilitate a cooperative team approach to homework and to learning new adaptive executive-functioning skills. This team notion is very important because in many families homework and other school-related issues are turned into battles. With the teaming-up skills in parent book Chapter 16, it is best to work primarily with the parent who will be working with school officials on the child's behalf. Ultimately the practitioner should seek input from the child and parent as to how to work with the family to enhance the child's academic development.

Tailoring within the Child Academic Development Module

Review the *Overview of the Child Academic Development Module* chart at the end of this chapter to give the parent an overall impression of the strategies that will be taught to promote academic success in children. Tell the parent that the focus of Chapter 15 is the promotion of "school survival skills" and that Chapter 16 is focused mostly on how the parent can effectively collaborate with school officials and advocate for the child at school. If properly implemented, these chapters together have great potential to turn around a struggling child at school.

Specific Procedures for Applying Parent Book Chapter 15

This chapter offers many ideas for teaching a child to be more productive with schoolwork. Children who have difficulty with completing schoolwork could have problems related to time management, organizational skills, planning, reviewing, and/or staying on task. This chapter focuses on teaching the child these executive functioning–type behaviors using standard behavioral training methods. The strategies described in this chapter are appropriate for children in elementary or older grades if adjusted accordingly. Parents are advised to set up a consistent time for homework each school night and to use this as a springboard for not only helping the child to get work done but also for teaching and coaching school survival skills.

> **Note:** *The forms and charts referred to in the discussion below are in parent book Chapter 15 and also at the end of this chapter unless otherwise noted.*

Discussing School Survival Skills with Parents

Explain to the parent that ability is only one part of the success equation at school. Note that a child who does not get the work done will not succeed no matter how capable he or she is. Many parents are now familiar with the term *executive functions,* so you can frame problems that interfere with academic performance—difficulties with working memory, sustained attention, and organization—as executive functioning problems. Such children can benefit from learning concrete strategies pertaining to organization, staying on task, checking work, planning, and so forth.

Children who are struggling at school also need empathic but firm guidance and motivation from parents because these children are often demoralized and want to avoid academic endeavors. It might actually be a relief to parents, who undoubtedly have been embroiled in conflicts with the child over schoolwork, to shift their attention to motivating the child along with teaching school survival skills (see parent book Chapter 3 for more ideas on motivating the child).

Getting Parents Started and Focused

Ask the parent to rate and check off items on the *Parent Checklist for School Survival Skills* that are going well and identify areas needing continued parenting effort. Because this checklist is a summary of the approach described in the chapter, it's important to answer any questions the parents have about the content and to stress how important it is for the parents to fully understand the information summarized on this checklist and detailed in parent book Chapter 15.

It is best to work on one or two school survival strategies/skills at a time, so the parent may need help narrowing down his or her list. Encourage the parent to stick with one skill until it is mastered and to proceed to other strategies/skills only at that point. Make sure that the parent understands, however, that the mandatory homework strategy and learning of school survival skills go together. **Explain that one objective of mandatory homework is to complete schoolwork and another objective is to facilitate the child's development of school survival skills.** Make sure that the parent understands and agrees to both functions of the mandatory homework method before going further.

Training the Child and Parent in Mandatory Homework Time

Begin by **defining homework** with the parent and child. Suggest a definition of homework that focuses on present, future, and past goals. The **present goal** is to get work done that is due tomorrow. The **future goal** is to plan and organize for tasks that need to be accomplished down the road. Finally, the **past goal** centers on reviewing what has already been learned in order to master it. Encourage the parent and child to structure mandatory homework accordingly, with some time devoted to each goal and brainstorm how to do this. This process might entail specifying a certain amount of time for present, future, and past goals during a routine evening of homework.

It is also important to focus on **defining the parent's role in the child's homework process.** Most parents think their role is to make the child sit down to do homework and that then it is up to the child to get it done on his or her own. Parents need to make a shift to being very involved with the child's completion of mandatory homework initially and then gradually fading out as the child learns and masters school survival skills. Caution the parents that it may take weeks or months to accomplish this transition, so they need to commit to making it a priority.

Brainstorm practical matters for implementing the completion of mandatory homework by delineating where, when, and for how long the homework will take place. Make sure that parent and child are working on homework as a team (see parent book Chapter 3 for more ideas for garnering parent–child teamwork). Also stress the importance of mutual cooperation. The parent should agree to maintain a positive tone, and the child has to agree to cooperate with the parent. Once the practical matters have been resolved, you can assign the homework of doing homework! Have parent and child report back in later sessions about how it is going so that strategies can be adjusted.

Training Child and Parent in School Survival Skills

Many school survival skills can be explained and then practiced in a simulated manner during meetings with the family. For example, for demonstration purposes, lead the development of a "session checklist" that identifies what the family wants to accomplish during the meeting that day. It might have items on it such as checking in on progress, problem solving about improving the child's motivation, and discussing the parent's follow-through with previously agreed-upon skills or strategies. Each task could have an estimate of how much time will need to be devoted to it. Then check off the items on that session checklist as tasks are accomplished. This not only keeps the meeting focused and productive but also demonstrates the use of a checklist that is similar to a homework checklist. Get the child actively involved in this application of the checklist method. Explain that a similar process can be used during mandatory homework.

Whenever possible, try to assist the family in constructing checklists and schedules and using planners in session for later use at home. For example, a homework checklist to be used that very evening might be created. Ideally, it would have sections for (1) getting things done that are due, (2) organizing and planning, and (3) reviewing. Tasks can be listed under each section, along with estimates of how much time each will take. Another example might be to fill out a weekly schedule of different activities and plan for when specified school-related tasks would be accomplished. Perhaps it would be fruitful to examine the child's paper or electronic calendar method and brainstorm how to use it best.

Organizational strategies could be worked on live in the meeting. It can be helpful, for example, to ask the child to bring in his or her backpack to the meeting to get it organized. This process could entail throwing out miscellaneous papers, organizing assignments into folders, designating a spot for assignments needing to be handed in, etc., within the backpack. It is also productive to facilitate a discussion between parent and child about organizing the child's desk and homework area at home.

Practice staying-on-task skills during a session or two. First describe, model, and role-play to demonstrate off- and on-task behavior for a simulated homework assignment. Then do a simulated homework assignment while practicing self-monitoring of on-task behavior using the *Staying on Task* form. You can conduct this training with the child and then invite parents in for a demonstration or train the child and parents together.

Parent and child may also benefit from having a training opportunity to use the staying-on-task child self-monitoring method during a live meeting. This is accomplished by defining tasks for the meeting, such as participating in discussion, role-playing, asking questions, looking at who is talking, etc. Then pause every 10–15 minutes to use the *Staying on Task* form for those session tasks.

Developing a Home Implementation Plan to Be Led by the Parent

Discuss details of how the family will implement a home plan. Ask family members to commit to a regular yet flexible time for doing mandatory homework during the week (e.g., begin homework 15 minutes after supper on Sunday–Thursday). Ask them to identify one or two school survival skills to work on (e.g., task checklists, self-monitoring of on-task behavior) during mandatory homework.

Also prompt the parent to set goals and perhaps even write them down on the ***Parenting Goals*** form (see parent book Chapter 3 and the end of Chapter 4 in this book). For example, the parent might write down a goal of assisting the child in developing a homework checklist each night. Another goal could be to coach the child in utilizing the ***Staying on Task*** form during mandatory homework time. Still another goal might be to "Stay calm when helping [child's name] during mandatory homework time."

Devising a structured method to monitor the child's personal progress can improve outcomes too. Lead the child to declare school-related goals such as using a planner each day, use the ***Staying on Task*** form during homework, etc. Encourage the child to write such goals on the ***Personal Goals (Basic*** or ***Advanced)*** form (see parent book Chapter 3 and the end of Chapter 4 in this book) and monitor progress by reviewing the goals now and then.

Specific Procedures for Applying Parent Book Chapter 16

This chapter provides ideas and strategies that parents can use to effectively collaborate and advocate with school officials on their child's behalf. The focus of this chapter is on the parent, who will put forth the most effort in teaming up with school personnel. The child will benefit by the adults' efforts at home and school to work together to make his or her school experience more positive and helpful.

Note: *The forms and charts referred to in the discussion below are in parent book Chapter 16 and also at the end of this chapter unless otherwise noted.*

Discussing the Child's School Challenges with Parents

Parents whose children have had ongoing academic problems can usually recite a long list of negative incidents and numerous failed attempts at correcting those problems. Unfortunately, some parents will also relate that they now have an adversarial relationship with the school. They may feel that working with the school is hopeless—in which case the practitioner will have to stress the importance of persevering, since the emotional effects of school problems can snowball to the point where the child does not like school and tries to avoid attending. Empathize with the parent and suggest that there are many things that can be done to help the child get on a more successful course at school. Define the goal as working effectively with the school to make that happen.

Getting Parents Started and Focused

Ask the parents to rate and check off items on the ***Parent Checklist for Teaming Up at School*** that are going well and identify areas needing continued parenting effort. Since this checklist summarizes the approach presented in the chapter, it's important to answer any questions the parents have to ensure that they fully understand the information on the list and the content of parent book Chapter 16.

Tell the parent that collaborating and advocating with school personnel are often needed to help a child succeed in his or her academic development. Define the primary goal of collaboration as identifying problems at school and coming up with solutions, while the primary goal of advocacy is to make sure that the child receives needed school-based services in accordance with his or her needs. Explain that if the parent collaborates and advocates with school personnel effectively, it will pay off for the child in the long run.

Training Parents in Collaborating Effectively with School Personnel

Review the **collaborating** section in parent book Chapter 16 with the parent and elaborate on different points as needed. It is a good idea to brainstorm methods by which the parent can facilitate ongoing communication with the teacher and/or other school personnel (by e-mail, phone, face-to-face meetings, etc.). If the parent is amenable, it can be helpful to do some role-play practice of communicating with a teacher about an important topic. For example, a role play might entail reviewing and practicing asking a teacher to cooperate with the parent in developing and using a school–home note. Be sure to underscore the advantages of maintaining ongoing contact with teacher(s) and school personnel rather than contacting them as an unknown entity when a crisis emerges.

Also tell the parent that it is most effective to communicate with school personnel by going beyond describing problem behaviors to thinking about replacement behavior(s) for the child. Tell the parent that many of the social–emotional skills described in the parent book (especially in Chapters 8–15) could serve as replacement behaviors for the child at school. Brainstorm how parents could inform school personnel of the skills the child has been learning and ways that teachers and other staff could support the use of those skills at school. For example, many of the forms and charts throughout the parent book could also be used by teachers at school.

A key strategy for direct collaboration with teachers is the utilization of a *School–Home Note,* like the two examples (one for younger and one for older children) provided in parent book Chapter 16 (and shown at the end of this chapter). Help the parent who chooses this strategy to pinpoint specific goals and target behaviors for the child on a *School–Home Note*. Then plan with the parent how to communicate those expectations to teachers and other school faculty. Discuss whether or not it is desirable and feasible to make daily home privileges contingent on daily school behavior and/or whether bonus rewards should be used. Come up with the specific details for this part of the plan, such as having the child earn tokens for good days (e.g., 80% "good" evaluations by teachers on the *School–Home Note*), which can then be turned in for rewards, such as a movie or pizza party on the weekend.

Training the Parents in Advocating Effectively at School

Review the **advocating** section in parent book Chapter 16 with the parent and elaborate on different points as needed. The main goals are to increase the parent's awareness of different types of categorical services that might be accessed at school and figure out the best way to work with school officials in creating a school-based plan for the child to get extra help.

The parent of a child with behavior problems should be advised to be assertive in asking the school for a specific plan to help the child succeed at school. Review the ***Behavior Improvement Strategies That Might Be Used at School.*** Make sure that parents understand that they do not need to know how to implement these interventions themselves because they are not experts in school-based behavior management. Rather, explain that the goal is to make the parent more knowledgeable about strategies that might be used at school. Suggest further that they could share this list of school strategies with behavior specialist staff at the school. These techniques could be part of an IEP, and/or a behavior specialist staff member could consult with a teacher on how to use them.

The ***Accommodations That Might Be Used at School*** chart can help parents understand what the school can do to alter the school environment and/or expectations for the child in an effort to help him or her succeed at school. Brainstorm with the parents about accommodations they might lobby the school to make on behalf of the child, but be sure to emphasize the importance of making such requests in an assertive yet respectful manner.

One or more school meetings might be needed to get the child the necessary help. For parents who have been frustrated by their communications with the school in the past, it can be very helpful to strategize with them ahead of time, planning what to say and how to say it. Role playing, if the parent is amenable, can ease nerves and reduce defensiveness.

Helping Parents Implement a Plan

Suggest that the parent consider writing down specific goals for teaming up on the ***Parenting Goals*** form (see parent book Chapter 3 and the end of Chapter 4 in this book). Goals might include the parent's weekly contact with a teacher or talking with school district officials about special education options for his or her child. Suggest that the parent periodically review the ***Parent Checklist for Teaming Up at School*** and/or specific related goals on the ***Parenting Goals*** form until the child is doing better at school.

Modifications for Using the Child Academic Development Module in Parent Groups

Present the ***Overview of the Child Academic Development Module*** chart in the parent group as a way of summarizing techniques and strategies that promote children's academic competency. Then ask parents to talk about typical academic and school-related challenges that are measures they have seen in their children and what they have tried to surmount them. Ask parents to elaborate on both their successes and frustrations in working with school officials. One cautionary note, however, is that sometimes one or more parents can adversely impact the climate of the group so that it turns into a complaining session about schools. Be sure to intervene and gently redirect the group if the discussion continues for too long in that unproductive direction. Inform parents that the main goal of this module is to come up with **solutions** by teaching the child school survival skills and by productively working with the school to obtain services if needed.

The charts and forms found in parent book Chapters 15 and 16 can be used to convey information and approaches for improving a child's academic functioning and school standing in a parent group. Encourage parents to also give each other ideas and suggestions. The role plays described in the preceding training sections for parent book Chapters 15 and 16 can be used in parent groups by having parents take turns, if they are comfortable doing so. Help each parent individually pinpoint specific academic goals and strategies to work on and designate them on the *Parenting Goals* form (see parent book Chapter 3 and the end of Chapter 4 in this book). This module is brief, so it can usually be introduced and covered in one meeting. Nonetheless, it is a good idea to revisit this general topic area in subsequent parent group meetings to follow up on successes or continuing challenges.

Chapter 15. Surviving School:
Teaching Your Child to Manage Time, Organize, Plan, Review, and Stay on Task

Establishing a Mandatory Homework Time

- Define homework as an activity in which the child is (1) getting things done that are due the next day, (2) organizing and planning ahead, and (3) reviewing things that have already been learned

- Set aside about 10 minutes per grade for homework (e.g., 50 minutes for a fifth grader) five times per week (often Sunday–Thursday)

- Parent involvement is crucial, but the goal is to fade out. At a minimum it is good to "check in" at the beginning and "check out" at the end

- Keep track of the minutes with a timer (breaks do not count as homework time)

- It might be a good idea to reward the child for doing mandatory homework the first few weeks to establish a routine

Teaching Basic Homework Organizational and Time Management Skills

- Begin each mandatory homework session by creating a "Homework Checklist" that indicates what needs to be done for tomorrow, what needs to be organized and planned, and what needs to be reviewed

- Ask your child to estimate how much time should be devoted to each task on the checklist

- Then check off items as they are accomplished

Teaching Broader Organizational and Planning Skills

- *Keeping environment organized*—use labeled bins, a bulletin board, a calendar for easy reference. Occasionally clean up and discard papers, etc., to avoid distracting clutter

- *Using folder system*—have "To School" and "To Home" folders in the backpack of a young child or "In Progress" and "Needs to Be Turned in" folders for each class in the backpack of an older child or teen

- *Using task checklists*—create a "Big Assignment To-Do List" (older child or teen)

- *Using reminder notes*—place little notes strategically to help remember things

Teaching On-Task Behavior

- *Teaching on-task behavior*—define and model on-task behavior

- *Using self-monitoring for on-task behavior*—keep track of on-task behavior to help child increase on-task behavior

See **Staying On Task** chart.

(cont.)

Chapter 16. Teaming Up: Collaborating and Advocating for Your Child at School

Collaborating Effectively at School

- Find out the best way to communicate with the teacher(s) and other school personnel (by phone, e-mail, face-to-face meetings, etc.)

- Ask school officials to go beyond just talking about the child's problems to defining "target behaviors," teaching/reinforcing "replacement" behaviors, and using other behavioral strategies at school

- Use a school–home note system to maintain communication about child's school behavior(s)

- Maintain ongoing contact with the teacher(s) and school personnel

See **School–Home Note for a Child** and **School–Home Note for an Older Child or Teen.**

Advocating Effectively at School

- Actively work with school officials to develop and implement a plan for child's success at school

- Become familiar with federal laws and related procedures to get the public education system to provide services for child

- Keep in close contact with the teacher(s) and school personnel while trying to have a friendly and cooperative attitude

- Be assertive (not aggressive) as needed in advocating for child at school

See **Behavior Improvement Strategies That Might Be Used at School** and **Accommodations That Might Be Used at School** charts.

Training Child in Academic Development Skills (Chapters 15 & 16)

- Focus on the family "team" working together

- Guide child to choose and then work on academic development skills and goals

- Identify parenting goals related to promoting child's academic development at home

- Learn, practice, and monitor progress with academic development skills and goals

See **Parent Checklist** for each chapter, as well as the **Personal Goals (Basic** or **Advanced)** form for the child and **Parenting Goals** form for the parent (both in Chapter 3 and also at the end of Chapter 4 in this book).

Forms from Parent Book Chapter 15

Parent Checklist for School Survival Skills

Name: _____ Date: _____

In the blanks below, indicate a score for **how well** you make use of that parenting behavior at this time.

Not too well	Okay	Very well
1	2	3

Parent's Efforts in Using Mandatory Homework Time with Child

A. _____ Using a mandatory homework time that focuses on getting things done that are due, organizing and planning for future assignments, and reviewing past school material

B. _____ Checking in with the child as homework begins and checking out with the child as homework ends

C. _____ Incorporating some stress management techniques into a mandatory homework session

D. _____ Providing assistance in a calm manner to make sure that things get done during mandatory homework time

Parent's Efforts in Teaching School Survival Skills to Child

E. _____ Teaching time management skills, like writing down tasks and estimating time during homework; and/or using a weekly schedule, calendars, or planners

F. _____ Teaching organization and planning skills, like creating an organized study area at home and/or using a folder system and/or using task checklists and/or using reminder notes

G. _____ Teaching reviewing by facilitating a habit of checking work for accuracy during homework time and developing a routine of reviewing different academic subjects each day

H. _____ Teaching on-task behavior, like self-monitoring, to improve on-task behavior during homework time

Staying on Task

Name: _____ **Date:** _____

Indicate below what task you will be doing (e.g., schoolwork, cleaning up your desk, a special project) and the time period you will be working on the task. After you have completed the task, or after the time period is over, rate yourself as to how well you stayed on task. Next a parent should rate how well you stayed on task.

Task to Be Completed and Time Period

1. I will work on this task during this time:

Child Evaluation

2. How well did I stay on task? (Circle one.)

1	2	3	4	5
Not at all	A little	Okay	Pretty well	Great

Parent Evaluation

3. How well did child stay on task? (Circle one.)

1	2	3	4	5
Not at all	A little	Okay	Pretty well	Great

Reward

4. If my rating matches my parent rating, I get this reward:

OR

5. If my parent rates me as a *3, 4,* or *5,* I get this reward:

Forms and Charts from Parent Book Chapter 16

Parent Checklist for Teaming Up at School

Name: _____ **Date:** _____

In the blanks below, indicate a score for **how well** you make use of that parenting behavior at this time.

Not too well	Okay	Very well
1	2	3

Parent's Efforts in Effectively *Collaborating* at School

A. _____ Finding out the best way to communicate with teacher(s) and other school personnel (phone, e-mail, face-to-face meetings, etc.)

B. _____ Asking school officials to go beyond just talking about the child's problems to defining "target behaviors," teaching/reinforcing "replacement" behaviors, and using other behavioral strategies at school

C. _____ Using a school–home note system about the child's school behavior(s)

D. _____ Maintaining ongoing contact with teacher(s) and school personnel, not just when problems arise

Parent's Efforts in Effectively *Advocating* at School

E. _____ Actively working with school officials to develop and implement a plan for the child's success at school

F. _____ Becoming familiar with federal laws and related procedures to get the public education system to provide services for the child

G. _____ Staying in close contact with teacher(s) and school personnel while trying to have a friendly and cooperative attitude

H. _____ Being assertive (not aggressive) as needed in advocating for the child at school

School–Home Note for a Child

Name: _____ Date: _____

Morning

Behavior Goals   **Circle one**

	☹	😐	☺

_____   Poor   Fair   Good

_____   Poor   Fair   Good

_____   Poor   Fair   Good

Comments: _____

Teacher's signature: _____

Afternoon

Behavior Goals   **Circle one**

	☹	😐	☺

_____   Poor   Fair   Good

_____   Poor   Fair   Good

_____   Poor   Fair   Good

Comments: _____

Teacher's signature: _____

Today's homework assignments are:

_____

_____

_____

School–Home Note for an Older Child or Teen

Name: _____ **Date:** _____

First Class

Behavior Goals	Circle one		
_____	Poor	Fair	Good
_____	Poor	Fair	Good
_____	Poor	Fair	Good

Comments: _____

Teacher's signature: _____

Second Class

Behavior Goals	Circle one		
_____	Poor	Fair	Good
_____	Poor	Fair	Good
_____	Poor	Fair	Good

Comments: _____

Teacher's signature: _____

Third Class

Behavior Goals	Circle one		
_____	Poor	Fair	Good
_____	Poor	Fair	Good
_____	Poor	Fair	Good

Comments: _____

Teacher's signature: _____

(cont.)

Fourth Class

Behavior Goals	**Circle one**		
_____	Poor	Fair	Good
_____	Poor	Fair	Good
_____	Poor	Fair	Good

Comments: _____

Teacher's signature: _____

Fifth Class

Behavior Goals	**Circle one**		
_____	Poor	Fair	Good
_____	Poor	Fair	Good
_____	Poor	Fair	Good

Comments: _____

Teacher's signature: _____

Sixth Class

Behavior Goals	**Circle one**		
_____	Poor	Fair	Good
_____	Poor	Fair	Good
_____	Poor	Fair	Good

Comments: _____

Teacher's signature: _____

Behavior Improvement Strategies That Might Be Used at School

Relationship Building and Catching 'Em Being Good: Disciplining a student is much more effective if the adult has a good relationship with him or her. Avoid critical comments and a frustrated voice tone when talking to the student. Make an extra effort to establish rapport with the child and be sure to praise positive behavior. Strive to make three or more positive comments for every one correction or reprimand.

Behavioral Contracting: Clearly specify behavioral expectations and rewards/consequences associated with meeting behavioral expectations. Devise a behavior progress form with behavioral goals stated, a method for evaluating progress (e.g., one to five ratings), and contingent rewards/consequences for indicated behaviors. It is best to get student input into the selection of reinforcers.

Check-In/Check-Out with Adult Mentor at School: Define behavioral goals with the student and teacher(s) and designate them on a goal chart. Mentor monitors behavioral progress at school. Mentor checks in with student for 5–30 minutes at the beginning of day and checks out with the student for 5–30 minutes at end of day regarding progress with behavioral goals. Mentor forms a positive relationship with the student and uses their relationship to give feedback and engage the student in problem solving about reaching behavioral goals.

Individualized "School Survival Skills" Training:

- *Time Management Skills:* Provide instruction on time budgeting with tasks and creating and following a daily or weekly schedule. Encourage/reward the student for using the skills.

- *Organizational and Planning Skills:* Provide instruction on using calendars to keep track of dates, using task checklists to monitor task completion, and using a folder system to organize schoolwork. Encourage and reward the student for using the skills.

- *Staying On-Task:* Define task-specific indicators of on-task behavior and provide instruction on self-monitoring of on-task behavior. Encourage and reward the student for using the skills.

Management of Noncompliant Behavior: When compliance is needed, give an *effective command* (clear, specific, one-step with eye contact and voice tone raised slightly). If there is no compliance with an effective command, then give a *warning* in the form of an "if . . . then" statement ("if you don't [command], then [time-out chair or time-out room or loss of small privilege]"). If there is no compliance after the warning, *follow through* with what was stated in the warning. Avoid power struggles and deescalate if needed. This procedure works best if the adult doing it has a good relationship and rapport with the student.

Management of Angry Outbursts:

- *Proactive Maintenance of Calm in Student.* Have predictable classroom routines and clearly stated rules and expectations.

- *Proactive Redirecting with Increasing Agitation in Student.* Use calming strategies such as guiding use of stress management, allowing the student to go to "cool down" area.

- *Reactive Management of Outbursts in the Student.* Isolate and remove others from the angry/acting-out student and get help. After calming down, the student should restore the environment and/or make restitution.

Deescalate to Avoid Power Struggles: When the student is agitated, stay calm, minimize verbal commands and directives, reduce eye contact, turn away, and walk away. Do not add consequences. Once calm, reengage the student regarding behavior expectations.

Note: *An educational and/or behavior specialist may need to be involved in implementing these strategies at school.*

Accommodations That Might Be Used at School

Place the student in a low-distraction location in the classroom.

- Use multimodal instruction by presenting information in a variety of ways (auditory, visual, and tactile)

- Fully explain what will be graded for each assignment and what should be focused on before starting an assignment (e.g., spelling, creativity, neatness, showing work).

- Provide instructions for assignments orally and in writing.

- Provide prompt and frequent positive reinforcement for desired behaviors, including beginning tasks, staying on task, and completing assignments.

- Give corrective statements in a brief, immediate, calm, and matter-of-fact tone of voice.

- Provide opportunities to move around the classroom.

- Structure class time to include frequent breaks contingent upon reaching short-term goals.

- Allow extra time to complete tasks and exams/tests in the classroom.

- Shorten some assignments.

- Allow time and provide assistance for the child to do homework at school.

9 Using the Parent Well-Being Module

The parent book section "Enhancing Your Well-Being as a Parent" (Chapters 17 & 18) is the focus of this chapter. It provides parents with strategies for enhancing their own ability to recognize and change unhelpful parent thinking and cope with stress that can affect their parenting. Cognitive-behavioral therapeutic skills training methods are emphasized in this module, but the focus is on parenting more than on the parent's personal functioning per se. **The practitioner should read and fully understand the *content* in parent book Chapters 17 and 18 before using the related *procedures* described here.**

Obviously this module is focused on the parent, so the practitioner will primarily work with the parent in it. In addition, there is a possibility that the parent's personal struggles will be discussed, and many parents prefer those issues to be private. There may be exceptions to this general guideline. Sometimes it can be productive to work with the child using the emotional development module while simultaneously assisting the parent with the parent well-being module. As long as personal boundaries are respected, it can be fruitful for child and parent to work on similar skills. The practitioner should seek input from the parent as to how to proceed with the parent well-being module.

Tailoring within the Parent Well-Being Module

Parents seeking help for a child's behavioral–emotional problems naturally expect the child to be the focus of intervention, so some parents balk at the idea that their own well-being is relevant. Most will readily admit that they are under stress (particularly the stress of the child's problems), but they may not immediately see how their stress level can impact their child. Success with the methods in this module rest on parents' understanding that the child's problems can increase parental stress and that parental stress can exacerbate the child's problems. For this reason it's important to introduce the parent well-being module by reviewing the ***Parent Stress Cycle*** (reproduced from parent book Chapter 18, at the end of this chapter).

Provide psychoeducation about how parent stress, parent thoughts, parenting, and child struggles are linked, as shown in the bullet points on the chart. Note that when parents are stressed out, they are more likely to think unhelpful thoughts, and vice versa. Explain further that stressed-out parents who have unhelpful thoughts are prone to reactive and often ineffective parenting responses to their child. State that subpar parenting can have a negative impact on the child's behavior or feelings, which in turn stresses out the parent. Suggest that the parent could intervene within any of the boxes in the *Parent Stress Cycle* but that the focus of this module are the components in the top two boxes. Answer any questions that arise and ask parents if they can recognize the existence of this cycle in their own life.

To head off defensiveness or unproductive guilt, indicate that although parent stress levels can have a powerful impact on the child, it is often an indirect impact and hardly intentional on the parent's part. Empathize with the parent and explain that intense or chronic problems will tax anyone. Suggest that in moments of stress it is understandable that parents may not always be effective in their interactions with their child. It may be useful to review strategies for fostering helpful thinking early on with parents who are blaming themselves for their child's problems.

Then present the *Overview of the Parent Well-Being Module* chart at the end of this chapter to summarize the main concepts and skills in this module. Note that Chapter 17 focuses on helpful thoughts and Chapter 18 centers on stress management for parents. Emphasize the overarching message that parents need to take care of themselves by working on these skills in order to be better parents to the child. The initial discussion should conclude in broadly stated options to pursue in skills training within the parent well-being module.

Specific Procedures for Applying Parent Book Chapter 17

In this chapter parents are educated to become more aware of their parenting-related thoughts. The chapter provides instructions for restructuring unhelpful parent thoughts to make them more helpful. Parents are also advised to stay calm so that they can think in a more helpful manner while interacting with their child.

Note: *The forms and charts referred to in the discussion below are in parent book Chapter 17 and also at the end of this chapter unless otherwise noted.*

Discussing Unhelpful Parental Thinking with Parents

Ask the parent to reflect on a recent difficult interaction with the child and then describe what happened and what he or she was thinking. Tune in to any unhelpful parent thoughts as the incident is recalled, such as "He was acting up on purpose" or "I felt like a worthless parent." Then ask if these thoughts affected how the parent responded to the child and, if so, how. Solicit other examples when such thoughts led to behavior that the parent can see was unproductive. The more examples you can bring into the discussion, the more quickly the parent will realize that parent thoughts influence parenting behaviors directed at the child.

Refer to the *Parent Stress Cycle* again to point out that the arrow goes both ways between the Parent Stress and Unhelpful Parent Thoughts boxes. That is, parental stress can lead to unhelpful thoughts, and vice versa. Addressing both will exert the greatest positive effect on parenting behaviors. Tell the parent that this chapter focuses on unhelpful thoughts and the next focuses on stress.

Getting Parents Started and Focused

Ask the parent to identify areas on the *Parent Checklist for Helpful Parent Thoughts* that are going well and others that need some work. Because the overall approach to helpful parent thinking is summarized on this checklist, it's important to answer any questions the parent may have about the skills content presented on the checklist. It is also important to make sure that the parent understands the information summarized on the list and presented in the text of parent book Chapter 17.

Training Parents in Helpful Thinking Skills

To facilitate a personal awareness and understanding in the parents, review the *Unhelpful Parent Thoughts* form. Ask the parents if they often have any of the listed unhelpful parent thoughts. Help the parents pinpoint which unhelpful thought(s) on the list are typical for them. Then ask the parents to review the questions at the bottom of the form that relate to how the identified unhelpful thoughts might make the parents feel and act in a parenting context. Keep reviewing these questions until the parents understand their own typical unhelpful parent thoughts and also know that these thoughts negatively impact their feelings and parenting behaviors.

Next review the *Helpful Parent Thoughts* chart with the parents. Ask them to "counter" previously identified unhelpful thoughts with a corresponding helpful thought on this list. Ask the parents to answer the questions at the bottom of this chart. Draw a contrast between the answers to the *Unhelpful* form and the *Helpful* chart. Keep discussing this until the parents see that these countering helpful thoughts are associated with less stress and more productive parenting behaviors. Make the general observation that these helpful parent thoughts can have a positive impact on how the parents feel and behave in relation to their parenting.

Discuss the *Helpful Thoughts Worksheet for Parents*. Explain that this worksheet can be used to structure the process of identifying unhelpful parent thoughts and changing them to be more helpful. It can be quite helpful to conduct role-play practice to illustrate using the worksheet and the broader concept of helpful thinking. The practice exercise described in parent book Chapter 17 will work nicely as the basis of a role play to practice helpful parent thinking (e.g., "I'm sick and tired of that brat" scenario). Generate other scenarios with the parent for additional discussion and/or role-play practice of helpful thinking. Explain that the parent can use a similar helpful parent thinking strategy at home.

Be sure to reiterate that stress and related negative emotions can disrupt helpful thoughts. Tell the parent that it is important to stay calm to think helpful thoughts. Staying calm can be accomplished by stepping away, taking deep breaths, etc. (see parent book Chapter 18 for more ideas). Then repeat the same role plays as above, but this time incorporate a brief cooling-down period before trying to think helpful thoughts. In other words, have the parent practice first calming down and then using the helpful thoughts strategies during the role plays.

Unfortunately, many children's behavioral–emotional struggles are chronic, which can be quite demoralizing for parents. It can be constructive to introduce the concept of **middle path parent thinking** as a framework for parents who are dealing with persistent difficulties in their child. Discuss the notion of a "middle path" view of the parents' situation in which they simultaneously seek to make changes and also accept the child and themselves as they are. Review the examples of middle path parent thinking described in Chapter 17. Ask the parents if this type of thinking makes sense to them and whether or not it might help them cope better. It can be beneficial to help the parents generate and write down a list of personal middle path thoughts that they can look at now and then as a reminder.

Briefly review two other ideas in the text of parent book Chapter 17 pertaining to **avoiding hopelessness** and **focusing parent worries with the funnel technique.** These helpful thoughts strategies are also useful for the parent who is dealing with chronic child and family stress. Both of these ideas orient the parent toward thinking less and taking more action. Explain that by being conscious of hopeless-type thinking and using the funneling technique, the parent will be less likely to get overwhelmed and more likely to cope actively and/or to solve problems.

Developing a Home Implementation Plan for the Parent

Ask parents to indicate which helpful thoughts skills they will emphasize at home. In ensuing meetings, review the *Parent Checklist for Helpful Parent Thoughts.* Ask the parents to evaluate how well they are following through with helpful thinking. Use the checklist as a tool to remind them what they should work on.

Also suggest that parents consider writing down specific goals to help them develop helpful thinking on the *Parenting Goals* form (see parent book Chapter 3 and also the end of Chapter 4 in this book). They might set a goal to fill out a *Helpful Thoughts Worksheet for Parents* form at least once a day. Another goal could be to become more aware of a middle path way of thinking and review it each day. Finally, parents might set a goal to try to stay calm when interacting with their child so that their thoughts remain helpful. Periodically, parents should review their progress toward their goals until their thoughts seem helpful most of the time.

Specific Procedures for Applying Parent Book Chapter 18

In this chapter parents are counseled on several effective ways to manage their own stress, from reducing global stress to preventing parenting challenges that arise in the moment, from causing stress to being more mindful and present in the moment with their child.

Note: *The forms and charts referred to in the discussion below are in parent book Chapter 18 and also at the end of this chapter unless otherwise noted.*

Discussing Parent Stress with Parents

Go back to the *Parent Stress Cycle* that you introduced at the beginning of this module, but tell parents that now you are going to focus on the parent stress box. Review how the parents' own personal stress impacts their parenting thoughts and behaviors and, as a result, the child's functioning. Stress how important it is for parents to take care of themselves to be better parents to their child.

Solicit information about the stress the parents feel they are experiencing by explaining that it may include personal stress, marital/relationship stress, parenting stress, and/or having little or no social support from family or friends. Point out that stress management can reduce the negative impact of any of these forms of stress.

Note. *If this discussion reveals that the parents' stress level or personal problems are serious, a referral for personal mental health treatment might be in order. Therapy for themselves can reduce the parents' stress in the process and in turn have a positive impact on their parenting.*

Getting Parents Started and Focused

Ask the parents to rate and check off items on the *Parent Checklist for Parent Stress Management* that are going well and pinpoint areas needing some work. Because this checklist summarizes the overall approach of the chapter, it's important to answer parents' questions so that they thoroughly understand the items on the list as well as the text of parent book Chapter 18.

The parent stress management chapter has several components that each needs to be reviewed and taught separately. Some parents will be able to go through them all in one session, whereas others will need several sessions to cover this material. Either way, the ultimate goal is for the parent to develop a personalized parent stress management plan.

Training Parents in Stress-Reducing Lifestyle Changes

Talk to parents about how difficult it can be to engage in "damage control" with stress and then point out how much less energy and time stress prevention can require. One fundamental area where changes can prevent stress is lifestyle. Brainstorming can reveal that the parents might be willing and able to improve their diet, exercise regularly, develop better sleep habits, etc. (a list of possibilities appears in parent book Chapter 18). Note that scheduling occasional pleasant events can also build parents' resilience and thus lessen general stress.

Obviously parents are not likely to follow through on such changes unless they have made these choices themselves and are committed to following through, which is not easy to do for anyone and is even more difficult for those already under stress. Collaborate by brainstorming to choose one or two stress-reducing lifestyle habits to work on and then set up a concrete plan, such as deciding when and where to exercise or making a list of pleasant events and starting to schedule them. Practitioners should follow through in subsequent meetings not only to see if the changes have taken place but also to get the parents' feedback on whether their stress level has declined and, if so, whether the reduced stress had any positive effect on their parenting. It can be useful to review the stages of change, prioritizing, and goal attainment methods discussed in parent book Chapter 3 for parents who know it would be good to make lifestyle changes but think they cannot manage to do so.

Training Parents in Mindfulness

Mindfulness, a state of being that allows people to shed preconceived notions and worries and focus on the here and now, being fully present with the child in the moment, can definitely prevent stress from occurring in that moment. As a regular practice, it can also reduce parents' stress level in general. Another benefit is that mindful parenting, which reduces parent stress, can improve parent–child interactions, as noted in the ***Parent Stress Cycle.***

Review how to be a mindful parent, as detailed in Chapter 18 of the parent book: calming down to be present, accepting oneself and the child, listening to the child, and attending to what is occurring. Discuss these four techniques until the parent has a rudimentary grasp of them. Note, however, that mindfulness does not come naturally to many people, and it can be a difficult concept to explain. Parents may benefit from reading other sources of information and instruction on mindfulness or from some instruction in a class.

Then try some mindfulness exercises in the session. You could model, and then role-play, mindfulness at that moment. One simple exercise is to simply focus on breathing for a minute. Ask the parent to breathe normally and focus all of his or her attention on inhaling and exhaling. Tell the parent to bring his or her attention back to breathing if the mind wanders. Another exercise could be done with the child and parent together. Perhaps they could build a tower together with blocks or draw a picture for 5 minutes. While doing this, prompt the parent to use the four techniques of mindful parenting. Afterward, ask the parent to report on the experience.

Suggest that the parent try similar mindfulness exercises at home. In later meetings ask the parent to report how this mindful approach is going.

Training Parents in Staying Calm

Parents know very well how tough it can be to stay calm in the moment when a child is stressing them out. Staying calm when a child is violating a house rule, throwing a tantrum, or otherwise acting out involves recognizing stress, relaxing the body, using calming self-talk, using imagery, and taking effective action. These five steps are detailed in the *Parent Staying Calm* chart.

Train parents to **recognize stress signals,** first by reviewing the examples of signals from the body, thoughts, and actions in parent book Chapter 18. Then ask parents to recall an incident where their child stressed them out and ask them to list the body, thought, and action signals that came up for them during that stressful moment.

Now train the parents to **control their reactions** within the same areas of functioning (body, thoughts, and actions). **Relaxation** methods include taking deep breaths, muscle tension–release, and counting to 10. These can be followed by a good presentation of the essence of **coping self-talk.** Ask parents to make a list of personal coping self-statements that they could think during stressful interactions with the child. For example: "Don't let her get you," "Take some deep breaths," "Chill out." Next discuss the use of **imagery or visualization** to help reduce stress. For example, many parents seem to like the imagery of a robot. The robot has no feelings, is therefore always calm, and can execute behavior in a calm manner. Suggest that the parent in "robot mode" can take a similar sort of detached approach to parenting in the moment of a high-stress incident. Finally, the idea of taking **effective action** when stressful events arise should be discussed. Remind the parent that such actions include walking away, ignoring, taking a walk, expressing feelings, etc. These actions not only calm the parent down but can also disrupt any parent–child conflict that may be occurring.

It is a good idea to do some modeling and role-play exercises to help the parent learn and consolidate these skills. Tell the parent that it would be rather naïve to expect to use these skills in the moment under pressure without having practiced them beforehand. Guide the parent through discussion and role-play practice of a typical scenario. For example, a situation to which many parents can relate is when the child is procrastinating with homework and it is getting late. First model how to cope with this situation while referring to the *Parent Staying Calm* chart. Go through each step, narrating it out loud. Then have the parent practice the same way with the procrastinating child. Have the parent also refer to the *Parent Staying Calm* chart during the role-play(s) for guidance. Keep discussing and role-playing this important parent coping skill until the parent seems to have mastered it.

Developing a Home Implementation Plan for the Parent

Ask the parents to indicate which parent stress management skills they will emphasize at home. In subsequent meetings, review the *Parent Checklist for Parent Stress Management.* Ask the parents to indicate how well they are following through with techniques for managing parent stress. The checklist can be used to remind the parents about what they need to keep working on.

Also suggest that the *Parenting Goals* form (see parent book Chapter 3 and also at the end of Chapter 4 in this book) can be used to write down specific goals related to stress management. For example, the parent might set a goal to exercise more to reduce global stress. Another goal could center on being more mindful in interactions with the child. The parent might set a third goal to review the *Parent Staying Calm* chart on a daily basis and refer to it when disciplining the child.

Recommend that parents periodically review the *Parent Checklist for Parent Stress Management* and/or specific related goals on the *Parenting Goals* form until parent stress management skills become routine.

Modifications for Using the Parent Well-Being Module in Parent Groups

A great way to introduce this module is to first have group members examine and discuss the *Parent Stress Cycle* chart. Then encourage parents to talk about their own personal stress and what they have tried in the past to reduce it. This topic typically elicits a lot of lively discussion.

The *Overview of the Parent Well-Being Module* chart can then be reviewed with parent group members to generate ideas for using helpful thoughts and stress management skills. Inform parents that the main goal of this module is to foster their well-being so that they can be better parents. Then brainstorm with parents about specific chapters and/or techniques they would like to learn more about in upcoming weeks within this module.

The parent well-being module can be introduced over one meeting, but two or more meetings will usually be required to cover all of the topics. The charts found in parent book Chapters 17 and 18 can be used, as needed, to convey information and approaches for improving parents' emotional well-being. The role plays described in the preceding training sections for parent book Chapters 17 and 18 can be used in parent groups by having parents take turns if they are comfortable doing so. Help each parent individually to pinpoint specific parent stress management goals and strategies to work on and designate them on the *Parenting Goals* form.

Overview of the Parent Well-Being Module

Understanding Parent Stress Cycle

- *Parent Stress Cycle (see below)*—shows how parent stress, parent thoughts, parenting, and child struggles are all related and can become a vicious cycle that is hard to stop

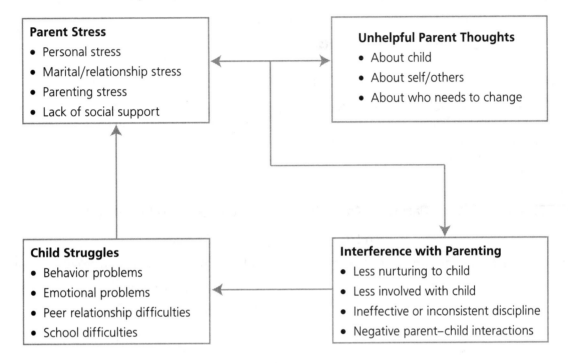

Parent Stress
- Personal stress
- Marital/relationship stress
- Parenting stress
- Lack of social support

Unhelpful Parent Thoughts
- About child
- About self/others
- About who needs to change

Child Struggles
- Behavior problems
- Emotional problems
- Peer relationship difficulties
- School difficulties

Interference with Parenting
- Less nurturing to child
- Less involved with child
- Ineffective or inconsistent discipline
- Negative parent–child interactions

- *Take-home message*—parents can reduce stress to be better parents.

Chapter 17. You Parent The Way You Think: Thinking Helpful Thoughts to Enhance Parenting

Increasing Awareness of Unhelpful and Helpful Thinking

- Be aware of unhelpful thoughts about your child, self/others, and who needs to change that are related to negative feelings and unproductive behaviors

- Make a goal to have more helpful thoughts about your child, self/others, and who needs to change to have more positive thoughts and productive behaviors

See **Unhelpful Parent Thoughts** form and **Helpful Parent Thoughts** chart.

Using Helpful Parent Thinking Steps

1. Am I thinking unhelpful parent thoughts and, if so, what are they?

2. How do my unhelpful parent thoughts make me feel about and act toward my child and family?

(cont.)

3. Why is it unhelpful to keep thinking this parent thought?

4. What are different or more helpful parent thoughts I can think?

5. How do my helpful parent thoughts make me feel about and act toward my child and family?

6. Why is it helpful to keep thinking this new parent thought?

See **Helpful Thoughts Worksheet for Parents.**

Dealing with Parent Thoughts Related to Chronic Parenting Stress

- *Avoiding hopeless thoughts*—have a can-do attitude and keep on trying
- *Focusing parent worries with funnel technique*— funnel worries down into one or two focus areas of effort at a time
- *Middle path parent thinking*—seek change and at the same time accept your child and self

Chapter 18. Cool Parents: Managing Your Own Stress to Enhance Parenting

Making Stress-Reducing Lifestyle Changes

- Take time away from family responsibilities
- Take time to be with your child
- Seek out social support from friends and/or family
- Schedule pleasant events and enjoyable activities
- Develop good health habits
- Join a parent support group

Being a Mindful Parent

- Calm down so you can be present
- Accept yourself and your child
- Listen to your child
- Pay attention to what is occurring

Handling High-Stress Episodes

- *Learn to recognize stress*—recognize "signals" from body, thoughts, and actions
- *Relaxation*—deep breathing, count to 10, relax muscles, etc.
- *Visualization*—"see" self as calm; imagine being a robot
- *Helpful self-talk*—say statements like "Take it easy," "Stay cool," "Don't let him bug me," "I'll be okay," etc.
- *Take effective action*—walk away, use effective discipline, solve the problem, etc.

See **Parent Staying Calm** chart.

Training Parent in Parent Well-Being Skills (Chapters 17 & 18)

- Identify skills and goals related to promoting well-being of parent
- Learn, practice, and monitor progress with parent well-being skills and goals

See **Parent Checklist** for each chapter and **Parenting Goals** form (in Chapter 3 and at the end of Chapter 4 of this book).

Forms from Parent Book Chapter 17

Parent Checklist for Helpful Parent Thoughts

Name: _____ Date: _____

In the blanks below, indicate a score for **how well** you make use of that parenting behavior at this time.

Not too well	**Okay**	**Very well**
1	2	3

Parent's Efforts in Fostering Helpful Parent Thinking Skills

A. _____ Having awareness of parenting-related thoughts

B. _____ Making a conscious effort to change unhelpful parent thoughts to helpful parent thoughts in day-to-day family life

C. _____ Staying calm while interacting with the child to promote more helpful thinking

Parent's Efforts in Fostering Own Middle Path Parent Thinking

D. _____ Striking a balance between seeking change and fostering acceptance of child and self

Unhelpful Parent Thoughts

Listed below are common thoughts that parents of children with behavioral–emotional problems may have. Read each thought and indicate how frequently that thought (or a similar one) typically occurs for you over an average week. There are no right or wrong answers to these questions. Use the 3-point rating scale to help you answer these questions.

1	**2**	**3**
Rarely	**Sometimes**	**Often**

Unhelpful Thoughts about My Child

1. ____ My child is behaving like a brat.

2. ____ My child acts up on purpose.

3. ____ My child is the cause of most of our family problems.

4 ____ My child's future is bleak.

5. ____ My child should behave like other children. I shouldn't have to make allowances for my child.

Unhelpful Thoughts about Self/Others

6. ____ It is my fault that my child has a problem.

7. ____ It is his/her fault (other parent) that my child is this way.

8. ____ I can't make mistakes in parenting my child.

9. ____ I give up. There is nothing more I can do for my child.

10. ____ I have no control over my child. I have tried everything.

Unhelpful Thoughts about Who Needs to Change

11. ____ My child is the one who needs to change. All of us would be better off if my child would change.

12. ____ I am the one who needs to change. My family would be better off if I would change.

13. ____ My spouse/partner needs to change. We would all be better off if he/she would change.

14. ____ The teacher needs to change. We would be better off if he/she would change.

15. ____ Medications are the answer. Medications will change my child.

For each thought you rated a *3*, ask yourself the following questions:

1. How does this unhelpful thought make me **feel** about my child and family?

2. How does this unhelpful thought make me **act toward** my child and family?

3. Is this an unhelpful thought that I should be more aware of and try to change?

Helpful Parent Thoughts

Listed below are counterthoughts that parents can think instead of unhelpful thoughts. Unhelpful Thought #1 corresponds to Helpful Thought #1, and so on. Compare the unhelpful thoughts to the helpful thoughts.

Helpful Thoughts about My Child

1. My child is behaving positively too.

2. It doesn't matter whose fault it is. What matters are solutions to the problems.

3. It is not just my child. I also play a role in the problem.

4. I have no proof that my child will continue to have problems. I need to wait for the future.

5. I can't just expect my child to behave. My child needs to be taught how to behave.

Helpful Thoughts about Self/Others

6. It doesn't help to blame myself. I will focus on solutions to the problem.

7. It doesn't matter whose fault it is. I will focus on solutions to the problems.

8. My child is perhaps more challenging to parent than others, and therefore I will make mistakes. I need to accept the fact that I am going to make mistakes.

9. I have to parent my child. I have no choice. I need to think of new ways to parent my child.

10. My belief that I have no control over my child might be contributing to the problem. Many things are in my control. I need to figure out what I can do to parent my child.

Unhelpful Thoughts about Who Needs to Change

11. It's unhelpful to think of my child as the only one needing to change. We all need to change.

12. It's unhelpful to think of myself as needing to change. We all need to change.

13. It's unhelpful to think of my spouse/partner as being the only one who needs to change. We all need to change.

14. It's unhelpful to think that only the teacher needs to change. We all need to work together.

15. Medications may help but will not solve the problems. We will also need to work hard to cope with the problems.

Ask yourself the following questions about each of these helpful thoughts:

1. How does this helpful thought make me **feel** about my child and family?

2. How does this helpful thought make me **act toward** my child and family?

3. Is this a helpful thought that I should be more aware of and try to keep?

Helpful Thoughts Worksheet for Parents

Name: _____ Date: _____

Fill out the worksheet during or after you have experienced unhelpful parent thoughts.

1. Am I thinking unhelpful parent thoughts, and if so, what are they?

2. How do my unhelpful parent thoughts make me feel about and act toward my child and family?

3. Why is it unhelpful to keep thinking this parent thought?

4. What are different or more helpful parent thoughts I can think?

5. How do my helpful parent thoughts make me feel about, and act toward, my child and family?

6. Why is it helpful to keep thinking this new parent thought?

How Well Did It Work?

(Circle *1, 2, 3,* or *4.*)

1. **I didn't really try too hard.**
2. **I sort of tried, but it didn't really work.**
3. **I tried hard, and it kind of worked.**
4. **I tried really hard, and it really worked.**

Forms from Parent Book Chapter 18

Parent Checklist for Parent Stress Management

Name: _____ Date: _____

In the blanks below, indicate a score for **how well** you make use of that parenting behavior at this time.

	Not too well	**Okay**	**Very well**
	1	2	3

Parent's Efforts in Making Stress-Reducing Lifestyle Changes

A. _____ Taking time away from family responsibility

B. _____ Taking time to be with spouse/partner (if applicable)

C. _____ Taking time to be with your child

D. _____ Seeking out social support from friends and/or family

E. _____ Scheduling pleasant events and enjoyable activities

F. _____ Developing good health habits

G. _____ Joining a parent support group

Parent's Efforts in Mindful Parenting

H. _____ Mindfully focusing attention on being fully present with the child in "good" moments

I. _____ Mindfully focusing attention on being fully present with the child in "bad" moments

Parent's Efforts in Staying Calm with the Child

J. _____ Being attentive to body, thought, and behavior signals of stress

K. _____ Controlling your reactions and staying calm by relaxing your body, thinking coping thoughts, using imagery, taking effective action, etc.

Parent Staying Calm

1. **Recognizing Stress**—be aware of stress "signals."

   Body Signals:

   - Breathing/heart rate increases
   - Tense muscles
   - Increased sweating
   - Face turns red
   - Body feels hot

   Thought Signals:

   - "That brat! I'm not going to take any more!"
   - "I'm a worthless parent."
   - "I give up."
   - "I can't handle this!"
   - "I hate him/her."

   Behavior Signals:

   - Yell/threaten
   - Cry
   - Tremble
   - Withdraw

2. **Relaxing Your Body**—do deep breathing, tense and release muscles, count to 10, and so forth.

3. **Using "Coping Self-Talk"**—examples of coping self-talk include the following:

   - "Take it easy."
   - "Don't let it bug you."
   - "I can handle this."
   - "I'm going to be okay."
   - "Stay cool."
   - "Relax."
   - "I'll try my best."

4. **Using Imagery**—imagine yourself as a robot when your child is stressing you out. Robots execute behavior but have no feelings. Like a robot, execute the behavior of parenting your child while staying cool.

5. **Taking Effective Action**—walk away, ignore it, take a walk, try to discuss it, express feelings, think of new ways to solve the problem.

10 Using the Family Well-Being Module

The parent book section "Enhancing Your Family's Well-Being" (Chapters 19 & 20) examines broader family relationships that impact the child's functioning. Chapter 19 focuses on the parent's efforts to improve the parent–child relationship and to shore up family organization. The primary goal of Chapter 20 is to improve familywide interactions in relation to communication, problem solving, and conflict management. This module is useful for families with children of all ages but may be especially helpful for families with older children or teens. **The practitioner should read and fully understand the *content* in parent book Chapters 19–20 before using the related *procedures* described here.**

Clearly this module is focused on the family, so most often the practitioner will want to work with the child and parent together regardless of age. Additional considerations center on whether, when, and how to involve other family members like siblings, coparents, divorced parents, and extended family members. The practitioner will need to use general practice judgment and seek input from the parent as to who should be involved in the family well-being module.

Tailoring within the Family Well-Being Module

The *Overview of the Family Well-Being Module* chart at the end of this chapter can be used to give parents a succinct review of the skills targeted in this module. It can also be used as the basis of a psychoeducation-focused discussion with the parent about strategies to promote better parent–child and broader family relationships. Tell the parent that these chapters help to facilitate bonding, organization, and day-to-day interactions in the family. Review the different bullet points and answer any questions. The discussion should conclude by zeroing in on specific skills or strategies the parent thinks are most needed by the family.

Specific Procedures for Applying Parent Book Chapter 19

In this chapter parents plan and then execute strategies for enhancing family cohesion and organization. Parents will be exposed to numerous ideas and learn methods for building parent–child bonds through activities, enhancing family connections via rituals, and improving family organization through routines. Practitioners should help the parent and child narrow down the choices to work on one or two strategies/skills at a time.

Note: ***The forms and charts referred to in the discussion below are in parent book Chapter 19 and also at the end of this chapter unless otherwise noted.***

Discussing Family Bonding and Organization with Parents

Time has often taken its toll on families who have a child with behavioral–emotional problems. The parent–child bond can deteriorate and broader family relationships can become strained over the years. Likewise, over time children sometimes develop "bad habits," such as procrastinating on homework, watching TV late at night, and getting little exercise, especially when the family's attention has been commandeered by more urgent behavioral–emotional problems. Ask the parents whether these patterns sound familiar. Do they think it would be useful to rekindle the parent–child relationship and/or strengthen family connections? Could the child develop better habits with more structured, predictable routines in the family? It takes commitment and intentional actions within daily family life, but armed with those prerequisites, parents can use the ideas in Chapter 19 to improve family bonding and family organization.

Getting Parents Started and Focused

Ask the parents to identify areas on the ***Parent Checklist for Family Bonding and Organization*** that are going well and areas that need strengthening. Because the checklist summarizes the main ideas and techniques for Chapter 19, it's important to answer all questions about the list and to ensure that parents understand it and the contents of Chapter 19.

Training the Child and Parent in Family Bonding Skills

Begin by discussing parent- versus child-directed activities. Typically parents direct many task-oriented activities within the family and some fun activities as well. But family bonds can be strengthened when the child directs a lot of the fun activities instead.

Parents may wonder how this shift to child direction promotes bonding and why the parents are needed at all if the child is in charge. Explain that it is the parent's "job" to be present and available to the child during that activity. This means that the parent is to **follow the child's lead** during the activity. For a **younger child** this might mean the child picks certain toys and the parent plays with those toys just like the child. For an **older child or teen** this could mean the child chooses an activity, like baking a cake, playing catch, or going for a bike ride, and the parent and child engage in the activity together.

Following the child's lead can start with brainstorming to generate a list of possible child-directed activities calibrated to the child's age. Caution parents, however, that parents can still guide the selection process and exercise veto power. They should, for example, avoid passive activities like TV or noninteractive activities like some video games. A list of suggested activities appears in the parent book. It is also a good idea to schedule these activities on the family calendar if possible.

It's crucial that the parents be truly present and available to the child during these child-led activities. The goal is to describe the child's actions and praise the child during the activity, to let the child know that he or she has the parents' full attention. Reviewing the examples of describing and praising comments provided in parent book Chapter 19 will clarify what this entails and help parents pick a speaking style with which they are comfortable. Use the analogy of a play-by-play sports announcer who describes events as they unfold.

Then model and conduct role-play practice of child-directed play using the describing and praising comments. First the practitioner can act as the parent while the parent acts as the child. Later these roles can be reversed. Once the parent gets good at it, he or she should be encouraged to practice these techniques with the child in the meeting. Later be sure to emphasize that the parent should use these techniques at home during scheduled child-directed fun activities.

One idea for an activity with a **younger child** might be playing with a toy train set. The child would lead this play activity, and the parent would describe what the child is doing and offer praise (e.g., "You are driving the train with the people in it," "You are good at being a conductor," "I like the way you tell the passengers about the train stops"). Encourage the parent to follow the child's lead in the play and use similar describing and praising commentary.

For an **older child or teen**, the activity might be playing a card game. The child would select a specific type of card game, and while the cards are being played, the parent would describe the activity and praise the child (e.g., "You shuffle the deck very well," "I did not realize you were such a good card player," "You seem to enjoy this," "We should do this again"). Also encourage the parent to follow the child's lead in the activity and use similar describing and praising commentary.

Brainstorm when and how to engage in special conversations with the child or teen. Prompt the parent to think about opportune moments that come up when the child or teen might be receptive to conversation (dinnertime, riding in the car, etc.). Suggest that the parent talk about what is going on in the child's life and not about chores, homework, tasks, or other "musts." **Also encourage the parent to do a lot more listening than talking during these special conversations.** It might be useful to do some role playing with the parent to demonstrate and practice the give-and-take of a back-and-forth conversation with the child or teen. Then it might be good to have the parent actually try this with the child or teen in the session.

Discuss the importance of family rituals. Note that family rituals are symbolic and indicate that the family as a unit is important. Brainstorm with family members about when and how to have more family rituals. Perhaps they would like to incorporate regular meal-times into their busy weekly schedule. Ask them to be concrete and indicate on the calendar when these meals will take place. Perhaps the family would like to emphasize "tradition-oriented" family rituals such as annual summer vacations, going to holiday concerts, etc. Make sure all family members have their say about these family rituals.

Training the Child and Parent in Family Organization Skills

Ask the parents about daily routines around the house. Does the family typically accomplish what needs to get done on a daily basis? Does everyone get to school on time, complete homework, get enough sleep, etc.? If there are concerns in any of these areas, ask if the parent would like to develop more consistent routines as one way to improve them.

Review the section in parent book Chapter 19 that illustrates different types of family routines. Communicate that the main idea behind family routines is to establish order, predictability, and structure in everyday family life. Note that this will help the child also establish more structure and order in his or her daily functioning.

Brainstorm how to develop routines and use checklists with the parent like the ones depicted in Chapter 19. Develop a checklist or two for the family in the meeting by identifying tasks and generating steps toward accomplishing those tasks. The checklists could center on the entire day or on narrower activities such as getting ready for school in the morning, homework, dinnertime, bedtime, expectations of responsibility or chores, etc. Discuss with the parent whether these routine checklists might be posted and, if so, where. Talk about how the parent might review the checklists with the child on a regular basis.

Developing a Home Implementation Plan to Be Led by the Parent

Ask parents to identify which family bonding and/or family organization strategies they will work on. Discuss specific ways in which the parents can implement those ideas at home, including details about when (evenings, weekends, etc.), where (usually home), and how often (once per day or week, several times per day or week, etc.) to engage in specified family bonding and/or family organization methods. Ask the parents to consider designating these specific ideas as goals to accomplish on the *Parenting Goals* form (see parent book Chapter 3 and the end of Chapter 4 in this book). For example, the parent might state a goal of scheduling and doing 30-minute child-directed activities with the child on Monday and Thursday evenings for the next month. Another goal might be to develop a bedtime reading ritual (with a younger child) or a Saturday breakfast ritual (with an older child or teen). Still another goal might be for the parent to develop and use an evening checklist to get the family more organized on school nights so that homework gets done and the child gets to bed at a decent time.

In later meetings, review the ***Parent Checklist for Family Bonding and Organization*** until progress is made. Ask the parents to evaluate how well they are following through with different elements of family bonding and/or family organization. Use the checklist as a tool to remind the parents about what areas they should work on.

Specific Procedures for Applying Parent Book Chapter 20

This chapter addresses familywide interaction skills by giving the parent and child (and often, other family members) strategies to facilitate communication, problem solving, and conflict management skills. Family members learn to recognize when family interactions are not going well and to employ these adaptive interactional skills. This approach not only helps the family but also provides an opportunity for the child to learn important skills that can help him or her in other relationships—with siblings, peers, teachers, coaches, etc.

Several sessions may be needed to initially train family members in effective communication, problem-solving, and family conflict resolution skills. Typically the sessions are directed at the family unit as a whole. The parent is still in the lead for guiding the family to use the skills at home, however, and therefore much attention and planning needs to be directed toward the parent.

> **Note: *The forms and charts referred to in the discussion below are in parent book Chapter 20 and at the end of this chapter unless otherwise noted.***

Discussing Family Interaction Skills with the Parent and Child

Discuss with the parent and child that sometimes families develop unhelpful interaction habits. They may keep experiencing the same problems over and over, often due to poor communication habits and inability to resolve conflicts that arise. Ask the parent and child how well their family deals with day-to-day challenges at home and whether they are able to work out their conflicts in a productive way. Note that family interaction difficulties can be harmful to family relationships and negatively affect each family member. Ask if it might be a good idea for the family to work on communication, problem-solving, and conflict resolution skills.

If a child or parent has a propensity to blame the other, or does not see the relevance for him or her to work on family interactions, it can help to reframe problems within an interactional context. This entails discussing how the child and parent mutually affect one another. Explain that if someone interrupts a lot, the other may yell in reaction. Likewise, when someone talks too long, the other may not listen. Ask for examples involving different family members where someone's way of interacting affected the other. Note too that everyone can benefit from work on family interactions regardless of who may need to work on it the most.

Explain to the parent that the methods in Chapter 20 are good for a family with any-age child, but they are particularly well suited for the family of an older child or teen. Children should participate more in family decisions and exert increasing autonomy within the family as they get older. It is also often the case that an older child or teen's struggles impact other family members, and these emerging problems need to be solved within the family. For these reasons a focus on familywide interaction skills can be productive, particularly with the older child or teen.

Getting Parents Started and Focused

Ask the parents to rate and check off items on the *Parent Checklist for Family Interactions* form that are going well for the family and other areas needing some work. Because the checklist summarizes the overall approach of this chapter, be sure to answer any questions the parent may have about the skills content presented on the checklist and stress the importance that the parent understand the content detailed in parent book Chapter 20.

Training the Child and Parent in Family Interaction Skills

Chapter 20 presents three interrelated family interaction skills, which ideally should be taught separately before the parent, child, and other family members are taught how to use them all together.

Family Communication Skills

Communication is fundamental, and good communication skills will both facilitate fruitful problem solving and reduce family conflict, so it's best to start with family communication skills. Note, however, that mutual cooperation among family members is critical. If anyone in the family resists working on communication skills—believing, for example, that everyone already has these skills—spend some time on psychoeducation before teaching the skills. Review the *Family Communication Skills* chart. Ask family members to look at the "DON'Ts" and ask generically if a family whose regular communication style included a lot of the DON'Ts might have family interaction problems. No doubt most family members would be able to see that the DON'Ts might be related to family strife.

Now ask family members to identify their own personal DON'Ts on the *Family Communication Skills* chart. If everyone has bought in to the need for working on communication skills, this process should go reasonably well. On the other hand, some family members might prove more interested in someone else's DON'Ts than in their own and will need to be encouraged to help the family as a whole by owning up to a DON'T or two.

After each family member has identified personal DON'Ts, ask family members if it is okay to give each other constructive feedback. Don't push this step too hard if it is clear that one or more family members are feeling defensive or put on the spot. If that is the case, then it may be best to focus only on the self-identification of DON'Ts.

Suggest that each family member consider using the corresponding DOs related to his or her personal DON'Ts. **Note that each DO is an opposite and more helpful way of communicating than the corresponding DON'T.** Ask family members to think about specific DOs that they may want to work on.

Note that each family member's way of communicating interacts with other family members' ways of communicating. For example, a parent who is giving a long lecture might elicit poor listening in a child—but poor listening from a child might elicit a parent's long lecture too. Observe that one family member's working on his or her communication skills can impact other family members. Discuss how DOs can also be interactive. For example, if a parent is brief and to the point, the child may listen better, or if the child is listening (eye contact, leaning toward, nodding, etc.), the parent might be briefer. Ask family members for other examples of how one family member's communication can affect others.

Next do some modeling and role playing related to family communication. Begin with an easy topic, such as what to have for dinner that evening. For illustration purposes only, ask family members to intentionally use the DON'Ts while trying to discuss dinner plans. This can be amusing while also getting across the point of how the DON'Ts can interfere with effective family communication. Then state that the goal of the next role play is to use the family communication DOs while avoiding the DON'Ts to discuss dinner. If that goes well, then introduce a more difficult real-world issue such as when homework will be done that evening. Again for fun, it might be useful to discuss the homework issue using the DON'Ts first and then contrast that with the same discussion employing the DOs. Be sure to note that the role plays involving intentional use of DON'Ts are "pretend" and should not be taken personally as if they were real discussions. During these exercises, the practitioner's job is to coach and direct the family to look at the *Family Communication Skills* chart and use the identified communication skills.

Later help each family member identify specific communication DOs that he or she will work on at home and use the *My Family Communication Goals* form to monitor progress. For example, a father might work on being direct and specific instead of sarcastic; a mother might work on making briefer statements instead of going on and on; and a child or teen might work on expressing feelings instead of keeping them in and sulking. Discuss how the family will periodically review their progress on the *My Family Communication Goals* form. Perhaps they will discuss their progress daily for a while and then once a week after some progress has been made.

Family Problem-Solving Skills

Follow a similar process to introduce and discuss family problem-solving skills. Review the *Family Problem Solving* chart and then ask family members if it would be helpful for them to solve ongoing family problems more effectively. Note that it is far more productive to do so while also using good communication skills.

Go back and do modeling and role playing with the same scenarios, now adding family problem solving to guide the process. Prompt and guide family members to use effective communication skills along with family problem solving to deal with problems related to dinner and homework (in the examples above). The practitioner's job is again to coach and direct family members to use communication and problem-solving skills simultaneously.

Make sure that the child understands that everything is not open for negotiation via family problem solving. Counsel the parent to state clearly when family problem solving is or is not acceptable. For example, family problem solving may be okay when figuring out when the child will do a homework assignment over the weekend, but it is not okay in determining a curfew time. Forewarn the child to expect that sometimes his or her version of family problem solving may not work for the parent and that the parent is in charge.

Discuss ways in which the family will use family problem solving at home. Note that it may help to post the *Family Problem Solving* chart (along with the *Family Communication Skills* chart). Suggest that perhaps family members agree that it is okay for any one of them to request the use of family problem solving if a disagreement emerges (sometimes after a family cool-down, as discussed next).

Family Conflict Management Skills

Ask family members if they get upset with each other too often and what effect that has on their communication and problem solving. Suggest that they work on cooling down so that they can communicate better and solve their problems effectively. Note that it is important for all family members to cooperate and agree to use the **family cool-down** before learning it and trying it at home. Ask the parents to consider providing a reward to the child for trying it (see parent book Chapter 3 for more ideas on motivating the child).

Suggest that family members become aware of "family conflict signals." Help family members recognize their own personal body signals, personal thought signals, and broader family action signals that are present during conflict (see parent book Chapter 20 for examples). It is a good idea to write down the signals that are generated by family members and review them to create more awareness.

Conduct modeling and role playing of managing family conflict in a manner similar to the communication procedures. Refer to the *Family Cool-Down* chart while doing so. Be sure to choose the *Family Cool-Down* chart with younger or older children to match the age of the child. Go through the earlier scenarios of dinner and homework, but ask family members to first "act" getting angry. Caution them that this is "pretend" and not to go too far. The practitioner's job is to again coach and direct them to use the *Family Cool-Down* steps to resolve the problem that caused the original conflict.

Discuss specific ways in which the family will use family conflict management at home.

It may be helpful to post the *Family Cool-Down* chart in the home. It may also be of benefit to review the *Family Cool-Down* chart periodically. Make sure that everyone agrees that another family member can call for a family cool-down of a few minutes as long as the person intends to come back and try to solve the problem in good faith.

Putting It All Together

Describe, model, and do role playing of all steps together. For example, the same dinner and homework scenarios could be recycled briefly, this time using all family interactions skills. The family, having a conflict over dinner or homework, would first separate to cool down for a while and then come back to solve the problem using good communication skills. Then it is useful to practice all the skills with a real-life problem during a session with the assistance of the practitioner. For example, the issue might center on possibly changing a Friday night curfew because a friend of the child is having a party. The practitioner should again guide the family in using all family interaction skills together (family cool-down, problem solving, and communication) as they attempt to discuss and resolve this common family dilemma.

Developing a Home Implementation Plan to Be Led by the Parent

As mentioned earlier, the parent should lead the family's efforts in using family interaction skills. Discuss concrete ways in which the parent will do this. For example, the parent can plan and lead occasional brief 10-minute family meetings (see parent book Chapter 3) to discuss and review progress with family interaction skills. When doing so, it would be advisable for the parent to have the selected family interaction skills charts handy to serve as a reference. Brainstorm with the parent about when and how often these family meetings might take place.

Also suggest that the parent consider writing down specific ideas to accomplish this plan on the *Parenting Goals* form (see parent book Chapter 3 and the end of Chapter 4 in this book). For example, the parent might declare a goal of organizing brief family meetings on Monday evening, Wednesday evening, and Saturday morning for the next 3 weeks. Another goal might be for the parent to specify communication DOs that he or she will personally work on and monitor progress by using the *My Family Communication Goals* form. Still another goal might be to motivate the child by providing a tangible reward for completing a certain number of *My Family Communication Goals* forms (see parent book Chapter 3 for more details on motivating the child).

Suggest that the older child or teen also set goals and monitor his or her progress. Accordingly, the child might also utilize the *My Family Communication Goals* form or the *Personal Goals (Basic* or *Advanced)* form (see parent book Chapter 3 and the end of Chapter 4 in this book) to declare specific goals to work on pertaining to family interaction.

Modifications for Using the Family Well-Being Module in Parent Groups

Present the ***Overview of the Family Well-Being Module*** chart to parent group members as an introduction to skills within this family-oriented module. Ask the parents to discuss ongoing challenges for their family as they relate to parent–child bonding, family organization, and family interactions. Ask the parents to reveal their perceptions of their family's well-being. Encourage parents to share how they have attempted to shore up family operations and relationships in the past. Parents normally have tried many things to improve their family and sometimes feel frustrated by the lack of results. Sharing with other parents can provide some support and awareness that they are not alone in facing family challenges.

Also allow parents to process their positive feelings about how their family used to be and negative feelings about how it might be currently. Suggest that this module may help parents make improvements within the family, thus perhaps motivating them to work on the family well-being domain. Inform parents that the main goal of this module is to get the family back on track through the parents' guiding family members to make changes in day-to-day operations and to use family interaction skills. Help parents in the group jointly identify areas within the family well-being module that should be emphasized for that meeting and/or over several meetings to come.

This module can be introduced over one meeting, but several more meetings will be needed to cover the topics of facilitating parent and child motivation/commitment and reviewing new family-oriented skills. The charts found in parent book Chapters 19 and 20 can be used to convey information and approaches within the family well-being module. The role plays described above in the preceding training sections for parent book Chapters 19 and 20 can be used in parent groups by having parents take turns acting out different family roles if they are comfortable doing so. Help each parent identify specific family-related goals and strategies and designate them on the ***Parenting Goals*** form. Check in regarding progress parents are achieving with their family-related goals during later meetings.

Overview of the Family Well-Being Module

Chapter 19. Let's Get Together: Strengthening Family Bonds and Organization

Building Parent–Child Bonds through Activities

- Make time for positive child-directed activities
- Make time for special conversations
- Get more involved in child's activities

Building Family Bonds through Rituals

- Daily family rituals (e.g., regular dinner time)
- Special family rituals (e.g., holiday traditions)
- Community rituals (e.g., everyone helping in the community)

Enhancing Family Organization through Routines

- Daily schedule for school days
- Task list for getting ready for school in the morning
- Task list for homework
- Task list for dinnertime
- Task list for bedtime
- Other task lists

Chapter 20. We Can Work It Out: Strengthening Family Interaction Skills

Learning and Practicing Family Communication Skills

- Family members evaluate dos and don'ts of family communication
- Practice role plays of communication dos

See **Family Communication Skills** chart.

Using Family Communication Skills at Home

- Use new communications skills at home
- Set communication goals and monitor progress

See **My Family Communication Goals** form.

(cont.)

Learning and Practicing Family Problem-Solving Skills

- Family members evaluate effective family problem-solving methods
- Practice role plays of effective family problem solving

See **Family Problem Solving** chart

Using Family Problem Solving at Home

- Use new family problem-solving skills at home
- Don't use family problem solving unless parent is truly open to compromise/negotiation

Learning to Recognize Family Conflict

- *Personal body signals*—breathing rate, heart rate, sweating, increased muscle tension, flushed face
- *Personal thought signals*—"she's making me mad," "I hate her!," "I wish she were dead," "He is so unfair," etc.
- *Family action signals*—raised voices, angry facial expressions and body postures, put-downs and interruptions

Reducing Family Conflict via Family Cool-Down at Home

- Family members agree that anyone can call for family cool-down
- Separate for 5 or 10 minutes
- Each member reduces his or her own anger and frustration
- Family members come back together to work out the problem, using good communication and problem-solving skills

See **Family Cool-Down** chart.

Disengaging and Deescalating When Child Is Highly Agitated

- *Emotional level*—stay calm
- *Verbal level*—minimize talking
- *Physical level*—minimize eye contact and try to walk away

Training Family Members in Family Well-Being Skills (Chapters 19 & 20)

- Focus on the family "team" working together
- Guide child to work on family well-being skills and goals
- Identify parenting goals related to promoting family well-being skills at home
- Learn, practice, and monitor progress with family well-being skills and goals

See **Parent Checklist** for each chapter, as well as **Personal Goals (Basic** or **Advanced)** form for child and **Parenting Goals** form for parent (both in Chapter 3 and also at the end of Chapter 4 of this book).

Forms from Parent Book Chapter 19

Parent Checklist for Family Bonding and Organization

Name: _____ Date: _____

In the blanks below, indicate a score for **how well** you make use of that parenting behavior at this time.

	Not too well	Okay	Very well
	1	2	3

Parent's Efforts in Building Parent–Child Bonds Through Activities

A. _____ Making time for positive child-directed activities

B. _____ Making time for special conversations

C. _____ Getting more involved in activities and at school

D. _____ Other (specify): _____

Parent's Efforts in Strengthening Family Bonds through Rituals

E. _____ Making time for regular family rituals

F. _____ Making time for special family rituals

G. _____ Making time for community rituals

H. _____ Other (specify): _____

Parent's Efforts in Enhancing Family Organization through Routines

I. _____ Getting ready for school in the morning

J. _____ Having regular homework time

K. _____ Having regular dinnertime

L. _____ Having regular bedtime

M. _____ Other (specify): _____

Forms and Charts from Parent Book Chapter 20

Parent Checklist for Family Interactions

Name: _____ Date: _____

In the blanks below, indicate a score for **how well** you make use of that parenting behavior at this time.

Not too well	**Okay**	**Very well**
1	**2**	**3**

Parent's Efforts in Promoting Family Communication Skills

A. _____ Reviewing and practicing family communication skills

B. _____ Guiding the family to use the family communication skills at home, including reviewing the charts

Parent's Efforts in Promoting Family Problem-Solving Skills

C. _____ Reviewing and practicing family problem-solving skills

D. _____ Guiding the family to use the family problem-solving skills at home, including reviewing the charts

Parent's Efforts in Promoting Family Conflict Management Skills

E. _____ Reviewing and practicing family conflict resolution skills

F. _____ Guiding the family to use the family conflict resolution skills at home, including reviewing the charts

Family Communication Skills

DON'Ts

- Long lectures or "sermons"

- Blaming (e.g., "You need to stop _____," "It's your fault")

- Vague statements (e.g., "Shape up," "Knock it off," "I don't like that")

- Asking negative questions (e.g., "Why do you do that?" or "How many times must I tell you?")

- Poor listening—looking away, silent treatment, crossing arms, etc.

- Interrupting others

- Not showing that you understand someone

- Put-downs (e.g., "You're worthless," "I'm sick of you"), threats, and so forth

- Yelling, screaming, and so forth

- Sarcasm

- Going from topic to topic

- Bringing up old issues, past behavior

- Keeping feelings inside

- Scowling facial expression

- "Mind reading" or assuming you know what other people think

DOs

- Brief statements of 10 words or less

- "I" statements (e.g., "I feel _____ when _____")

- Direct and specific statements (e.g., "Stop teasing your sister [brother]," "I really don't like when you _____")

- Be specific about what you want (e.g., "Do the dishes now," "Please talk calmly")

- Active listening—good eye contact, leaning forward, nodding, etc.

- Let person completely state his or her thoughts before stating yours

- Paraphrase what the other person said to you

- Constructive comments (e.g., "I'm concerned about your grades," "Something is bothering me; can we discuss it?")

- Neutral/natural tone of voice

- Say what you mean, be specific and straightforward

- Stay on one topic

- Focusing on here and now

- Verbally expressing feelings

- Neutral facial expressions

- Let people speak for themselves; ask questions to make sure you understand

My Family Communication Goals

Name: _____ **Date and time:** _____

Indicate which family communication "DOs" you will be working on below. Designate a time period for using this chart. At the end of the designated time period, rate how well you accomplished your goals. It may be helpful to get feedback from other family members as to how well they think you are accomplishing your goals.

Self-Awareness Monitoring

1. I am working on increasing family communication DOs of:

2. How well did I accomplish my goal(s)? (Circle one.)

1	2	3	4	5
Not at all	A little	Okay	Pretty well	Great

Family Members' Feedback (optional)

3. How well did family members think I accomplished my goal(s)? (Circle one.)

1	2	3	4	5
Not at all	A little	Okay	Pretty well	Great

Comments: _____

_____

_____

_____

_____

Family Problem Solving

1. Stop!! What is the problem we are having?

- Try to avoid blaming individuals.

- Focus on how family members are interacting and causing problems together.

- State specifically what the problem is so that everyone agrees.

2. What are some plans we can use?

- Think of as many alternative plans as possible.

- Don't evaluate or criticize any family member's ideas.

- Don't discuss any one solution until you have generated many alternatives.

3. What is the best plan we could use?

- Think of what would happen if the family used each of the alternatives.

- Think about how each alternative would make each family member feel.

- Decide which alternative is most likely to succeed and make most family members feel okay.

- Reach an agreement by as many family members as possible.

4. Put the plan into effect.

- Try the plan as well as the family can.

- Don't criticize or say, "I told you so."

5. Did our plan work?

- Evaluate the plan.

- Determine whether everyone is satisfied with the way the problem was solved.

- If the solution didn't work, repeat the entire family problem-solving process.

Try to stay focused on the here and now. Do not bring up old issues when trying to do family problem solving.

Family Cool-Down

1. Are we too angry at each other?

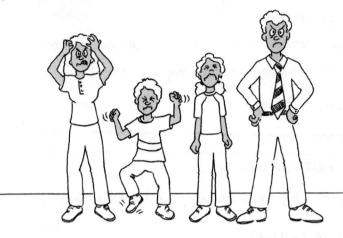

2. Briefly separate to cool down.

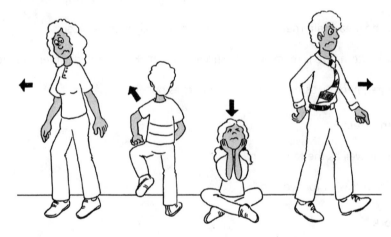

3. Come back together to solve the problem.

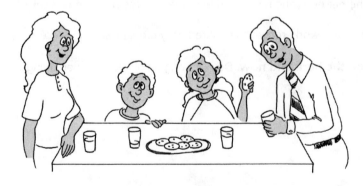

Family Cool-Down

1. Are we too angry at each other?

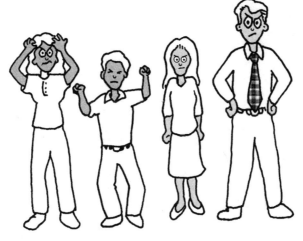

2. Briefly separate to cool down.

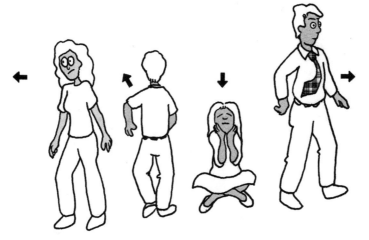

3. Come back together to solve the problem.

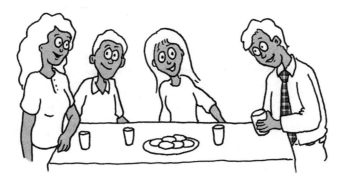

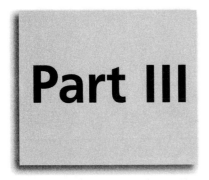

Part III

Case Examples

11

Practice Illustrations of the "Struggling Kids" Program

In this chapter specific cases and group models are presented to illustrate how the "Struggling Kids" program can be used in real-world practice. These examples show how evidence-based practice parameters can be applied in typical practice settings with typical cases and how services often unfold. These practice examples reflect my personal experience in providing the "Struggling Kids" program to thousands of children and their families in a variety of settings, as well as the lessons learned from training and supervising hundreds of aspiring practitioners in this type of approach.

First, three case studies illustrate one-family-at-a-time interventions provided in mental health and in-home settings (see pp. 261–294). Although the cases are fictional and any similarity between them and real families is purely coincidental, the cases are aggregated from many real cases and accurately show how skills training is provided using the "Struggling Kids" approach.

Then, three parent group models are described, one applied within the context of a conduct problem prevention initiative, another used in a psychiatric partial hospitalization program, and finally one model of parent and child programming conducted as an intensive outpatient program (see pp. 294–301).

Note: *References to chapters in the following text are from the parent book unless otherwise noted.*

Individual Case: Gabriela, Age 7

> **Diagnoses:** Oppositional defiant disorder; anxiety disorder not otherwise specified
> **Number of sessions:** 10
> **Setting:** School-based mental health clinic
> **Practitioner:** Dr. Susanne Jones, licensed clinical psychologist

Background Information

Gabriela lives with her parents, two older brothers, and one younger sister in a large city. Her father, Joseph, works full-time (with frequent overtime) as a shipping clerk, and her mother, Belinda, works part-time as a health aide in a nursing home. Gabriela attends the second grade at a local elementary school.

Joseph and Belinda would like Gabriela to get some help for her frequent displays of defiant, angry, and sometimes aggressive behavior. Although Gabriela has always been an exuberant and expressive child who at times is difficult for her parents to manage, her behavioral and emotional outbursts have intensified dramatically over the last 2 years. She exhibits these behavioral and emotional problems primarily at home but also at school, to some extent. Fortunately, Gabriela loves school and does well academically.

Gabriela attends an elementary school that has a school-based mental health clinic. A school social worker informed her parents about the clinic, and at his recommendation they decided to take Gabriela to the clinic for help. A clinical psychologist, Dr. Jones, performed an initial assessment and then provided 10 sessions of parent and family skills training to Gabriela and her family. Gabriela received other school-based services during the intervention.

Brief Review of History and Presenting Problems

As mentioned above, Gabriela has been an intelligent and independent child from the start, but she increasingly challenges her parents with arguments and stubborn refusals. Recently, Gabriela developed a quick temper and now becomes easily frustrated when interacting with peers and siblings. As a result she is involved in many conflicts and occasionally exhibits reactively aggressive behaviors such as yelling, pushing, hitting, and so on, when things don't go as she wants them to go. During one emotional outburst she shoved one of her siblings down for not giving in to her wishes, causing bruises and family turmoil. Her parents have tried punishing her, using sticker charts, and even letting her have her way, but "nothing works." School officials have been frustrated in their efforts to manage Gabriela's behavior and outbursts at school and have been pressuring her parents to do something.

Unfortunately, Gabriela has gradually alienated many of her peers and now is rejected by some of them. Although she is aware of this and feels bad about it, she lacks the skills and motivation to make changes. During the past year, on occasion, several girls have excluded her from their group on the playground and have called her names. This makes her feel sad and lonely.

The family lives in a high-crime neighborhood that is also plagued by gang activity. There have been reports of violent crimes nearby, and sometimes gunshots can be heard at night. Gabriela has become increasingly upset and bothered by these incidents over the last year or so and has become a "worry wart." She frequently worries about family members' safety and well-being when they're not at home, especially her mother.

Despite behavioral and social problems at school, Gabriela enjoys being there. Her teachers have always considered her bright. When calm, she actively participates in classroom learning activities.

Belinda feels continually stressed and exhausted by her responsibility for parenting and running the household. All of her children are very active, and often noisily argue with one another, creating an aggravating atmosphere in which Belinda can barely think straight. She is particularly worn down by the difficult and determined Gabriela. Joseph helps out, but the fact that he often works late limits his availability. Belinda finds herself losing patience and ends up yelling at Gabriela, which she immediately regrets. On top of all this, the family is struggling financially and does not have reliable transportation, which causes many daily hassles.

The family has a bundle of strengths too. The entire extended family has close bonds with one another. Belinda and Joseph value education and do their best to ensure that the children are ready for school, do their homework, and are well fed and rested. Grandparents, uncles, and cousins, on both sides, are involved and supportive of Gabriela and her family.

Family Readiness and Strategies Used to Promote Engagement over 10 Sessions

Dr. Jones initially placed the family in the "D" category of **family readiness to engage** (see Figure 3.1 in Chapter 3 of this book). This rating was based on the moderate to high severity of Gabriela's behaviors, and although the parents are internally motivated, it is likely that numerous daily stressors faced by the family might make it difficult for them to engage, placing them in the moderate to low category of capacity. Indeed Joseph attended sessions sporadically due to his demanding work schedule. In addition, because he drove their only car to work each day, his wife had problems getting to the school for meetings with the practitioner because she lived several miles away. The cost of public transportation limited her ability to attend.

During the course of the skills-building intervention, Dr. Jones utilized many engagement strategies with the family. To facilitate attendance, Dr. Jones worked with the family's health maintenance organization (HMO) to obtain transportation vouchers so that Belinda could come to school for family sessions. The school also had a day care setting, and so Belinda could drop off her youngest child while she attended sessions with Gabriela. Finally, whenever possible, sessions were scheduled during the lunch hour so that Joseph could attend. He was able to do so on four occasions.

The parents did not initially follow through with homework assignments (described later). At several points during the course of intervention it was necessary to revisit skills-building strategies to ensure mastery and competence. To accomplish this, role playing was used to make sure that the skills were developed by both the parents and Gabriela (described later). During the fourth and fifth sessions Dr. Jones implemented the *Parent Checklist* forms (described later) to review progress with skills acquisition. This increased the parents' awareness of how they could guide Gabriela in social and emotional skills development. Dr. Jones found that periodically reviewing the selected *Parent Checklist* form significantly stimulated the parents' accountability and follow-through, particularly with Belinda.

One time when Belinda was asked about some worksheets, she honestly exclaimed, "I feel like this is too hard! By the time I find out that Gabriela has caused trouble with her brothers or sister, it's already turned into a huge fight. Besides, I don't have time!" Dr. Jones implemented strategies that are consistent with parent book Chapter 3 in an attempt to increase Belinda's motivation. Through discussion Dr. Jones guided Belinda to figure out that Gabriela's behavior was a top priority and nudged her to pledge more effort. Dr. Jones also brainstormed with Belinda about ways to fit brief skills practice homework into her busy daily schedule. Gradually Belinda became motivated, and as she did the homework, she later expressed the gradual sense of empowerment that each small success brought her.

Content for Session 1: Collaboration and Initial Functional Assessment

- *Getting Back on Track:* Coming Up with a Skills-Building Plan for Your Child and Family *(primary focus)*

During the first intervention session, Dr. Jones went through the questions on the *Getting to Know You* form with the parents (see this book, Chapter 4). Although the parents, feeling desperate, preferred a quick remedy, they were assured that determining the best areas to focus on first would make the treatment shorter and more effective in the long run. The session revealed their strong family bond, but the parents were at a loss about how to handle Gabriela's aggressive behavior and outbursts.

A functional assessment was used to determine areas of focus for Gabriela and her family. Joseph and Belinda completed the *Examining How Your Child and Family Are Doing* form (parent book Chapter 2). Dr. Jones guided the parents, also providing some input, to reach a consensus in rating the functional areas below (using the rating format of 1–2 = struggling/stressed, 3–4 = is in progress, 5–6 = successful/coping). The ratings produced by the parents (along with the associated characteristics that are consistent with the ratings *in italics*) are summarized below:

_2_ Child behavioral development—*Gabriela exhibits defiant and aggressive behavior both at home and at school and protests when held accountable for her misbehavior.*

_2_ Child social development—*Conflicts with peers have alienated them from Gabriela, and now she is experiencing rejection. She is also not getting along too well with siblings.*

__1__ **Child emotional development**—*Gabriela exhibits quick temper and frustration when interacting with peers and siblings (related to reactive aggression), outbursts at home and school with adults who attempt to discipline her, and she worries about family members' safety and well-being.*

__5__ **Child academic development**—*Gabriela loves school, participates when calm, does well academically, and is considered bright by her teachers.*

__2__ **Parent well-being**—*Belinda is stressed by parenting, household responsibilities, and numerous daily stressors related to financial struggles, and loses her patience with the children. Joseph helps out, but work limits his availability.*

__3__ **Family well-being**—*Although there are close extended family ties, and the parents work hard to ensure that the children get a good education, there are also a lot of negative parent–child and sibling–child interactions in daily family life.*

The ratings showed that Gabriela's parents believed that she had significant behavioral, social, and emotional problems. Their low rating on parent well-being was a reflection of their stress, particularly how overwhelmed Belinda often felt. Family well-being was viewed as somewhat compromised too. Dr. Jones suggested that the areas with lower scores might be good places to focus. It is noteworthy that Gabriela's academic development is a relative strength. Dr. Jones noted that Gabriela's academic strengths are something that she can build on for the future.

Dr. Jones and Gabriela's parents then reviewed the *Selecting Skills-Building Strategies to Work On* form (in parent book Chapter 2) and determined that the intervention should focus on all three of the domains of concern for Gabriela. Joseph and Belinda agreed to read Chapter 2 before the next session to get a better idea of what they would be doing to help their daughter. Because they believed that improvements in Gabriela's behavior would lessen their stress, they decided to work on Gabriela's behavioral development first with the idea that improvements in her behavior would also improve their parent well-being. Dr. Jones agreed, and Joseph and Belinda expressed relief and optimism that a plan was beginning to take shape.

Content for Sessions 2–4: Focus on Behavioral Development

- *Doing What You're Told:* Teaching Your Child to Comply with Parental Directives (*primary focus*)
- *Staying Cool under Fire:* Managing Your Child's Protesting of Discipline and Preventing Angry Outbursts (*primary focus*)
- *Teaming Up:* Collaborating and Advocating for Your Child at School

The parents reported that, after reading Chapter 2 and discussing it at home, they were even more certain that the first area needing to be addressed was Gabriela's behavior. Dr. Jones showed them the *Overview of the Child Behavioral Development Module* chart (see Chapter 5 in this book) and used it to lead a collaborative discussion about all that the behavioral improvement methods entail. Together they decided the initial focus would be on Gabriela's disobedient behavior and angry outbursts.

Several sessions were conducted with the parents only. Gabriela did not attend because the focus was on behavior management as opposed to child skills. Chapters 4 and 7 (of the parent book) were the primary focus of these meetings. During the sessions the *Parent Checklist for Child Compliance* (parent book Chapter 4) and then later the *Parent Checklist for Child Protests and Angry Outbursts* (parent book Chapter 7) were reviewed and discussed step by step, with Belinda and Joseph evaluating their proficiency with the skills noted on the checklists and thereby identifying goals on which to work. They agreed that both of them needed to pay particular attention to giving clear and concise commands and to avoid getting caught up in power struggles and arguments with Gabriela. Dr. Jones asked them to read Chapters 4 and 7 (parent book) between sessions to reinforce and expand on the information presented via the checklists.

All of the steps for using time-out and managing protests were reviewed thoroughly, with role-play exercises used to practice procedures. Dr. Jones first modeled the "catching 'em being compliant" technique by praising "Gabriela" (played by Belinda) for in-session behavior. Dr. Jones demonstrated statements such as "Gabriela, you are doing a great job paying attention and contributing to the discussion today, and I appreciate it." Belinda was asked to generate a list of "catching 'em being compliant" statements that she could use with Gabriela at home and rehearsed making them in the session with Dr. Jones.

Time-out was also the subject of behavior rehearsal. Dr. Jones modeled the use of time-out with Gabriela, as played by Belinda, and then asked Belinda to demonstrate the same method with her, playing Gabriela. During the initial modeling and role playing, Dr. Jones suggested that Gabriela comply with time-out without protesting. Later the same modeling and role playing was repeated but with Gabriela exhibiting moderate protesting. This time Dr. Jones modeled how to stay calm and use the patient standoff method, followed by Belinda doing the same.

Joseph was reluctant to do role playing but said he understood the steps and methods. He did, however, have a problem with the procedure for handling protesting behavior when disciplining a child for noncompliance. The procedure calls for ignoring the protesting but patiently following through with time-out or removal of privileges when a child exhibits non-compliant behavior (parent book Chapter 7). Joseph felt that talking back to parents under any circumstance, including when protesting, was unacceptable, and that it was important to send the message that it would not be tolerated in their family. So with Dr. Jones's help, they modified the procedure so that if Gabriela talked back to her parents, she would **double** her time-out period (a 7-minute time-out would be 14 minutes, etc.). Joseph agreed to ignore any protesting that occurred after a **double-time** procedure was implemented. This modification accomplished Joseph's goal to send a direct message to Gabriela that talking back was not accepted but also thereafter reduced potentially escalating power struggles derived from her protesting.

During the fourth and fifth sessions Dr. Jones reviewed the *Parent Checklist* forms from Chapters 4 and 7 (parent book), which revealed that it was difficult for Belinda to maintain composure, let alone think straight, when Gabriela pushed her buttons. So she committed to trying to be consistent in giving clear warnings and then verbally disengaging from Gabriela's protests against time-out. Dr. Jones reinforced the integrity of the time-out procedure through additional modeling and role playing.

Belinda had a chance to use time-out in a real situation when, during the fourth session, Gabriela attempted to leave the room—to which her mother responded by stating a command to "stay in the room." Gabriela opened the door and Belinda then gave a warning that if she did not return, she would have a time-out right there. Gabriela burst into an explosive tantrum and stormed out of the office. Belinda was coached and encouraged to use the protest managing and compliance strategies she had previously learned. Dr. Jones and Belinda followed Gabriela into a hallway where she sat on the floor sulking. Dr. Jones asked Belinda, as they were approaching Gabriela, if the patient standoff procedure would be useful here, to which Belinda replied in the affirmative. Belinda told Gabriela that she would not be able to watch TV until she did her time-out either now, in Dr. Jones's office, or later at home. Since Gabriela was moderately protesting, and there were no imminent safety concerns, Dr. Jones suggested that they return to her office, but they kept the door cracked open to watch and listen just in case. About 5 minutes later Gabriela returned to Dr. Jones's office, and then Belinda told her "Now you have to go to time-out." It was difficult, but Belinda followed through and was able to eventually, and calmly, put Gabriela in time-out in a corner chair in Dr. Jones's office. As a result of this spontaneous incident, Belinda felt more confident in her ability to use these strategies with Gabriela at home or in public.

As the sessions progressed, the parents reported that Gabriela's behavior was gradually improving at home. They said that recently Gabriela had been following directions more at the command or warning stage and that her protesting was shorter and shorter when it occurred. Belinda gave a recent example of when she gave a command, and then a warning, to Gabriela about turning off the computer to begin the bedtime routine. Gabriela pouted, which Belinda ignored, but she turned off the computer and went to put on her pajamas. Belinda then praised Gabriela for following directions and getting ready for bed. The parents also noted some slight improvement in their stress levels. Belinda indicated that since Gabriela's behavior had improved, she had more energy and was exercising more.

Since Dr. Jones worked in the school, she was able to also briefly consult with Gabriela's teacher about effective ways of managing her noncompliant behavior in the classroom that were consistent with methods being used by the parents (with parental permission to do so). In addition, a parent–teacher meeting was set up and facilitated by Dr. Jones. During the meeting a school–home note (parent book Chapter 16) was devised for the teacher to complete and Gabriela to take home each day. The target behaviors at school were "Follow classroom rules" and "Listen and obey teacher." Dr. Jones urged Belinda to provide a small reward (special snack) for days on which Gabriela's school–home note indicated her good school behavior. Gabriela was not punished for bad behavior days, but her mother would discuss what went wrong and how she could do better the next day. The teacher reported to Dr. Jones that Gabriela's classroom behavior was steadily improving.

In Session 4, Dr. Jones asked the parents to fill out the *Parent Checklist* forms from Chapters 4 and 7 (parent book). The scores were mostly "3's," but Belinda became aware that she needed to keep working on giving warnings, and Joseph determined that it would be good for him to disengage more by talking less during Gabriela's protesting moments. Dr. Jones congratulated them on their success and encouraged them to keep working on the areas that needed continued tweaking.

Content for Sessions 5–7: Focus on Social Development

- *Making Friends:* Teaching Your Child Social Behavior Skills *(primary focus)*
- *Keeping Friends:* Teaching Your Child Social Problem-Solving Skills *(primary focus)*
- *Doing What's Expected:* Teaching Your Child to Follow Rules
- *Teaming Up:* Collaborating and Advocating for Your Child at School

Gabriela and Belinda attended all three of these sessions. Joseph, unfortunately, was able to make it to only one of them due to work commitments. During Sessions 6 and 7 two of the older siblings were also included in the meetings.

The primary focus during these sessions was on assisting Gabriela in developing social behavior and social problem-solving skills. The parents were asked to read Chapters 8 and 9 (parent book) before coming in for Session 5. Dr. Jones reviewed the *Parent Checklist* forms for the two chapters to facilitate learning, practicing, and then reviewing of the skills.

During Session 5, Dr. Jones asked Gabriela and Belinda to examine the *Identifying Social Behaviors to Work On* form in Chapter 8 (parent book). After careful discussion "cooperating" and "respectfully disagreeing with others" were the skills targeted for Gabriela. These social behaviors were explained, then modeled, and then practiced via role-play exercises. Gabriela played herself while Belinda and Dr. Jones "played" other children or siblings. Belinda agreed to utilize the *Personal Goals (Basic)* form with Gabriela (parent book Chapter 3) for a week to facilitate learning and generalization of the skills to the home environment. Gabriela was to practice them while playing or talking with her siblings, cousins, or friends at home. Her mother agreed to listen and pay attention to her interactions as much as possible to monitor and coach her. Gabriela admitted that she wanted to have more friends and that she did not like being made fun of, and Dr. Jones assured her that learning to get along with others would help.

During Sessions 6 and 7, held immediately after school, the focus shifted to social problem solving. The **Basic Social Problem Solving** chart (parent book Chapter 9) was used to structure the teaching of social problem-solving skills for Gabriela and her two older siblings. The sibling problem-solving mediation procedure was emphasized. Belinda practiced serving as a mediator between the siblings to guide them to work out their problems. Again, specific modeling and role-play exercises were used to teach skills, and all of the siblings enjoyed this part. A disagreement over which show to watch on TV provided a typical example of how to work out conflicts between the siblings.

During Session 7 Belinda reported that once during the week she had prompted the children to use social problem solving but they more or less ignored her and kept on loudly arguing about which movie to watch. Dr. Jones suggested that, in addition to social problem solving, a house rule could be established that "siblings must work out their problems in a respectful manner." This meant that threatening, throwing things, or physical contact would be a rule violation that would lead to an automatic time-out for any of the siblings involved. Belinda was asked to briefly review Chapter 5 regarding setting up house rules. The overall plan then was for parents to guide the children to work out their differences using social problem-solving skills (via mediation), but if the siblings engaged in any kind of fighting, they would be automatically sent to time-out. Dr. Jones reminded Belinda to set the length of time-out according to each child's age, but when she noted that it would be too hard to keep track if they all acted out at once, Dr. Jones agreed that giving everyone the same agreed-on amount of time (7 minutes) would make time-out easier to enforce. Dr. Jones noted that the combination of social problem solving with this house rule would likely be effective, and Belinda agreed to give it a try.

At this point Dr. Jones suggested that Belinda might benefit from using the **Parenting Goals** form (parent book Chapter 3) to identify and keep track of specific parenting goals. Belinda liked the idea and wrote down "Use time-out for noncompliance and the sibling rule violation," "Patiently follow through with time-out," and "Remind Gabriela to work on cooperating and working out problems." Dr. Jones was impressed with how confident Belinda had become and reminded her how important it was to continue listening to and watching Gabriela to catch her being good and intervening promptly, if possible, before disagreements turned into fights.

By the seventh session Belinda reported achieving most of her parenting goals at a level of "some progress." She was using time-out for noncompliance and sibling fighting and doing so in a patient manner if there was protesting. She thought she should be more attentive to prompting Gabriela to focus on cooperating and working out problems. Belinda committed herself to working even harder on her parenting goals. Dr. Jones recommended that the family celebrate their progress with an outing to get ice cream cones.

Dr. Jones consulted with the teacher about effective ways of guiding Gabriela's social behavior and social problem-solving skills in the classroom. The teacher agreed to be more immediately aware of and responsive to social interaction problems with Gabriela in the hope of preventing a potential escalation and to encourage her to get along better with peers. Specifically, the target behavior of "cooperating with peers" was added to the school–home note procedure (in addition to "follow classroom rules" and "listen and obey teacher," which were already on the note). The teacher and Gabriela began filling out the School–Home Note together at the end of the day so that the teacher could congratulate Gabriela on her successes and encourage her to keep working on her behavioral and social goals.

The teacher later reported to Dr. Jones that Gabriela was getting along better with classmates and even made friends with a new girl who had recently enrolled in the school. As the teacher and Dr. Jones discussed the situation, they speculated that Gabriela's improved classroom behavior drew less negative attention from her classmates. This, combined with Gabriela's more cooperative approach with others, was making her better liked by other children.

Content for Session 8: Focus on Emotional Development

- *Let It Out!*: Teaching Your Child to Understand and Express Feelings (*primary focus*)

The focus of the eighth session shifted to Gabriela's emotional development. Dr. Jones met with Gabriela for most of the session. The **Advanced Feelings Vocabulary Chart** and **Feelings Diary** form (parent book Chapter 12) guided the training process. Dr. Jones defined different feelings and asked Gabriela to chime in with what she knew about the feelings words. They also did the feelings charades game that involved taking turns making facial expressions and the other one stating what feeling was being portrayed. Then Dr. Jones asked Gabriela to fill out a **Feelings Diary** form based on events that had occurred that day. Gabriela wrote down that she felt sad and mad at recess when some kids would not take turns on the swings, but also felt happy when a friend talked to her at lunch. Toward the end of this session, Belinda was informed of these methods and was asked if she could coach and reinforce Gabriela for expressing her feelings. Dr. Jones asked Gabriela to show her mother the **Advanced Feelings Vocabulary Chart** and **Feelings Diary** form. The three of them discussed how they would fill out the **Feelings Diary** form at home on a daily basis for a while. Belinda was asked to read Chapter 12. Dr. Jones explained to Belinda that talking about her feelings would help Gabriela understand how she feels, which in turn may ease some of her frustration in getting along with other people.

Belinda thought that helping Gabriela understand and express her feelings was very important because otherwise she would bottle them up, making her grumpy around the house. Belinda decided to write down the goal "Help Gabriela talk about her feelings" on the **Parenting Goals** form. Belinda took the "Avoid power struggles" goal off the **Parenting Goals** form (because it was going so well) to make room for this new parenting goal.

It was a pleasure to observe the decreased tension between mother and daughter, and Dr. Jones encouraged them to make a little fun of themselves once in a while. They all smiled when Gabriela teased her mother for stammering and speaking in Spanish whenever she was upset with the kids, and Belinda laughed but reminded her daughter good-naturedly that no one is at their best when everyone is yelling or mad at one another!

Content for Sessions 9 and 10: Maintenance Phase and Final Functional Assessment

- *Doing What You're Told:* Teaching Your Child to Comply with Parental Directives
- *Let It Out!:* Teaching Your Child to Understand and Express Feelings

At the beginning of Session 9 Belinda reported that each day for a week, Gabriela had written down many of her worries and concerns related to her family's well-being on the **Feelings Diary** form, allowing her to express her concerns and also providing Belinda with opportunities to reassure her. For example, when Gabriela indicated, on the **Feelings Diary,** feeling sad about being teased at school or worried about a recent robbery in the neighborhood that was on the news, Belinda was able to discuss it with her and to reassure her. This shared process resulted in decreased worry and more confidence for Gabriela.

The last two sessions occurred 3 weeks apart. These sessions served as a chance to review skills with a particular emphasis on Chapters 4 and 12. Gabriela continued to be defiant and irritable on occasion, and so the resulting discussion provided an opportunity to review and practice skills related to behavior management and emotion expression with Gabriela and her parents.

Belinda, Joseph, and Gabriela all attended the last meeting. With the guidance of Dr. Jones, the parents completed the **Examining How Your Child and Family Are Doing** form (parent book Chapter 2) together and came to a consensus in rating the functional areas over the past several weeks (using the rating format of 1–2 = struggling/stressed, 3–4 = is in progress, 5–6 = successful/coping). The ratings produced by the family (along with the associated characteristics that are consistent with the ratings *in italics*) are summarized below:

__4__ **Child behavioral development**—*Gabriela's behavior has gradually improved in that she exhibits more compliance and far less protesting whenever disciplined. She still presents challenging behavior on occasion, but the parents think it is going in the right direction.*

__4__ **Child social development**—*Gabriela is getting along better with classmates and* *made a new friend at school, although some girls still exclude her from their social clique on occasion. She is working out social problems with her siblings under the guidance of her parents.*

__5__ **Child emotional development—***Gabriela worries much less and is much less volatile when she doesn't get her way. Gabriela reportedly talks more about challenges with friends and at school, and if prompted, will verbally express specific feelings. Plus her parents believe that she exhibits more confidence of late.*

__5__ **Child academic development—***She still loves school and participates even better because she is calmer.*

__5__ **Parent well-being—***The parents note some improvement in their stress levels. Belinda feels more confident as a result of learning new parenting techniques, and she is exercising more.*

__4__ **Family well-being—***There is decreased tension between mother and daughter, and the siblings are getting along a little better. Family members are joking around more like they used to.*

They were all proud to see that there had been progress from the initial rating. In particular, they are happy that family life is more harmonious and that Gabriela seems happier. The parents were less stressed out and feeling more confident in being able to assist Gabriela in her behavioral, social, and emotional development.

During the final session Dr. Jones noted that everyone slips up once in a while, and she stressed the importance of being alert to the possibility of relapse. She encouraged Joseph and Belinda to keep working on goals designated on the ***Parenting Goals*** form, especially those that relate to Gabriela's social and emotional development, since those had the lowest ratings at this point. They were also advised to pay attention to Gabriela's behavior at home to recognize the reemergence of old problems or the appearance of new ones. Given that Gabriela is in progress in a lot of areas, Dr. Jones encouraged them to keep working at it and to schedule a long-term follow-up meeting in 6 weeks to check in and troubleshoot any problems that might reemerge.

Case Management over 10 Sessions

During the course of the intervention, Gabriela's teacher was consulted in the manner described above (centering on use of a school–home note and prompting Gabriela to use specified social skills). In addition, given Belinda's high stress level, a referral was made at a community mental health center for her to receive a mental health assessment. She followed through and eventually joined a young mothers' support group in her neighborhood.

Individual Case 2: Michael, Age 12

> **Diagnoses:** Attention-deficit/hyperactivity disorder, combined type; oppositional defiant disorder; mood disorder not otherwise specified
>
> **Number of sessions:** 14
>
> **Setting:** Outpatient mental health clinic
>
> **Practitioner:** Mr. Louis Smith, licensed independent clinical social worker

Background Information

Michael lives with his mother, 14-year-old sister, and 11-year-old brother. At the time of the initial appointment the family was living in an apartment in a first-ring suburb of a large city. Michael was a sixth grader at a nearby middle school. His mother, Charlotte, was in the process of looking for a new residence because she was having difficulty paying the rent on her salary as a full-time office assistant.

Charlotte sought intervention services for Michael's behavioral, emotional, and school-related struggles after a recent mental health assessment revealed the diagnoses indicated above. Charlotte has tried a variety of treatments since Michael's problems began in preschool, including psychiatric medications, and has worked with the school to develop an individualized education program (IEP) for behavioral and emotional problems, but Michael continues to manifest significant difficulties at home and school. Charlotte is now "at her wit's end" with Michael and wants help for him and the family.

The family participated in 14 sessions of parent and family skills training with Mr. Smith. Michael also received other mental health and school services during the time of this intervention. He was followed by a child psychiatrist, who prescribed and managed medications targeting ADHD and mood symptoms. The school provided services to Michael in accordance with his IEP, including a daily behavioral contract whereby he could earn extra privileges for staying on task and following classroom rules.

Brief Review of History and Presenting Problems

A primary concern was Michael's display of physical and verbal aggression at home with his mother and siblings. A reasonable request by his mother to assist with household chores often sends Michael into a hostile verbal outburst. Charlotte's bedtime rule is viewed by Michael as a personal affront deserving of angry insults. Charlotte reported that last week Michael frightened her with his angry and intense reaction when she asked that he get off the Internet. He has frequent conflicts with both of his siblings that sometimes result in pushing and shoving. They too get very upset, along with Michael, which only increases family conflict. Michael frequently complains of being treated unfairly by family members, saying that his mother favors his siblings.

School is difficult for Michael because he is regularly disruptive and defiant in the classroom. He has trouble getting along with peers because he is impulsive and sometimes believes other kids are out to get him. When there is less structure, such as at lunchtime or during programs, Michael has gotten himself into trouble by instigating troublemaking behavior such as goofing around, roughhousing, and generally being a disruptive influence on his peers. He has an above-average IQ but struggles academically, largely due to not completing homework and accumulating many missing assignments.

Michael generally reports feeling out of sorts and unhappy. He seems sad at times, and being the recipient of continuous negative feedback at school or home is taking a toll on his self-esteem. It does not take much to trigger an angry outburst. He is aware at times of how his behavior affects others but feels sorry for himself because "no one understands me." Occasionally he makes passive suicidal comments about wishing he was dead or stating that the family would be better off without him. He usually makes these statements immediately after getting into trouble for his misbehavior.

Charlotte is a "no-nonsense" kind of parent who expects her children to follow her rules and also do well at school. Nonetheless, she and Michael have numerous battles about his not meeting those expectations, resulting in her frequently shouting at him out of frustration. She acknowledges feeling depressed and overwhelmed at times. She is also having a hard time financially and is behind on paying the bills.

The family has strengths too. When things are going well, they enjoy one another's company. Michael can have a great sense of humor and is adept at mimicking celebrity comedians and entertaining the family when he is in a good mood. Charlotte has a close bond with all of her children and is not hesitant to express her affection and devotion. At times the siblings do get along well, and they stick up for each other at school and around the neighborhood.

Family Readiness and Strategies Used to Promote Engagement over 14 Sessions

Based on available information, Mr. Smith initially conceptualized the family within the "B" category of **family readiness to engage** (see Figure 3.1 in Chapter 3 of this book). The historical and current problems indicated that Michael and his family were on the high side of the family severity continuum. Michael's behavioral and emotional concerns were significant. The family had serious conflict, and Charlotte was experiencing considerable stress and financial difficulties. Nonetheless, Mr. Smith thought that the family's capacity was toward the high end of the continuum. Charlotte was estimated to have average intelligence, and she presented as highly motivated and wanting to make a difference for Michael and the family. Her no-nonsense parenting approach is a strength that could be further shored up with effective parenting skills to help her better manage Michael's behavior. There were few apparent external barriers to attending intervention as Charlotte has good insurance, reliable transportation, and child care is not an issue for the siblings.

Initially, however, attendance was somewhat sporadic, and the family canceled an appointment and did not show for another. During the next session, a practical barrier was identified that interfered with attendance. The main barrier was the relative unavailability of Mr. Smith during preferred evening hours and the inflexibility of Charlotte's work schedule. Finally, after several weeks, Mr. Smith's schedule cleared up during Tuesday evenings (the one night per week that he worked late) at the six o'clock appointment slot. Eight sessions were initially blocked out for that time spot. Thereafter attendance improved, and the siblings were also able to participate in several meetings. After this initial intensive phase, the remaining sessions were spread out and scheduled, week to week, at times that were doable for Charlotte and the family.

Charlotte did well in collaborating with Mr. Smith to determine specific strategies to use, learned them in the sessions, and appeared motivated, but follow-through with using skills-building strategies at home was minimal early on, and Charlotte felt discouraged. During many discussions with Charlotte and Michael about how to enhance their motivation, they discovered the obstacles and barriers that interfered with progress toward goals. Charlotte was very busy with work, finding a new apartment, and then moving. The rest of her children had demands as well, and because of her weight issues and stress, she lacked the energy required by a child like Michael. Charlotte remarked that it would be easier to manage Michael and get his respect if his father was involved, but she said that wasn't going to happen. She would often resort to old ways of disciplining and interacting with Michael out of sheer exhaustion without even thinking about it. Beginning with the third session, Mr. Smith routinely reviewed various *Parent Checklist* forms to assist Charlotte in becoming more aware of her parenting behaviors and the utilization of selected skills-building strategies at home (discussed below). During the fifth session the *Parenting Goals* form was introduced and then reviewed often subsequently to help keep Charlotte focused on her goals.

Content for Session 1: Collaboration and Initial Functional Assessment

- *Getting Back on Track:* Coming Up with a Skills-Building Plan for Your Child and Family *(primary focus)*
- *Taking Care of Business:* Getting Going and Following Through

During the initial intake prior to commencement of the skills-building intervention, Mr. Smith briefly oriented Charlotte to the "Struggling Kids" program and asked her to read Chapters 2 and 3 for the next meeting. During this first intervention session Mr. Smith guided a functional assessment by asking Charlotte to rate Michael and the family on the ***Examining How Your Child and Family Are Doing*** form (parent book Chapter 2). Charlotte rated the functional areas (using the rating format of 1–2 = struggling/stressed, 3–4 = is in progress, 5–6 = successful/coping), and those ratings (along with the associated characteristics that are consistent with the ratings *in italics*) are summarized below:

__2__ **Child behavioral development**—*Michael displays poor rule following and angry defiance at home and disruptive behavior and defiance at school.*

__3__ **Child social development**—*Michael has friends, but he gets into conflicts with them because he is impulsive and angry.*

__1__ **Child emotional development**—*Michael exhibits frequent hostile verbal outbursts, and he often views himself as being treated unfairly and misunderstood by family members and peers. He is sad and seems to have low self-esteem. Now and then his sense of humor shines through.*

__2__ **Child academic development**—*Michael is not achieving up to his abilities. He hates homework, and he has many unfinished assignments. He and Charlotte have conflicts over his lackadaisical approach to homework.*

__2__ **Parent well-being**—*It is stressful for Charlotte to be looking for a new residence, and she is stressed out with parenting Michael. She is inconsistent in parenting and frequently shouts at Michael out of frustration.*

__4__ **Family well-being**—*There are close bonds between family members, but also frequent conflicts involving Michael, which takes a toll on family cohesion. At times he is physically and verbally aggressive with his mother and siblings.*

Charlotte's primary concerns centered on Michael, especially related to his behavioral and emotional development. She also rated significant concerns for both parent and family well-being. Relative strengths appear to be in terms of Michael's potential social development and academic functioning, which are in progress. Even though he is aggressive and disruptive, he has satisfactory social skills when he is calm, and peers seem to like him. Likewise, he is intelligent and can do well at school if he is in a good mood.

Mr. Smith then led Charlotte to review the *Selecting Skills-Building Strategies to Work On* form (parent book Chapter 2), after which they decided to focus on behavioral and emotional development domains for Michael and overall family well-being. Charlotte expressed a preference to begin with a focus on behavioral development because Michael's behavior was stressing out the entire family. Mr. Smith agreed, knowing that when behavior is a concern, it is often best to begin there and later address other areas of concern once behavior has improved. A comment made by Mr. Smith seemed to resonate with Charlotte. He said that it is often most helpful to begin with "parent management of the child" so that the child can be in a better position to learn "self-management" skills later. They agreed to focus on behavior first and on Michael's emotional skills and broader family skills at a later date.

After some discussion they agreed that the biggest problem at the moment was Michael's rule following. He and Charlotte argue about the same things nearly every day, such as getting up in the morning, bedtime, and homework. Mr. Smith advised Charlotte to read Chapters 5 and 7 of the parent book before the next session.

Mr. Smith spent time building a rapport with Charlotte and Michael by encouraging them not to give up hope of getting along and feeling better, as many families show great improvement and success after learning and practicing new skills. Mr. Smith provided some psychoeducation about the "P's to success" (described in parent book Chapter 2), and at the end of the session he asked the family if the approach discussed seemed to be the right track for them. Charlotte said yes, but Michael said he wasn't sure. He was a bit reluctant to discuss his behavioral and emotional concerns. He wasn't sure the proposed strategies would make a difference.

Content for Sessions 2–4: Focus on Behavioral Development

- *Doing What's Expected:* Teaching Your Child to Follow Rules *(primary focus)*
- *Staying Cool under Fire:* Managing Your Child's Protesting of Discipline and Preventing Angry Outbursts *(primary focus)*
- *Cool Parents:* Managing Your Own Stress to Enhance Parenting

The initial focus was on Michael's rule-violating behavior at home. During each session in this sequence much of the time was devoted to Charlotte. Michael participated in parts of each session too.

Chapter 5 guided Charlotte to set up and enforce house rules. During Session 2, Mr. Smith reviewed the ***Parent Checklist for Child Rule Following*** in the chapter with Charlotte and then prompted her to generate a list of potential rules. Charlotte and Mr. Smith discussed the rules, and Charlotte settled on four of them: "Play video games up to 1 hour a day," "Go to bed by 9:00 P.M. on school nights," "Begin homework by 6:00 P.M. on school days," and "Help with dishes after supper." This was followed by a thorough examination of potential privileges that could be linked to Michael's following of the rules on a daily basis, using the framework of the ***Daily Privileges for Following House Rules*** form (parent book Chapter 5). If Michael followed all four house rules on a particular day, he would have access the **next day** to "screens" (including video games, computer, and TV), his personal music device, and books, magazines, and sports equipment. He would have access to fewer privileges the next day if he followed two or three house rules, including only his personal music device, books, magazines, and sports equipment (losing screens). The fewest privileges would be provided for Michael's following only one or no house rules because under that scenario he could have access only to books, magazines, and sports equipment for the next 24 hours (losing screens and personal music device).

Finally, Michael was invited to participate in the last part of the second session to inform him of the procedures and to get his input. He was calm and able to participate in a helpful manner and had a few good ideas about how to define the rules and his privileges. Michael wanted to start homework at 6:30, after a favorite TV show, and everyone agreed that would be okay. Charlotte set a goal to implement the house rules procedure for the foreseeable future.

Between Sessions 2 and 3, Charlotte used the house rules method. It went well for a few days, and Michael followed the rules for the most part. But he became testy and started protesting after Charlotte removed 24 hours of screen time and personal music device privileges for violating three of the four rules on a particular day. He swore at his mother and pronounced the house rules "stupid" and said that he "hated" his mother. During the next session Mr. Smith reviewed how it was going and tried to enlist Michael's cooperation by explaining that he too could benefit from house rules by having fewer conflicts and arguments with his mother. Mr. Smith explained to Michael that once he complied with the rules for an extended time, he would begin to feel better because there would be more harmony and less stress in the family. Michael gave a sour expression, but he seemed to be taking the concept under advisement.

Chapter 7 of the parent book was an additional focus over the next several sessions. The *Parent Checklist for Child Protests and Angry Outbursts* in that chapter served as a reference for Mr. Smith to discuss and review methods to handle protesting with Charlotte. It was also very helpful to utilize modeling and role playing to get points across and to facilitate skill acquisition. Mr. Smith modeled how to disengage, deescalate, and utilize a patient standoff method for when "Michael" (played by Charlotte) exhibited moderate protesting after losing privileges for not following house rules. Together they role-played Michael refusing to stop playing video games after they had been restricted; Charlotte did her best to represent Michael's persistent arguments, and Mr. Smith stayed cool with authority. Charlotte then replicated the same procedure as she role-played managing the moderate protesting of "Michael" (played by Mr. Smith). Charlotte indicated that she would continue with the house rules procedure and try her best to manage Michael's protesting at home. The look on Charlotte's face as she said this was doubtful and apprehensive.

Charlotte also admitted she still had a tendency to get rattled by Michael. As a result of her concerns and lack of confidence that she could maintain composure and hold her ground with Michael, sections of Chapter 18 were introduced during the fourth session. In particular, Charlotte found it helpful to review the *Parent Staying Calm* procedure. A modeling and role-play sequence followed, in which Charlotte incorporated strategies for staying calm (e.g., slow breathing, coping self-talk) into her efforts to manage Michael's protesting. Directed by Mr. Smith, she imagined herself coping and doing well step by step during a typical conflict with Michael.

It was also during the fourth session that the skills-building strategies used thus far were integrated and focused. Using the *Parenting Goals* form, Mr. Smith led Charlotte to identify several continuing goals. She wrote down these goals: "Follow through with house rules," "Stay calm and avoid power struggles with Michael," and "Catch Michael following rules and staying calm."

There were plenty of challenges along the way as Michael struggled with following the house rules. For several weeks he followed them sporadically. He frequently protested whenever he lost privileges for violating the rules. He would shout at his mother and describe her as "stupid," "unfair," and "so mean."

On one occasion he got on the computer and refused to get off, even though that privilege had been taken away for breaking house rules the day before. He yelled at his mother after she followed the procedure outlined in Chapter 5, so she informed him that the 24-hour screen restriction had to start over (because he had used a screen privilege that had been taken away). Charlotte also remembered what she had read in Chapter 7, and practiced with Mr. Smith, as it pertained to such a power struggle. She used self-talk coping statements such as "Don't let it get to you," "Stay calm and follow through," and "It will get better in the long run if you hang in there," and she disengaged by walking to the next room. Michael pouted and slammed a chair but turned off the computer. Charlotte followed through and did not give Michael his screen privileges until 24 hours later.

At the end of Session 4, Charlotte reported that Michael's rule-following behavior had improved and his protesting had decreased. Things were far from perfect, but they were on the right track. Mr. Smith asked Charlotte and Michael if they intended to celebrate their progress, and together they decided on a family movie night with special treats, and Michael was allowed to choose the movie.

Content for Sessions 5 and 6: Focus on Academic Development

- *Surviving School:* Teaching Your Child to Manage Time, Organize, Plan, Review, and Stay on Task *(primary focus)*
- *Doing What's Expected:* Teaching Your Child to Follow Rules

Charlotte came in complaining about how Michael wasn't keeping up with his schoolwork and that they had been arguing about homework. Mr. Smith asked if it might not be fruitful to focus on Michael's academic development. He noted that Michael's behavior problems at home and school might also improve if he was keeping up at school. Charlotte agreed, and then Mr. Smith led her and Michael to come up with a "school success plan," using Chapter 15 for guidance. During each of these sessions there was also review of how well Michael was following house rules and how well Charlotte was staying calm when interacting with Michael.

It was agreed that Michael would have a mandatory homework time on Sunday through Thursday evenings. During the mandatory homework time they used homework task checklists as described in parent book Chapter 5. Michael was also guided by his mother to work on using his planner and to organize his backpack each day during mandatory homework.

Mr. Smith encouraged Charlotte to provide scaffolding by checking in with Michael when he sat down for homework and checking out with him as he completed it. Charlotte agreed to take him to a movie and buy popcorn if he agreed to try it for five school nights over a week.

Charlotte also helped by communicating with Michael's teachers about making up missed assignments and tests, checking the school online class reports, and then helping Michael organize time to complete the assignments and study for tests during the mandatory homework sessions.

The mandatory homework went well for a week, but then Michael began to balk. He said it was "stupid to study so much" and became irritable whenever Charlotte brought it up. During Session 6 Mr. Smith encouraged Charlotte to PERCON and follow through. They also collaborated in making changes to the house rules. The house rule of "Help with dishes after supper" was removed (it was going well) and replaced with "Do 1 hour of mandatory homework on Sunday–Thursday evening." The next week Michael refused twice to do mandatory homework. Each time Charlotte followed through by noting that one house rule was violated, and he ended up losing screen time privileges as stipulated on the ***Daily Privileges for Following House Rules*** form (parent book Chapter 5). After another week the mandatory homework was going better, and Michael seemed to be accepting it as part of his routine. At one point Michael grudgingly admitted that mandatory homework was helping him because he was keeping up and even got a compliment from his teacher about handing in assignments on time.

Content for Sessions 7 and 8: Focus on Emotional Development

- *You Are What You Think:* Teaching Your Child to Think Helpful Thoughts *(primary focus)*
- *Stress Busters:* Teaching Your Child to Manage Stress

The procedures for mandatory daily homework were tweaked during the next session, but the primary focus of Sessions 7 and 8 was on emotional skills development with Michael. As determined in the initial functional assessment, Michael has some emotional concerns. Through the process of collaborative discussion, Charlotte, Michael, and Mr. Smith explored whether or not it would be useful to work on emotion coping skills development for Michael.

In particular, Charlotte noted that in her observation Michael was a "negative thinker." Mr. Smith reframed negative thinking as "unhelpful thinking." Mr. Smith stated that it is important to know that a negative thought is unhelpful because of how it makes someone feel and act. Mr. Smith reviewed the ***Feelings, Thoughts, and Behaviors Go Together*** chart (parent book Chapter 12) to show Michael how thoughts are related to feelings. As an example, Mr. Smith noted that a typical negative thought for Michael, "She [mother] just wants to run my life!" is admittedly negative, but it is more **unhelpful** than anything. Such a thought makes Michael mad and prone to yell at his mother. Furthermore, Mr. Smith observed that it is true that Michael's mother runs his life to some degree because that is part of a mother's job description, so to keep dwelling on it leads to frustration and acting out against her. Michael kind of agreed, though he wasn't quite sure.

Mr. Smith then asked whether Michael would like to set a goal to work on having more helpful thoughts. Michael was initially uncertain and sarcastically said "I'm not thinking anything." This quip prompted Mr. Smith to ask Michael to complete the **Thinking about Personal Goals** form (parent book Chapter 3). Michael reluctantly went through the steps on the form related to the idea of working on a goal of helpful thinking. His mother encouraged him and provided some examples of unhelpful thoughts he had exhibited in the past, such as believing that people are mean to him or that he hates his mother or sister. Michael eventually agreed that the pros outweighed the cons and that it would be good to work on helpful thoughts, so he agreed to cooperate with his mother and Mr. Smith. He still did not appear outwardly to be fully motivated, but at least he discussed and thought about his unhelpful thoughts and made a public commitment to examine the matter further.

Mr. Smith guided Michael to review the **Unhelpful Thoughts List** (parent book Chapter 13) and encouraged Charlotte to chime in with constructive feedback. Michael realized, and then Charlotte concurred, that he tends to be an unfriendly thinker (thinking people are unfair, that people are mistreating him, etc.). These unfriendly thoughts typify the way Michael sees others when interacting with them, especially his mother and his siblings. After reviewing the **Helpful Thoughts List,** Michael begrudgingly acknowledged that he might benefit from working on friendly thinking.

A procedure was established whereby Michael would talk through the **Advanced Helpful Thoughts** chart with his mother at home if she prompted him. Mr. Smith asked Charlotte to consider giving Michael a small reward for talking through the **Advanced Helpful Thoughts** steps five times so as to enhance his motivation. Charlotte agreed to allow extra video game access on the weekend if he would do this. Thereafter Charlotte would converse with Michael about whether he was being an unfriendly thinker and whether he could change his thoughts to be more like a friendly thinker.

One specific persistent unhelpful thought Michael had trouble with involved thinking that his mother was "unfair" and "mean" for establishing a bedtime on school nights. Eventually he was able to replace that thought with "My mom cares about me and makes me go to bed so I can do better in school." Over the course of several weeks Michael became more aware of his unhelpful thinking tendency, and tried to think more helpful thoughts. Charlotte noted that he was getting angry with people less often.

Some of the Stress Busters procedures (parent book Chapter 14) were also brought into these sessions. Mr. Smith taught Michael and Charlotte the diaphragmatic breathing method. At first Michael laughed at the prospect of something silly like breathing making him feel better, but he gave it a shot and was mildly impressed. He then practiced it for 5 minutes a day between sessions, at home with his mother. Thereafter Charlotte occasionally prompted Michael to "cool down" and do some breathing during mandatory homework whenever he seemed a bit rattled. Sometimes Michael resisted when she did this, but over time he began to cooperate and use the breathing strategy. Charlotte added "Coach Michael to practice and use breathing when stressed" to her **Parenting Goals** form. She removed "Stay calm and avoid power struggles with Michael" from the **Parenting Goals** form because that was going much better.

At the end of the eighth session Charlotte exclaimed that at times it was "like having my old Michael back" in reference to his improved mood. She noted, and Michael concurred, that he was joking around more with his mother and siblings. He was even playing his guitar more like he used to do.

Content for Sessions 9 and 10: Focus on Family Well-Being

- *We Can Work It Out:* Strengthening Family Interaction Skills
- *Let's Get Together:* Strengthening Family Bonds and Organization

After a several-week hiatus, Charlotte brought Michael and his siblings in for several family-focused sessions. A particular emphasis was placed on the **Family Cool-Down** strategy from parent book Chapter 20. After some modeling demonstrations, the family had fun doing role-play exercises depicting how they would use the family cool-down at home. Michael especially liked that he was able to go to his room and do some diaphragmatic breathing when the family arguments heated up. Charlotte was developing more skills and confidence, and subsequently she reported that she was successful in prompting her children to use the strategy on a number of occasions at home, although family conflict continued to some degree. She thought it was making a difference, and Michael said that he felt happier at home because there was less arguing between him and his siblings.

Charlotte complained that her family was very disorganized and frenzied in terms of its day-to-day operations and that they lacked dedicated family time. There was no consistent time for homework or bedtime, and sometimes chores like the dinner dishes didn't get finished. Therefore skills from Chapter 19 were introduced. Charlotte attempted to create and use a relatively flexible schedule for the weekdays that included times for waking up, getting homework done, going to bed, etc. Family members enjoyed coming up with ways that they could build in more rituals and bonding activities. Charlotte decided that they would have Sunday evening dinners, and the children organized a family movie night to occur after dinner.

Content for Sessions 11–14: Maintenance Phase and Final Functional Assessment

- *You Are What You Think:* Teaching Your Child to Think Helpful Thoughts
- *Doing What's Expected:* Teaching Your Child to Follow Rules
- *Surviving School:* Teaching Your Child to Manage Time, Organize, Plan, Review, and Stay on Task

These three sessions were spread out, with four to six weeks between them, and they were attended by Charlotte and Michael. During these meetings there was review of progress and brainstorming around emerging challenges that had come up, all with an aim toward helping Michael and Charlotte maintain the gains they had made. Charlotte was most diligent and focused on the house rules, mandatory daily homework, and continued dialoguing with Michael about helpful thinking. Mr. Smith coached and encouraged them to keep PERCONing and stay on course.

During the last meeting Charlotte and Mr. Smith discussed the ***Examining How Your Child and Family Are Doing*** form (using the rating format of 1–2 = struggling/stressed, 3–4 = is in progress, 5–6 = successful/coping; in parent book Chapter 2). The ratings they assigned after reviewing recent progress (along with the associated characteristics that are consistent with the ratings *in italics*) are summarized below:

4 **Child behavioral development—***Charlotte indicated that Michael was generally following her rules and although he still argued sometimes, it was mostly mild protesting that she could ignore.*

4 **Child social development—***Although not a direct focus of the skills-building intervention, Charlotte observed that Michael was having fewer arguments with his friends, and he was getting in trouble less for goofing around with peers at school.*

3 **Child emotional development—***Michael has become more aware of his unhelpful thinking tendency, and with his mother's prompting to calm down and think helpful thoughts, he is getting better at changing his thoughts to make them more helpful. Charlotte noted that Michael is in a better mood and not so irritable. He is joking around more with his mother and siblings. Michael's emotional functioning is far from perfect, but Charlotte thought it was going in the right direction.*

5 **Child academic development—***Michael made a lot of progress in this area. He was cooperating with mandatory homework and, as a result, had virtually no missing assignments. His teachers were recognizing him for his success and were observing less disruptive and more on-task behavior at school. Charlotte thought that Michael's keeping up at school also reduced his stress level.*

5 **Parent well-being—***Charlotte noted she was using more calming self-statements and that she was staying calmer with Michael. She was happy with her personal progress in developing more skills, which gave her a feeling of confidence.*

4 **Family well-being—***Charlotte thought that family members were getting along better, and Michael said he was feeling happier at home because there was less arguing between him and his siblings.*

As can be seen by the ratings above, Charlotte is reporting good progress in important child- and parent/family-focused domains. She readily admits that the family still needs to do some work, but she is satisfied that they are making progress. Mr. Smith encouraged Charlotte to periodically review progress on her *Parenting Goals* form. Mr. Smith advised her to call him if the family experienced a relapse and reemergence of problems. He congratulated Michael and Charlotte on all of the progress they had made.

Case Management over 14 Sessions

During the course of the intervention, Michael continued to receive psychiatric medication consultation, and he was the beneficiary of an updated IEP. Mr. Smith coordinated with a psychiatrist and school-based officials periodically to facilitate these services.

Although not a direct case management focus, Charlotte reported during each session on her progress with securing affordable housing for the family. Over the course of the intervention she was successful in renting a new, less-expensive apartment and coordinated the move with the help of extended family members. With the decreased financial strain and improved family relations in progress, Charlotte's health became more of a priority and she was able to begin a routine of walking with a friend.

Individual Case 3: Brian, Age 16

Diagnoses: Major depressive disorder, single episode; conduct disorder, adolescent-onset type

Number of sessions: 16

Setting: In-home family therapy

Practitioner: Ms. Cassandra Sanders, licensed marriage and family therapist

Background Information

Brian lives with his mother and father in a rural area just outside of a large city. Both his mother, Katie, and father, Robert, are elementary school teachers. Brian is a junior at a nearby public high school.

Brian is involved with the juvenile court system and on probation (for reasons described below). He is court-ordered to participate in therapy, which is to be provided by a contracted in-home family therapeutic services agency. Brian indicated to his parents that he didn't need therapy, but he would do it to satisfy the court.

The most immediate concerns center on Brian's continuing parent-reported "anger problem" and the fact that he frequently violates parental and school rules. Katie and Robert are afraid that Brian will get himself into trouble again and then be further involved in the court system. The probation officer is convinced that Brian has a significant mental health problem and that if treated effectively, Brian might be diverted from court.

Brian and his parents participated in 16 sessions of combined individual and family therapy that emphasized skills building within the "Struggling Kids" program. Brian also received additional mental health and court-ordered services. He was evaluated by a child psychiatrist, who prescribed and managed medications targeting depressive and agitation symptoms. The court ordered that Brian complete community service and check in with a juvenile officer every 2 weeks.

Brief Review of History and Presenting Problems

Brian was described by his parents as a "normal" child up until middle school, although he struggled some at school early on. He had mild articulation problems and was flagged as a slow reader in the first grade. He received speech/language and Title I services for reading during the first to fourth grades but eventually benefited enough to test out. His grades have since been mostly in the average range. He was always a bit shy but has had several good friends.

Brian developed increasing behavioral problems during early middle school and on into high school years. He got involved with the court due to truancy and curfew citations, an episode of shoplifting, and was charged twice with assault stemming from two incidents where he was violent with his parents. With the exception of the assaults at home, Brian typically gets in trouble while hanging out with his friends, and therefore peer affiliations are a primary concern.

Over the past 2 years Brian has become increasingly depressed. He is very irritable, increasingly withdrawn, and has lost interest in things he used to like doing. Athletically inclined, Brian got involved in sports early in his development, thanks to his parents. Brian was involved in football and baseball and displayed potential, but he dropped out of these sports in high school, according to his father, "because he'd rather play video games in his room." Brian acknowledged that he was tired of getting into trouble but felt discouraged and hopeless that things would ever get better.

Katie and Robert are obviously under a lot of parenting stress. Sometimes they are even afraid of Brian. Whenever they attempt to provide structure, guidance, or discipline Brian's misbehavior, he more often than not responds in an unpredictable and hostile manner. They generally agree on how to parent Brian but find themselves reluctant to do so, wanting to avoid his wrath. Both parents dread the day when Brian becomes an adult, because he could end up in trouble in the adult corrections systems.

The family also has strengths. Both parents are highly educated and are committed to Brian. They have a good marital relationship and mostly agree on child-rearing issues. In the past they all used to get along pretty well, but the parents and Brian have grown distant in recent years.

Family Readiness and Strategies Used to Promote Engagement over 16 Sessions

Based on the preceding information, Ms. Sanders conceptualized Brian and his family as "D" within the **family readiness to engage** framework (see Figure 3.1 in Chapter 3 of this book). This rating is based primarily on the severity of Brian's recent behavioral and emotional problems and his level of resistance to intervention. Although the parents are quite capable, they are struggling to manage and guide Brian, and even avoid doing so because he is so angry and unpredictable. It was obvious from the beginning that it would be difficult to get Brian on board to make changes. Brian tended to minimize problems and blame his parents.

Brian and his family did not present with external practical barriers or obstacles to engagement, but there were several internal factors that needed to be addressed. First, although the parents were motivated, they primarily wanted Brian to receive help. Robert did not see why the parents should be involved since "Brian is the one with the problems." Second, Brian was reluctant to get involved, and his motivation was tentative at best. Ms. Sanders recognized that these internal motivational issues needed to be dealt with at the outset and were likely to be a challenge throughout (examples of how she handled this area are provided below).

Ms. Sanders thought it was paramount to spend time establishing rapport with the family at the outset and to reframe problems to increase the family's buy-in (see Chapters 3 and 4 of this book). Ms. Sanders often reframed Brian's problems within an interactional context. For example, Katie reported that Brian "causes trouble at home." Ms. Sanders discussed how the parents' response to the "trouble he caused" (confronting him and getting into power struggles) exacerbated the problem. Katie began to realize that their responses to him tended to escalate his anger and perhaps there was another way to handle it. The parents gradually came to recognize their own role in the problem. Ms. Sanders also pointed out that the goal of intervention was not to blame anyone for problems but rather to share in responsibility for solutions, and that each of them had a part to play in getting Brian and the family back on track. Over time the parents, and to some extent Brian, increased their motivation.

Ms. Sanders employed motivational strategies from parent book Chapter 3 with both the parents and Brian as the intervention unfolded (described below). Setting goals, prioritizing, making a commitment, and committing effort were all discussed with the parents at one point when they were considering implementing a house rules strategy, and with Brian when he entertained the notion of working on his "stress problem" (elaborated on below).

Katie and Robert recognized that they had a long road ahead of them. Ms. Sanders asked them how they were coping. After a short discussion the couple decided that going out to dinner on occasion would help them maintain the energy for the parenting challenges ahead.

Content for Session 1: Collaboration and Initial Functional Assessment

- *Getting Back on Track:* Coming Up with a Skills-Building Plan for Your Child and Family *(primary focus)*
- *Taking Care of Business:* Getting Going and Following Through

An initial session focused on building rapport with Brian and both of his parents. During the session, Brian was somewhat defensive but acknowledged that he and his family had problems to work on. Robert and Katie both admitted that they were at a "parenting dead end" and not sure what to do.

Toward the end of this session, the parents and Brian were guided by Ms. Sanders to evaluate current functional concerns using the ***Examining How Your Child and Family Are Doing*** form (using the rating format of 1–2 = struggling/stressed, 3–4 = is in progress, 5–6 = successful/coping; parent book Chapter 2). The ratings they produced (along with the associated characteristics that are consistent with the ratings *in italics*) are summarized below:

1 **Child behavioral development**—*Brian frequently violates parent and school rules. He exhibits dishonesty in the form of sneakiness (e.g., truancy, curfew citations) and shoplifting.*

2 **Child social development**—*Brian is able to make friends but tends to get in trouble while hanging out with them.*

1 **Child emotional development**—*There have been many mild and serious episodes of hostility and anger from Brian, especially directed at his parents. He has been increasingly depressed over the last 2 years.*

3 **Child academic development**—*Brian's grades are average, but he misses school a lot and so is at risk for falling behind.*

3 **Parent well-being**—*The parents have a happy marriage and generally agree about parenting, but they are stressed out by Brian's volatile behavior and have been avoiding setting limits on him. They worry a lot about his future.*

2 **Family well-being**—*The family is not too cohesive, and the parent–child bond has grown distant in recent years.*

There was some not too surprising discrepancy in how the parents and Brian rated the problems. Brian did not fully agree with his parents' assessment of the problems and said that the parents needed to change more than he did. Ultimately, Ms. Sanders permitted the ratings above to reflect the parents' point of view, but she did acknowledge that Brian had a different perspective.

Ms. Sanders and the family then reviewed the *Selecting Skills-Building Strategies to Work On* form (parent book Chapter 2) to collaborate on coming up with an initial plan. They all acknowledged that family relations were strained. Ms. Sanders encouraged them to begin with family interaction skills in part because Brian thought that the family was all "messed up," and therefore he might cooperate with this approach at the outset. The parents agreed to start there, but Katie was adamant that Brian also eventually receive some "therapy for his anger problem."

Brian said that he might agree to participate in individual sessions later. Ms. Sanders agreed to revisit the notion of some individual work for Brian later, knowing that motivational engagement can develop slowly over time. She thought that at least he had agreed to a family-focused intervention, and that was a good first step.

Ms. Sanders recommended that the parents read specific chapters from the parent book. They were asked to read Chapter 20 prior to the next session. They were also encouraged to eventually read Chapter 3 whenever it was convenient. Ms. Sanders noted that additional chapters would be suggested later.

Content for Sessions 2–4: Focus on Family Well-Being

- *We Can Work It Out:* Strengthening Family Interaction Skills (*primary focus*)

The second and third sessions were tense and stressful for all involved. During Session 2, Ms. Sanders introduced the *Family Communication Skills* chart from parent book Chapter 20, stating that it might be more productive to work on problems if everyone used good communication skills. They all agreed with that premise, but at first they were most interested in pointing out one another's DON'Ts in family communication skills. They tended to blame each other more than reflect on their own communication style. Brian presented as sullen, and at times Robert was sarcastic.

Ms. Sanders persistently redirected family members to focus on themselves initially and pointed out that they could give each other feedback later. Eventually each family member identified family communication DON'Ts to decrease and family communication DOs to increase for themselves. Several role-play exercises were utilized to assist family members in learning the skills during Session 3. For example, they discussed options for a family vacation next summer while practicing good family communication. The tone became more upbeat as Robert had to laugh at himself when everyone remembered how he fell asleep in the sun and got sunburned. At times the family seemed to enjoy these role-play exercises, which apparently broke the ice and enabled them to examine family communication skills in earnest.

Each of them set family communication goals and then attempted to monitor progress using the *My Family Communication Goals* form from parent book Chapter 20 for several weeks. The specific communication goals set were "Active listening and neutral/natural voice" for Brian, "'I statements' and focusing on here and now" for Katie, and "Brief statements and say what you mean" for Robert. By the end of the third session, family members reported progress in family communication skills. To his credit, Brian admitted that he needed to work harder on his family communication goals, and he appeared to do so.

In Session 3, Ms. Sanders observed that the family had better communication skills and that family members were more motivated to work on their own communication patterns. All of them would occasionally self-correct, pointing out a DON'T in themselves and then restating something as a DO. For example, Robert was going on and on to make the point that Brian should help out more around the house when he stopped, pointed out that he was "lecturing again," and then simply said, "I expect you to help with dishes and trash every day."

During the fourth session, the focus turned toward family conflict resolution. The *Family Cool-Down* method was the focus (parent book Chapter 20). A lot of time was spent in role-playing contrived and then realistic situations of family conflict. Typical conflict resolution role playing included discussion of times for parent-enforced curfew and parents' insistence that Brian tell them where he was going when out of the home.

The family issue of curfew brought on an actual disagreement between Brian and his father during the session. Brian thought his parents' setting a curfew and then waiting up for him was unreasonable, treating him like a baby. Robert began raising his voice and said, "I wish I could trust you to come home on time, but you seem to think that showing your parents some respect and consideration is beneath you!" Ms. Sanders asked if this would be a good time to use the family cool-down method of taking a break from the subject, and everyone agreed. Robert stepped outside of the room briefly, while Brian and Katie chatted for a few minutes. When Robert returned they were able to discuss the curfew issue. It was not fully resolved, but at least they discussed it in a calmer manner.

In later sessions, the family reported moderate success in reducing family conflicts at home. One episode at home was particularly noteworthy. Katie called for a family cool-down when Brian became angry at her for giving him the "fifth degree" when he said he was going out with friends. Brian, Katie, and Robert complied with it, and they were able to come back together after 5 minutes to discuss it. In that instance Brian agreed to call his mother if he left the house of the friend that he had said he was going to visit that evening.

Ms. Sanders encouraged the parents to monitor the family's progress. Katie and Robert planned to hold occasional 10-minute family meetings after dinner. They also said that they would review the *Parent Checklist for Family Interaction Skills* several times per week for a few weeks. Robert found it difficult not to be sarcastic when challenged by Brian because it had become such a habit. It became evident that Brian responded with less anger when his father was able to consistently say what he wanted in a clear and specific manner. These methods helped keep the family on track in their efforts to improve family interaction skills by motivating each member to notice the effect of his or her own behavior.

Content for Sessions 5–8: Focus on Behavioral Development

- *Doing What's Expected:* Teaching Your Child to Follow Rules (*primary focus*)
- *Staying Cool under Fire:* Managing Your Child's Protesting of Discipline and Preventing Angry Outbursts (*primary focus*)
- *Hanging with the "Right Crowd":* Influencing Your Child's Peer Relationships
- *Taking Care of Business:* Getting Going and Following Through

Unfortunately, just prior to the fifth session the parents found out that Brian had sneaked out in the middle of the night to attend a party with friends. Further parental investigation revealed that Brian had also skipped school with friends on two recent occasions. The parents told Brian that they were restricting him from driving the family car until further notice. This resulted in a loud confrontation in which Robert and Brian said some hurtful things to each other. Everyone was discouraged, and it was a major setback. When Ms. Sanders found out about this incident, she suggested that the parents work on behavior management strategies at this juncture, to which the parents wholeheartedly agreed.

Brian's parents were the focus of these four sessions, but Brian did participate in some parts of these sessions too. Consistent with parent book Chapters 5 and 11, Ms. Sanders helped Robert and Katie set up three house rules to monitor Brian better. The house rules centered on setting a specified curfew time, following the four W's when away from home (i.e., telling his parents who, what, where, and when), and limiting his visits to households with parents at home. They also planned to check up on him more to make sure he was in the house at night and was attending school. In accordance with methods outlined in parent book Chapter 5, if any of the house rules were violated, Brian would lose the use of his cell phone for the next day.

Ms. Sanders was aware that the parents were sometimes reluctant to discipline Brian due to his angry responses. She spent some time reviewing motivational ideas consistent with parent book Chapter 3 and dialoguing with the parents about their priorities, commitment, and the effort they would commit to, in effect, clamp down on Brian. It was a good discussion in which the parents voiced their trepidations and then their resolve to follow through with house rules and monitoring.

In the coming weeks, Brian repeatedly violated the four W's house rule, and each time severely protested when his parents asked for the cell phone. Through discussion and role playing, Ms. Sanders taught the parents to use the patient standoff method and to disengage/deescalate from Brian during his protesting moments (parent book Chapter 7) and encouraged them to PERCON with it (parent book Chapter 2). At one point, per the protocol in Chapter 7, Robert and Katie went "on strike"—stopped doing favors or extras for Brian (e.g., doing his laundry or buying requested snacks)—until he gave up the cell so that it could be restricted for 24 hours. Eventually, Brian began following the four W's house rule more consistently and also protested less.

His parents also encouraged Brian to get involved in positive peer activities. Brian agreed to volunteer with the theater production at his high school as a set builder because he was interested in carpentry. Brian made one new friend whom his parents believed had the potential to be a positive influence. Over about a month's time the parents noted that Brian's behavior and mood had improved, but they continued to monitor him and made sure that he was following the house rules by checking with the school and monitoring his comings and goings.

Content for Sessions 9–12: Focus on Child Emotional Development

- *You Are What You Think*: Teaching Your Child to Think Helpful Thoughts (*primary focus*)
- *Stress Busters*: Teaching Your Child to Manage Stress (*primary focus*)
- *Taking Care of Business*: Getting Going and Following Through

The parents requested that Brian learn skills to control his anger. Realizing that Brian was defensive about any focus on himself, Ms. Sanders reframed Brian's "anger problem" as a "difficulty dealing with stress" and suggested that Brian might benefit from "stress management skills training." Brian accepted that framework enough to agree cautiously to meet with Ms. Sanders individually.

During these sessions the format was for Brian and Ms. Sanders to meet for 30 minutes, and then the parents joined for the last 30 minutes. These sessions were anchored by parent book Chapters 13 and 14. The charts from those chapters were used in sessions with Brian, and his parents read the chapters to stay abreast of what Brian was learning, and to get ideas on how they could support the new skills.

Ms. Sanders remembered that Brian was initially not in favor of any individual sessions, and she reasoned that perhaps he was only half-invested in it now. She thought that it would be a good time to ask him to evaluate his priorities and motivation to work on the goal of learning to manage stress. She asked him to complete the **Thinking about Personal Goals** form (parent book Chapter 3) as it pertained to stress management skills. This procedure was useful in assisting Brian to recognize the benefits of such efforts. Through dialoguing with Ms. Sanders and using the worksheet as a catalyst, Brian realized that his stress level was related to his having conflict with family members, which was getting him into all sorts of trouble. After this careful consideration, Brian indicated a desire and motivation to work on stress, and this shift was later shared with his parents.

Ms. Sanders knew that Brian's thoughts were related to his stress. She asked Brian to look at the **Feelings, Thoughts, and Behaviors Go Together** chart (parent book Chapter 12) to learn about how thoughts can be related to stress, and she emphasized the **thoughts** component of the triangle in her psychoeducation with him. From this Brian was able to see that the way he thinks impacts the way he feels and behaves. Additionally, Ms. Sanders had Brian review the *Unhelpful Thoughts List,* and he found it to be an eye-opener. He acknowledged being an unfriendly and downer thinker. He grudgingly admitted this to his parents when they joined in on that session. In response Robert said that he too was sometimes an unfriendly thinker, and Katie noted that she had a tendency to be a downer thinker. Brian and then his parents were also familiarized with the *Helpful Thoughts List*, and the point was made by Ms. Sanders that helpful thinking is a good way to reduce stress. Brian agreed that if he had more friendly and upper thoughts, his stress would go down.

At this point Ms. Sanders led a motivationally focused discussion with Brian and his parents. The sum of it was that Brian made a commitment to fill out the *Advanced Helpful Thoughts Worksheet* five times to earn 5 points toward 10 points needed for a mountain biking trip with his father. His parents pledged to coach Brian at home to use helpful thoughts and to be a good role model of helpful thinking too.

Somewhere in the middle of these sessions the concept of stress management was broadened to include the behavioral component of the triangle on the *Feelings, Thoughts, and Behaviors Go Together* chart (parent book Chapter 12). Brian agreed to work on some additional skills for stress reduction (parent book Chapter 14), including resumption of jogging, which had fallen by the wayside. In addition, Ms. Sanders taught him diaphragmatic breathing to deal with intense higher-stress moments (parent book Chapter 14). Brian then practiced this breathing method for several weeks. It was fairly easy to get Brian to learn and use calming self-statements when stressed, given that he was already familiar with helpful thoughts. Ms. Sanders led several role-play exercises with Brian to simulate getting stressed out with a typical parent–child exchange at home or when a teacher might reprimand Brian at school. During these role plays Brian practiced staying calm by using deep breathing and calming self-statements.

At this point Ms. Sanders suggested that Brian consider declaring his goals on the *Personal Goals (Advanced)* form (parent book Chapter 3). Although he was a bit reluctant to be pinned down, Brian did eventually agree to write down several goals. One goal was to "Think helpful thoughts." After brainstorming with Ms. Sanders, Brian agreed to take the steps to reach that goal by posting the *Helpful Thoughts List* on the inside of his clothes closet door and reviewing it every day. Whenever he opened the closet door, he would see it and be reminded of helpful thoughts. A second goal was to "Get back in shape [to reduce stress]." Ms. Sanders pressed for specificity of this rather broadly stated intention. On the steps to reach that goal Brian indicated that he would "Jog on Monday, Wednesday, Friday, and Saturday mornings" and "Cut down on junk food." A third goal was to "Stay calm." With Ms. Sanders's prompting, Brian indicated he would take the steps of "Practice breathing each day for 5 minutes" and "Try to use calming talk when upset." Brian shared the *Personal Goals (Advanced)* form with his parents. Ms. Sanders encouraged the parents to verbally reinforce Brian's declaration of wanting to work on personal goals.

With the assistance of Ms. Sanders, Brian and his parents also worked out a deal that if he would sincerely review his progress on the *Personal Goals (Advanced)* form five times, he could earn 5 more points. Once he accumulated a total of 10 points his father agreed to take him to a nearby state park for a 1-day mountain biking excursion. This not only motivated Brian but also provided an opportunity for father and son to partake in an enjoyable bonding activity.

During each of these sessions Ms. Sanders made sure to check in with family members about how things were going in terms of family interaction skills and whether Brian was following the house rules (particularly the four W's). The family had their ups and downs, but generally they were making some progress.

Content for Sessions 13–16: Maintenance Phase and Final Functional Assessment

- *You Are What You Think*: Teaching Your Child to Think Helpful Thoughts
- *Stress Busters*: Teaching Your Child to Manage Stress
- *Doing What's Expected*: Teaching Your Child to Follow Rules
- *We Can Work It Out*: Strengthening Family Interaction Skills

During the maintenance phase Brian and his family met on a biweekly basis for Sessions 13–15 and then 1 month later for Session 16. The sessions focused on reviewing family interactions skills and assisting Brian in maintaining helpful thinking and staying calm. The parents continued to monitor Brian, especially in terms of activities when with peers, and primarily focused on two house rules.

During the last meeting the parents completed the ***Examining How Your Child and Family Are Doing*** form (using the rating format of 1–2 = struggling/stressed, 3–4 = is in progress, 5–6 = successful/coping; parent book Chapter 2). The ratings they generated by reviewing recent progress (along with the associated characteristics that are consistent with the ratings *in italics*) are summarized below:

3 **Child behavioral development**—*The parents said that Brian was following the four W's house rule better and his general protesting had declined to a manageable, milder level.*

4 **Child social development**—*Brian followed through with his commitment to be a volunteer set builder with his high school theater production and made a new friend that the parents thought could be a positive influence. Also, by following his parents' rules, Brian was getting into much less trouble with his peers in general.*

4 **Child emotional development**—*The parents thought that Brian was more aware of his downer and unfriendly thinking and was more receptive if they pointed it out to him. They thought he was making attempts to think in a more helpful manner. They noted that Brian had followed through with jogging three to four times per week. Additionally, the parents thought he was using deep breathing and calming* *self statements when stressed during parent–child discussions. Although he was still irritable at times, the parents noted that Brian seemed generally happier.*

5 **Child academic development**—*Brian exhibited increasingly better school attendance, and the parents were pleased that his grades had gone up a bit.*

5 **Parent well-being**—*The parents noted that their parenting stress was much less, and they attributed this to Brian's improved behavior and better family interactions.*

4 **Family well-being**—*The parents were actively practicing good family communication, and they thought Brian was making an effort too. There was much less family conflict, and Brian was responding to his parents' directives in a calmer manner. Brian reportedly enjoyed going mountain biking with his father.*

The parents were satisfied that many areas of child functioning were at least "in progress." Brian's behavior and emotional functioning improvements, along with work on family interactions, made home life bearable and even enjoyable at times!

The topic of relapse prevention was discussed. Ms. Sanders told the parents that there was risk of relapse and that the possible draw of negative-influence peers was particularly strong for Brian. The parents were encouraged to be vigilant in recognizing whether old problems were reemerging and to reread chapters from the parent book and/or call Ms. Sanders. Brian was reassured that he could contact Ms. Sanders at any point in the future.

Case Management over 16 Sessions

As mentioned early in this case example, Brian was being monitored by the juvenile court system and he met periodically with a probation officer. Brian and his parents also consulted with a local child psychiatrist. He received medication targeting mood symptoms. The school's liaison paraprofessional monitored Brian's school attendance and comportment, and notified the parents if any problems emerged. Ms. Sanders maintained regular contact with these professionals and coordinated with them when necessary.

Parent Group Model 1: Within a School- and Community-Based Prevention Program

Targeted children: Children in kindergarten–third grade with teacher-rated aggression

Number of Sessions: 10

Setting: Nonprofit neighborhood family services agency

Practitioners: Bachelor-degreed paraprofessionals with several previous years of experience in human services or educational settings. These individuals participate in extensive initial training and are well supervised as the program is delivered (see Appendix for more information on the training and supervision protocol for the "Struggling Kids" program).

Elements of the "Struggling Kids" program have been incorporated as one facet of services delivery within the "Early Risers" conduct problems prevention program. Early Risers is an empirically validated, multicomponent prevention program designed for early-elementary school-age children showing early aggression and disruptive behavior (Bloomquist et al., 2005). In Early Risers, children with behavioral–emotional problems receive interventions delivered by community- or school-based practitioners for up to 2 years. A "CHILD" component incorporates child skills training and school support interventions, and a "FAMILY" component consists of parent education/skills training and family support interventions. Early Risers has proven effective in reducing behavior problems and in promoting social, emotional, and academic progress in high-risk children (August, Realmuto, Hektner, & Bloomquist, 2001; August, Lee, Bloomquist, Realmuto, & Hektner, 2003; August et al., 2006; Bernat, August, Hektner, & Bloomquist, 2007; Bloomquist, August, Lee, Realmuto, & Klimes-Dougan, 2010).

In a recent iteration of Early Risers, conducted in a low socioeconomic, multiethnic urban setting, an earlier version of the "Struggling Kids" program was used within the FAMILY component. In that initiative, practitioners who worked for a nonprofit family services agency recruited aggressive children in kindergarten–third grade from local schools. Their families came to the agency setting on weekday evenings for 10 biweekly family nights that included a parenting group program (see Bloomquist et al., 2012, for details).

Family Nights

The parent groups are embedded within 90-minute family nights conducted at the community center. Children and parents participate in joint and separate activities, including a 15-minute assembly for all with snacks, a **60-minute parent group** with corresponding 60-minute fun child activity, and a 15-minute parent and child activity at the end of the evening. Typically 8–12 families are invited to the community center for a given family night.

To maximize attendance at family nights, they are scheduled in the early evening (usually 5:00 P.M.) and some provision is made for transportation and child care. Practitioners are encouraged to be as creative as possible to increase attendance, and they routinely send home flyers with the children (who are involved in Early Risers CHILD programming) that emphasize how much fun the children will have and make reminder calls the day before.

Skills Training in the Parent Group

Practitioners lead parent groups, usually with a coleader (student, volunteer, etc.). Parents are empowered as a group to select skills (previously referred to as "Success Plans" in Bloomquist et al., 2012) from the *Selecting Skills-Building Strategies to Work On* form (see parent book Chapter 2). Usually parents select one skills strategy per night. Parents are given a handout of the indicated skills-building strategy (similar to a *Struggling Kids* book chapter) to aid in the education and training process. The time sequence of events within the 60-minute parent group is:

- 15 minutes for introduction, check-in, and progress monitoring
- 30 minutes for didactic instruction, modeling, and role playing
- 15 minutes for parents to discuss and practice the skills presented in that session or to discuss any other pertinent parenting issues

Over time, the parents are exposed to a wide variety of skills-building strategies. They are encouraged to use skills-building strategies as they fit within the goals they have for their home and family. The practitioner encourages each parent to use newly acquired parenting skills at home, and each parent typically agrees to do so.

Although most of the group is focused on skills acquisition, the practitioners always allow enough time for the parents to discuss their own individual concerns and problems. A group climate of trust and open dialogue is promoted. Parents are encouraged to tell stories about difficult parenting moments and to give each other support and advice. Many parents comment that the emotional support they receive as part of the group experience is very important and helpful to them.

It is also important for parents to discuss successes and challenges in using the skills-building strategies at home. Parents are encouraged to support each other and give one another suggestions for following through. In addition, the *Parenting Goals* form is used to track use of and progress with the skills on which each parent is working.

Family Consultation

The practitioners also provide opportunities for parents to receive individual consultation, above and beyond the group program. The Early Risers practitioners offer parents one-to-one sessions to fine-tune the parents' skills repertoire. Sometimes the child is also included in these sessions. This additional component gives parents a chance to individualize training beyond the group. Parents can further refine and/or practice the skills on which they want to work.

In addition, some families are experiencing problems that are serious enough in nature to warrant extra attention of the Early Risers family support strategy within *family*. This extra support entails family-focused case management to help parents set practical goals (e.g., find better housing) and broader case management (e.g., help the child access other school, community, or mental health services).

Typical Outcomes

As one component of a comprehensive four-component Early Risers program, it is impossible to attribute specific effects to just the parenting groups. Nonetheless, anecdotal observations reveal that the parent groups are popular among those who attend. Parents routinely report that they like the practical skills-focused methods they learn. Those who follow through and employ the methods tell other parents in the groups that they are noticing improvements in their child and family. The families of the parents who attend the parent groups typically also attend other components at a higher rate than parents who do not attend the groups.

Parent Group Model 2: Within a Psychiatric Partial Hospital Program

Targeted children: Children (ages 6–11) and adolescents (ages 12–18) with serious mental health problems
Number of Sessions: 6, with an option for family therapy follow-up
Setting: Psychiatric partial hospital settings program with coordinated behavior milieu system
Practitioner: Licensed clinical psychologist

The "Struggling Kids" program is being used in the context of a psychiatric partial hospitalization program. This program provides short-term intensive mental health services to children and adolescents (ages 6–18) with major psychiatric illness during the daytime hours Monday–Friday. Services include psychiatric consultation, child group therapy, family therapy, public schooling, and a parent group that is held one evening per week. A behavior milieu system is used by staff to manage children's on-site behavior and to teach them basic social–emotional skills. The partial hospitalization program has separate program tracks for children ages 6–11 and adolescents ages 12–18. Likewise, there are separate parent groups for the same-age children.

Skills Training within the Parent Group

The parent group program was adapted to meet several logistical challenges. The average child is in the partial hospital program for approximately 6 weeks, which means that parents have the opportunity to participate in six weekly parent group sessions. Therefore, content for sessions is cycled every 6 weeks. The 6-week program cycle corresponds to the functional framework of the "Struggling Kids" program as follows:

- Week 1: Enhancing Your Child's Behavioral Development
- Week 2: Enhancing Your Child's Social Development
- Week 3: Enhancing Your Child's Emotional Development
- Week 4: Enhancing Your Child's Academic Development
- Week 5: Enhancing Your Well-Being as a Parent
- Week 6: Enhancing Your Family's Well-Being

In addition, material and strategies from the "Getting Started and Staying with It" module (parent book Chapters 1–3) that pertain to the tailoring of programming and motivation of the parent and child are discussed, to some extent, during each meeting.

One challenge is the rolling nature of admissions to the program. Parents join the parent group at different points in the 6-week cycle. It is therefore necessary to plug parents into the 6-week sequence based on when their child was admitted. For example, one parent might have joined at Week 1, whereas another came in at Week 5. Most parents are exposed to all six content topic areas over their child's admission in the program. A parent whose child is discharged early has the option of completing the full 6-week parent group program on an outpatient basis.

During each meeting, one of the **Overview** charts provided in Chapters 5–10 of this practitioner volume is used to give parents the "big picture" of the skills-building approach. For example, during Week 1 of the outline above, the **Overview of the Child Behavioral Development Module** chart is reviewed. Similar corresponding **Overview** charts are employed in subsequent weeks. Copies of the *Struggling Kids* book are made available to parents so that they can read corresponding chapters. The primary goal of the parent group is to help parents become familiar with skills-training approaches. The staff encourages parents to be open and share feedback about how the skills training is going with their child. If there is confusion, parents are encouraged to ask questions.

Modeling and role playing are an important part of the sessions. For example, many parents have difficulty managing the time-out procedure with their child. The group leader may role-play, using the parent playing the part of a child, with the leader in the parent role. The group leader may go on to explain the purpose of time-out as a learning tool, not as punishment, and that parents should stay calm and persistent for the most effective use of this tool.

In the parent group there is discussion about practical matters and a significant emphasis on parents supporting one another. These parents are feeling stressed out and sometimes discouraged. Consequently, these practical and support functions are very important. Parent-to-parent brainstorming about common challenges is also emphasized.

Family Consultation

Individual family consultation is available to build on skills-training methods introduced in the parent groups. This component occurs during family therapy sessions as part of the child's 6-week admission and/or on an outpatient basis once the child is discharged. This family consultation provides an opportunity to tailor, refine, and build on skills-building strategies introduced in the parent group. It is a big step for the child to return home after treatment for the entire family, and the more support the child receives, the likelier the program will be a success.

Typical Outcomes

Since the parent group is a portion of the overall comprehensive intervention provided within the partial hospitalization program, it is impossible to note its specific effects. Anecdotal information, however, indicates that attending parents are very satisfied with the information and support received during the parent groups. Those who also receive follow-up sessions just for their family show the best results in terms of skills acquisition and report that the skills training has helped their family.

Parent Group Model 3: Within an Intensive Outpatient Mental Health Program

Targeted Children: Children (ages 8–12) with diagnoses of attention-deficit/hyperactivity disorder and/or oppositional defiant disorder comorbidly with anxiety or depressive disorders

Number of Sessions: 12 parent sessions (1.5 hours) within the context of a 6-week intensive outpatient program that also includes child programming

Setting: Mental health center

Practitioner: Mental health providers under the supervision of a licensed clinical psychologist

A "Struggling Kids" parent group is being used as one component of an intensive 6-week outpatient program for children with behavioral–emotional problems. The program is offered Mondays through Thursdays from 3:30 to 6:30 P.M. over 6 weeks and has child and parent skills tracks. The size of each cohort being served is 8–10 children and their parents at a time. The program is for children ages 8–12 years old, but they are grouped into age cohorts within 2–3 years apart (e.g., 8–10 years).

Child Skills Component

On Mondays through Thursdays the children meet with two staff for 3 hours during the afternoons (72 hours over 6 weeks). The schedule each day is:

- Check-in and recreational activities (3:30–4:30) including snacks, discussion of the day so far, games, crafts, etc.
- Social–emotional skills training using "Second Step" curriculum (Committee for Children, 2011) (4:30–5:30), emphasizing structured skills instruction and practice
- Therapeutic activities (5:30–6:30) such as goals review, academic enrichment/homework, and parent–child activities (6:10–6:30 on Mondays and Wednesdays)

A "leader" and a "co-leader" are deployed, and the staff alternate in these roles. The leader delivers the content of the program (leads a recreational activity, "Second Step" lesson, etc.). The co-leader focuses on a token system, in which children earn points for adaptive behavior that can be exchanged later for rewards. Both staff work together in implementing other procedures of behavior management (time-out, interrupting and redirecting negative peer affiliations, etc.) and prompting skills use throughout all three hours of programming.

The social–emotional skills training hour is based on the "Second Step" program. "Second Step" is a well-regarded, commercially available program that teaches children social, emotion-management, and problem-solving skills with engaging materials and activities. It has programming materials that are calibrated for specific age groups. Skills are taught using presentation, discussion, behavior-rehearsal, and goal-attainment methods. Several randomized controlled studies indicate that "Second Step" increases social–emotional competencies and decreases behavioral–emotional problems in children (Frey, Nolen, Van Schoiack-Edstrom, & Hirschstein, 2005; Grossman et al., 1997). Figure 11.1 shows the content from "Second Step" that is used in the intensive outpatient program.

Parent Skills Component

On Mondays and Wednesdays the parents meet with one or two staff for 1.5 hours from 5:00 to 6:30 p.m. (18 hours over 6 weeks). Delivery of parent skills follows a specified sequence:

- 20 minutes for introduction, check-in, progress on parent goals, review of last week's skill(s), and discussion of any other pertinent parenting issues or topics
- 50 minutes for didactic instruction, modeling, role playing, and discussion of new skill(s)
  - Use the *Parent Checklist* form for that chapter
  - Adjust *Parenting Goals* form if indicated
- 20 minutes for parent–child activity to discuss and practice the skills with child and review progress on the child's goals

The practitioner tries to make the group experience as enjoyable and supportive as possible. Figure 11.1 shows the content from the "Struggling Kids" program that is used in the intensive outpatient program. Parents who miss a session receive an offer of phone consultation the next day to review the "Struggling Kids" chapter for the missed parent group.

There is also a significant emphasis on coordinating between the child skills and parent skills components. On Mondays and Wednesdays there are parent–child activities that center on practice of skills and planning how skills can be used or supported at home. The skills-building methods from the parent skills component are targeted during the parent–child activities. The charts from the "Struggling Kids" program serve to coordinate between child skills and parent skills components and are used to assist parents in transferring skills learned in the sessions to the home context. Figure 11.1 shows the focus of the parent–child activities that is drawn from the "Struggling Kids" program.

Typical Outcomes

Parents complete the ***Examining How Your Child and Family Are Doing*** form (parent book Chapter 3) every other week for a total of three times across the 6-week program. The ratings show improvements over the 6 weeks for most children. Since this is not a controlled research protocol, whether the program causes the ratings improvements or expectancy is at work cannot be determined. Likewise, since parent skills are one of two components being provided, it is not possible to impute specific effects on the parenting groups. Nonetheless, parents do report positive changes, and are pleased with the results, so there are some noteworthy clinical effects. In addition, parents routinely express satisfaction with the parent groups and the "Struggling Kids" program.

Child skills: "Second Step" lessons (delivered over 24 sessions on Mondays through Thursdays)	Parent skills: "Struggling Kids" chapters (delivered over 12 sessions on Mondays and Wednesdays)
1. Being Respectful Learners	1. The Struggling Child
2. Using Self-Talk	2. Getting Back on Track
3. Being Assertive	3. Taking Care of Business
4. Planning to Learn	4. Doing What You're Told
5. Identifying Others' Feelings	5. Doing What's Expected
6. Understanding Perspectives	6. Doing the Right Thing
7. Conflicting Feelings	7. Staying Cool under Fire
8. Accepting Differences	8. Making Friends
9. Showing Compassion	9. Keeping Friends
10. Making Friends	10. That Hurts!
11. Introducing Emotion Management	11. Hanging with the "Right Crowd"
12. Managing Test Anxiety	12. Let It Out!
13. Handling Accusations	13. You Are What You Think
14. Managing Disappointment	14. Stress Busters
15. Managing Anger	15. Surviving School
16. Managing Hurt Feelings	16. Teaming Up
17. Solving Problems, Part 1	17. You Parent the Way You Think
18. Solving Problems, Part 2	18. Cool Parents
19. Solving Classroom Problems	19. Let's Get Together
20. Peer-Exclusion Problems	20. We Can Work It Out
21. Negative Peer Pressure	
22. Reviewing "Second Step" Skills	

Parent–Child Activities (delivered over 12 sessions on Mondays and Wednesdays)
1. Create and discuss "Good Behavior Box" and **Time-Out**
2. Introduce, model, and practice house rules
3. Target, model, and practice social behaviors from **Identifying Social Behaviors to Work On**
4. Discuss, model, and practice **Basic** or **Advanced Social Problem Solving**
5. Discuss, model, and practice **Basic** or **Advanced Feelings Vocabulary** and **Helpful Thinking**
6. Discuss, model, and practice **Staying Calm** methods for child
7. Discuss, model, and practice ignoring and assertiveness with bullies
8. Discuss, model, and practice peer pressure coping skills
9. Review progress with **Basic** or **Advanced Helpful Thinking** and **Staying Calm** skills for child and parent
10. Review progress with **Basic** or **Advanced Helpful Thinking** and **Staying Calm** skills for child and parent
11. Brainstorm child-directed activities that parent and child can do together
12. Introduce, model, and practice **Family Problem Solving** and **Family Cool-Down**

FIGURE 11.1. Child and Parent Skills Training in a 6-Week Intensive Outpatient Program

Implementation Support Protocol for the "Struggling Kids" Program

It has been suggested that implementation support should be utilized in evidence-based practice (Beidas & Kendall, 2010; Bloomquist, August, Horowitz, Lee, & Jensen, 2008). This Appendix describes an implementation support protocol that I have used to train mental health professionals in the evidence-based "Struggling Kids" program at the University of Minnesota and in community mental health centers. This protocol serves as an example of implementation support protocol for an evidence-based practice initiative and also elucidates the skills in which a practitioner should be proficient to deliver the "Struggling Kids" program competently.

Implementation support is also a hallmark of the research validated child- and family-focused skills training programs reviewed in Chapter 2 of this practitioner book. Implementation support applies facilitation strategies designed to promote fidelity and effectiveness in a practitioner's delivery of services (Durlak & DuPre, 2008; Henggeler & Schoenwald, 1999; Weisz, 2004). The usual implementation support facilitation protocol minimally involves the use of manuals, training, technical assistance, supervision, and continuous performance feedback (Beidas & Kendall, 2010). Similar procedures are used in the implementation support for the "Struggling Kids" program.

The *Struggling Kids* Books as a Manual

A manual standardizes the delivery of services and assures that key procedures are utilized in an intervention. This practitioner book and the parent book serve as the manual for the "Struggling Kids" program. This manual gives practitioners explicit instructions for program delivery and suggests fidelity parameters that practitioners should strive to meet. This "Struggling Kids" manual should be used flexibly in delivering skills training to parents and children.

Formal Training

Effective training is considered a staple of evidence-based practice (Becker & Stirman, 2011). A training model for the "Struggling Kids" program is described briefly here. I conduct training up to

12 hours. It consists of a didactic presentation to provide practitioners with knowledge of all facets of the program. Video and live modeling/role-playing exercises are used to convey information and skills during the didactic training.

The training then shifts to practice-simulated role playing. During role plays, practitioners are observed and rated using the *"Struggling Kids" Observer Rating of Practitioner* form at the end of this Appendix. Practitioner trainees are "checked out" to ensure that they meet minimum fidelity standards of program delivery. Role plays are continued until practitioners demonstrate minimal fidelity standards (i.e., mostly "3's" on the *"Struggling Kids" Observer Rating of Practitioner* form).

Technical Assistance and Supervision

Training alone has limited and short-lived effects on practice (Lopez, Osterberg, Jensen-Doss, & Rae, 2011), and it is not as effective as training followed by ongoing technical assistance and supervision (Lochman, et al., 2009). Therefore, ongoing program-related technical assistance and supervision occur after training in the "Struggling Kids" program. Supervision focuses on the application of the program with specific cases under real-world care conditions (i.e., families seeking services). Practitioners meet every week as a group and also receive individual supervision. Cases are reviewed with peers and the supervisor. In addition, the supervisor routinely conducts cotherapy with trainees.

Performance in intervention is enhanced when practitioners receive ongoing feedback about it (Beidas & Kendall, 2010). Thus performance feedback methods—two fidelity-related forms pertaining to trainees' performance in delivering the "Struggling Kids" program—are incorporated into ongoing training and supervision activities.

First, practitioners independently complete the *"Struggling Kids" Fidelity Checklist*, found at the end of this Appendix, after each session. This form lists the most important practice and fidelity parameters, and filling it out allows the practitioner to self-monitor how well he or she is using those parameters in service delivery. The practitioner is also reminded of key fidelity parameters each time he or she fills it out. This checklist is incorporated into chart notes that practitioners make to document service provision for individual clients. The supervisor routinely reviews these checklists as the trainee documents service delivery.

Second, it can also be helpful to have a supervisor or peer observe sessions and complete the *"Struggling Kids" Observer Rating of Practitioner* form. The observer form is similar to the self-report of fidelity but uses another source of data. It gives information from an observer's view as to how well the practitioner is meeting key fidelity parameters. The rating of practitioners on important fidelity indicators during live observation can improve practitioners' fidelity performance (Lochman, Boxmeyer, et al., 2009; Weisman et al., 1998).

These fidelity-related forms are used as feedback methods in working toward proficiency with the "Struggling Kids" program. The practitioner strives to meet as many of the fidelity indicators as possible.

"Struggling Kids" Observer Rating of Practitioner

_____   _____
Child's Name   **Parent Name**

_____   _____
Practitioner's Name   **Date**

Observe the session in an unobtrusive manner. Look for indicators of behaviors pertaining to each of the items. Take notes and give specific examples. At the end of the session, rate the item on a 0–3 scale, as follows:

0	1	2	3
Not applicable	**Not accomplished**	**Partially accomplished**	**Successfully accomplished**

Built Alliance with Family:

____ Developed rapport/trust with parent(s)/guardian(s) through conversation, active listening, providing information, and answering questions

____ Developed rapport/trust with child through conversation, active listening, providing information, and answering questions

Comments: _____

Examined Functional Status:

____ Collaborated with family to determine child struggles and parent/family stresses

____ Collaborated with family to determine skills building

Comments: _____

Promoted Engagement:

____ Dialogued with parent(s)/guardian(s) about their views/concerns of child and/or family and whether skills-building strategies will address them

____ Dialogued with child and parent(s)/guardian(s) to enhance their motivation

____ Reviewed **Progress Monitoring** chart(s), a **Parent Checklist**, and/or the **Parent Goals** form with parent to check in on progress with implementing skills

____ Reviewed a specific chart or form and/or the **Personal Goals (Basic** or **Advanced)** form with the child.

(cont.)

_____ Discussed/brainstormed about obstacles/barriers to using skills and/or progress toward goals

_____ Discussed adapting skills to better fit the cultural background of family

_____ Asked family to evaluate usefulness of the session and skills-building strategies

Comments: _____

Trained Child and/or Family:

Which skills-building strategies (within parent book chapters) was the focus (specify):

_____

_____ Referred to the book and/or provided handout(s)/charts/forms to convey information and skills

_____ Explained skills

_____ Modeled, role-played, and/or practiced skills

_____ Homework assignment given and/or goal(s) were set

_____ Allowed for questions and discussion of procedures

Comments: _____

Provided Family Support and/or Case Management:

_____ Child health/mental health focus   _____ Parent health/mental health focus

_____ Child school focus   _____ Basic family needs focus

Comments: _____

Quality of Delivery

_____ Adequately prepared for the session

_____ Displayed enthusiasm and energy while interacting with parent(s)/child

_____ Asked questions to elicit participation and promote learning

_____ Utilized "fun" modeling and role playing

_____ Used verbal statements to reinforce/encourage parent(s)/child's ideas, comments, questions, etc.

_____ Used nonverbal gestures (e.g., nodding, eye contact) to reinforce/encourage parent(s)'/child's ideas, comments, questions, etc.

_____ Paused to summarize and/or check for parent(s)'/child's comprehension

Comments: _____

"Struggling Kids" Fidelity Checklist

Client Name:_____ **Date:**_____

Diagnostic Codes:_____ **Length of Session:**_____

Practitioner:_____ **Supervisor:**_____

Functional Status, Past Two Weeks (practitioner impression):

(1–2 = struggling/stressed, 3–4 = is in progress, 5–6 = successful/coping)

_____ Child Behav. Dev.   _____ Child Emot. Dev.   _____ Parent W-Being

_____ Child Social Dev.   _____ Child Academ. Dev.   _____ Family W-Being

_____ Other (specify): _____

Family Readiness to Engage Rating (designate one):

_____ A (low severity, high capacity)   _____ C (low severity, low capacity)

_____ B (high severity, high capacity)   _____ D (high severity, low capacity)

Promoted Engagement (designate all that apply):

_____ Reviewed a **Parent Checklist** and/or the **Parent Goals** form(s) with the parent.

_____ Reviewed a specific chart or form from the book and/or the **Personal Goals (Basic** or **Advanced)** form with the child.

_____ Dialogued with parent(s) about their views/concerns of child and/or family and skills-building strategies that will address them

_____ Dialogued with child and parent(s) to enhance their motivation

_____ Discussed/brainstormed about obstacles/barriers to using skills and/or progress toward goals

_____ Discussed adapting skills to better fit the cultural background of family

_____ Asked family to evaluate usefulness of the session and skills

Skills Focus of This Session (check all chapters that apply):

_____ 1. The Struggling Child   _____ 3. Taking Care of Business

_____ 2. Getting Back on Track   _____ 4. Doing What You're Told

(cont.)

_____ 5. Doing What's Expected

_____ 6. Doing the Right Thing

_____ 7. Staying Cool under Fire

_____ 8. Making Friends

_____ 9. Keeping Friends

_____10. That Hurts!

_____11. Hanging with the "Right Crowd"

_____12. Let It Out!

_____13. You Are What You Think

_____14. Stress Busters

_____15. Surviving School

_____16. Teaming Up

_____17. You Parent the Way You Think

_____18. Cool Parents

_____19. Let's Get Together

_____20. We Can Work It Out

_____Other (specify): _____

_____

Trained Child and/or Family (designate all that apply):

_____ Referred to the parent book and/or provided handout(s)/charts/forms to convey information and skills

_____ Explained skills

_____ Modeled, role-played, and/or practiced skills

_____ Homework assignment given and/or goal(s) were set

_____ Allowed for questions and discussion of procedures

Family Progress (rate below):

To what extent was the *parent(s)* attentive, cooperative, and participating during the meeting?

_____ 1 = Not at all _____ 2 = A little bit _____ 3 = Somewhat _____ 4 = Pretty good _____ 5 = Very much

To what extent was the *child* attentive, cooperative, and participating during the meeting?

_____ 1 = Not at all _____ 2 = A little bit _____ 3 = Somewhat _____ 4 = Pretty good _____ 5 = Very much

To what extent has the family worked on or made progress toward any *skills-building strategies* since last meeting?

_____ 1 = No work/progress _____ 3 = Some work/progress _____ 5 = Significant work/progress

_____ 2 = A little work/progress _____ 4 = Good work/progress _____ NA

(cont.)

To what extent has the family worked on or made progress toward any *other goals* since last meeting?
Specify goal: _____

_____ 1 = No work/progress   _____ 3 = Some work/progress   _____ 5 = Significant work/
                                                                                           progress

_____ 2 = A little work/progress   _____ 4 = Good work/progress   _____ NA

Provided Family Support and/or Case Management (designate all that apply):

_____ Child health/mental health focus   _____ Child school focus

_____ Parent health/mental health focus   _____ Basic family needs focus

Narrative Description of Session *(describe session or meeting)*:

_____

_____

_____

_____

_____

_____

_____

_____

_____

_____

_____

_____

_____

_____

_____

References

Alexander, J., Pugh, C., Parsons, B., & Sexton, T. (2000). Functional family therapy. In D. S. Elliott (Ed.), *Blueprints for violence prevention* (Vol. 3). Boulder, CO: Venture.

Allwood, M. A., & Bell, D. J. (2008). A preliminary examination of emotional and cognitive mediators in the relations between violence exposure and violent behaviors in youth. *Journal of Community Psychology, 36,* 989–1007.

American Psychological Association Presidential Task Force on Evidence-Based Practice. (2006). Evidence-based practice in psychology. *American Psychologist, 61,* 271–285.

Armbruster, P., & Kazdin, A. E. (1994). Attrition in child psychotherapy. In T. H. Ollendick & R. J. Prinz (Eds.), *Advances in clinical child psychology* (Vol. 16, pp. 81–108). New York: Plenum Press.

August, G. J., Bloomquist, M. L., Lee, S. S., Realmuto, G. M., & Hektner, J. M. (2006). Can evidence-based prevention programs be sustained in community systems-of-care?: The Early Risers advanced-stage effectiveness trial. *Prevention Science, 7,* 151–165.

August, G. J., Gewirtz, A., & Realmuto, G. M. (2009). Moving the field of prevention from science to service: Integrating evidence-based preventive interventions into community practice through adapted and adaptive models. *Applied and Preventive Psychology, 14,* 1–96.

August, G. J., Lee, S. S., Bloomquist, M. L., Realmuto, G. M., & Hektner, J. M. (2003). Dissemination of an evidence-based preventive innovation for aggressive children living in diverse, urban neighborhoods. *Prevention Science, 4,* 271–286.

August, G. J., Lee, S. S., Bloomquist, M. L., Realmuto, G. M., & Hektner, J. M. (2004). Maintenance effects of an evidence-based prevention innovation for aggressive children living in culturally diverse urban neighborhoods: The Early Risers effectiveness study. *Journal of Emotional and Behavioral Disorders, 12,* 194–205.

August, G. J., Realmuto, G. M., Hektner, J. M., & Bloomquist, M. L. (2001). An integrated components preventive intervention for aggressive elementary school children: The Early Risers program. *Journal of Consulting and Clinical Psychology, 69,* 614–626.

Baker, L. A., Raine, A., Liu, J., & Jacobson, K. C. (2008). Differential genetic and environmental influences on reactive and proactive aggression in children. *Journal of Abnormal Child Psychology, 36,* 1265–1278.

Baldwin, S. A., Christian, S., Berkeljon, A., & Shadish, W. R. (2012). The effects of family therapies for adolescent delinquency and substance abuse: A meta-analysis. *Journal of Marital and Family Therapy, 38,* 281–304.

Barkley, R. A. (1997). *Defiant children: A clinician's manual for assessment and parent training* (2nd ed.). New York: Guilford Press.

Barkley, R. A. (2006). *Attention-deficit hyperactivity disorder: A handbook for diagnosis and treatment* (3rd ed.). New York: Guilford Press.

Barkley, R. A., Edwards, G. H., & Robin, A. L. (1999). *Defiant teens: A clinician's manual for assessment and family intervention.* New York: Guilford Press.

Barlow, J., Coren, E., & Stewart-Brown, S. (2002). Meta-analysis of the effectiveness of parenting programs in improving maternal psychosocial health. *British Journal of General Practice, 52,* 223–233.

Barrera, M., Jr., & Castro, F. G. (2006). A heuristic framework for the cultural adaptation of interventions. *Clinical Psychology: Science and Practice, 13,* 311–316.

Becker, K. D., & Stirman, S. W. (2011). The science of

training in evidence-based treatments in the context of implementation programs: Current status and prospects for the future. *Administration and Policy in Mental Health and Mental Health Services Research, 38,* 217–222.

Beelmann, A., Pfingsten, U., & Losel, F. (1994). Effects of training social competence in children: A meta-analysis of recent evaluation studies. *Journal of Clinical Child Psychology, 23,* 260–271.

Beidas, R. S., & Kendall, P. C. (2010). Training therapists in evidence-based practice: A critical review of studies from a systems-contextual perspective. *Clinical Psychology: Science and Practice, 17,* 1–30.

Bernat, D., August, G. J., Hektner, J. M., & Bloomquist, M. L. (2007). The Early Risers preventive intervention: Six-year outcomes and meditational processes. *Journal of Abnormal Child Psychology, 35,* 605–617.

Biegel, G. M., Brown, K. W., Shapiro, S. L., & Schubert, C. M. (2009). Mindfulness-based stress reduction for the treatment of adolescent psychiatric outpatients: A randomized clinical trial. *Journal of Consulting and Clinical Psychology, 77,* 855–866.

Bierman, K. L., Greenberg, M. T., & Conduct Problems Prevention Research Group. (1996). Social skills training in the Fast Track program. In R. D. Peters & R. J. McMahon (Eds.), *Preventing childhood disorders, substance abuse, and delinquency* (pp. 65–89). Thousand Oaks, CA: Sage.

Blechman, E. A., Prinz, R. J., & Dumas, J. E. (1995). Coping, competence, and aggression prevention. *Applied and Preventive Psychology, 4,* 211–232.

Bloomquist, M. L. (2006). *Skills training for children with behavior problems: A parent and practitioner guidebook* (rev. ed.). New York: Guilford Press.

Bloomquist, M. L., August, G. J., Horowitz, J., Lee, S. S., & Jensen, C. (2008). Moving from science to practice: Transposing and sustaining the "Early Risers" conduct problems prevention program in a community service system. *Journal of Primary Prevention, 29,* 215–229.

Bloomquist, M. L., August, G. J., Lee, C.-Y. S., Realmuto, G. M., & Klimes-Dougan, B. (2010, June). *Going to scale with the Early Risers conduct problems prevention program.* Presentation as part of Going to Scale: Implementation of Sustainable District- and State-Level Prevention Infrastructure symposium presented at the 18th annual meeting of the Society for Prevention Research, Denver, Colorado.

Bloomquist, M. L., August, G. J., Lee, S. S., Berquist,

B. E., & Mathy, R. M. (2005). Targeted prevention of antisocial behavior in children: The Early Risers "Skills for Success" program. In R. G. Steele & M. C. Roberts (Eds.), *Handbook of mental health services for children, adolescents, and families* (pp. 201–214). New York: Kluwer Academic/Plenum.

Bloomquist, M. L., August, G. J., Lee, S. S., Piehler, T., & Jensen, M. (2012). Parent participation within community center or in-home outreach delivery models of the Early Risers conduct problems prevention program. *Journal of Child and Family Studies, 21,* 368–383.

Bloomquist, M. L., Horowitz, J. L., August, G. J., Lee, C.-Y. S., Realmuto, G. M., & Klimes-Dougan, B. (2009). Understanding parent participation in a going-to-scale implementation trial of the Early Risers conduct problems prevention program. *Journal of Child and Family Studies, 18,* 710–718.

Bloomquist, M. L., & Schnell, S. V. (2002). *Helping children with aggression and conduct problems: Best practices for intervention.* New York: Guilford Press.

Borntrager, C. F., Chorpita, B. F., Higa-McMillan, C., & Weisz, J. R. (2009). Provider attitudes toward evidence-based practices: Are the concerns with the evidence or with the manuals? *Psychiatric Services, 60,* 677–681.

Brondino, M. J., Henggeler, S. W., Rowland, M. D., Pickrel, S. G., Cunningham, P., & Schoenwald, S. (1997). Multisystemic therapy and the ethnic minority client: Culturally responsive and clinically effective. In D. K. Wilson, J. K. Rodriguez, & W. Taylor (Eds.), *Health-promoting and health-compromising behaviors among minority adolescents* (pp. 229–250). Washington, DC: American Psychological Association.

Brownlie, E. B., Beitchman, J. H., Escobar, M., Young, A., Atkinson, L., Johnson, C., et al. (2004). Early language impairment and young adult delinquent and aggressive behavior. *Journal of Abnormal Child Psychology, 32,* 453–467.

Burke, J., & Loeber, R. (2010). Oppositional defiant disorder and the explanation of the comorbidity between behavioral disorders and depression. *Clinical Psychology: Science and Practice, 17,* 319–326.

Carroll, K. M., Martino, S., & Rounsaville, B. J. (2010). No train, no gain? *Clinical Psychology Science and Practice, 17,* 36–40.

Castro, G., Barrera, M., & Holleran Steiker, L. K. (2010).

Issues and challenges in the design of culturally adapted evidence-based interventions. *Annual Review of Clinical Psychology, 6,* 213–239.

Chaffin, M., Funderburk, B., Bard, D., Valle, L. A., & Gurwitch, R. (2011). A combined motivation and parent–child interaction therapy package reduces child welfare recidivism in a randomized dismantling field trial. *Journal of Consulting and Clinical Psychology, 79,* 84–95.

Chaffin, M., Valle, L. A., Funderburk, B., Gurwitch, R., Silovsky, J., Bard, D., et al. (2009). A motivational intervention can improve retention in PCIT for low-motivation child welfare clients. *Child Maltreatment, 14,* 356–368.

Chorpita, B. F. (2007). *Modular cognitive-behavioral therapy for childhood anxiety disorders.* New York: Guilford Press.

Chorpita, B. F., & Daleiden, E. L. (2009). Mapping evidence-based treatments for children and adolescents: Application of the distillation and matching model to 615 treatments from 322 randomized trials. *Journal of Consulting and Clinical Psychology, 77,* 566–579.

Chorpita, B. F., Reise, R., Weisz, J. R., Grubbs, K., Becker, K. D., Krull, J. L., et al. (2010). Evaluation of the brief problem checklist: Child and caregiver interviews to measure clinical progress. *Journal of Consulting and Clinical Psychology, 78,* 526–536.

Chorpita, B. F., Taylor, A. A., Francis, S. E., Moffitt, C., & Austin, A. A. (2004). Efficacy of modular cognitive behavior therapy for childhood anxiety disorders. *Behavior Therapy, 35,* 263–287.

Chu, B., & Harrison, T. L. (2007). Disorder-specific effects of CBT for anxious and depressed youth: A meta-analysis of candidate mediators of change. *Clinical Child and Family Psychology Review, 10,* 352–372.

Chu, B., & Kendall, P. C. (2004). Positive association of child involvement and treatment outcome within a manual-based cognitive-behavioral treatment for children with anxiety. *Journal of Consulting and Clinical Psychology, 72,* 821–829.

Cicchetti, D., & Toth, S. L. (2009). The past achievements and future promises of developmental psychopathology: The coming of age of a discipline. *Journal of Child Psychology and Psychiatry, 50,* 16–25.

Coard, S. I., Wallace, S. A., Stevenson, H. C., Jr., & Brotman, L. M. (2004). Towards culturally relevant preventive interventions: The consideration of racial socialization in parent training with African American families. *Journal of Child and Family Studies, 13,* 277–293.

Coatsworth, J. D., Duncan, L. G., Greenberg, M. T., & Nix, R. L. (2010). Changing parents' mindfulness, child management skills and relationship quality with their youth: Results from a randomized pilot intervention trial. *Journal of Child and Family Studies, 19,* 203–217.

Committee for Children. (2011). *Second Step (rev.): A violence prevention curriculum.* Seattle: Author.

Connor, D. F. (2002). *Aggression and antisocial behavior in children and adolescents: Research and treatment.* New York: Guilford Press.

Crick, N. R., & Dodge, K. A. (1994). A review and reformulation of social information processing mechanisms in children's social adjustment. *Psychological Bulletin, 115,* 74–101.

Crick, N. R., & Dodge, K. A. (1996). Social information-processing mechanisms in reactive and proactive aggression. *Child Development, 67,* 993–1002.

Crick, N. R., Ostrov, J. M., & Werner, N. E. (2006). A longitudinal study of relational aggression, physical aggression, and children's social–psychological adjustment. *Journal of Abnormal Child Psychology, 34,* 131–142.

Crowe, S. L., & Blair, R. J. R. (2008). The development of antisocial behavior: What can we learn from functional neuroimaging studies? *Development and Psychopathology, 20,* 1145–1159.

Cummings, E. M., Davies, P. T., & Campbell, S. (2000). *Developmental psychopathology and family process: Theory, research, and clinical implications.* New York: Guilford Press.

Dane, A. V., & Schneider, B. H. (1998). Program integrity in primary and early secondary prevention: Are implementation efforts out of control? *Clinical Psychology Review, 18,* 23–45.

David-Ferdon, C., & Kaslow, N. J. (2008). Evidence-based psychological treatments for child and adolescent depression. *Journal of Clinical Child and Adolescent Psychology, 37,* 62–104.

Dawson, P., & Guare, R. (2010). *Executive skills in children and adolescents: A practical guide to assessment and intervention* (2nd ed.). New York: Guilford Press.

Deater-Deckard, K., Dodge, K. A., Bates, J. E., & Pettit, G. S. (1998). Multiple risk factors in the development of externalizing behavior problems: Group and individual differences. *Development and Psychopathology, 10,* 469–493.

de Graaf, I., Speetjens, P., Smit, F., De Wolf, M., & Tavecchio, L. (2008). Effectiveness of the triple P positive parenting program on behavioral problems in children. *Behavior Modification, 32*, 714–735.

de Haan, A. D., Prinzie, P., & Dekovic, M. (2010). How and why children change in aggression and delinquency from childhood to adolescence: Moderation of overreactive parenting by child personality. *Journal of Child Psychology and Psychiatry, 51*, 725–733.

DeRosier, M. E., & Gillione, M. (2007). Effectiveness of a parent training program for improving children's social behavior. *Journal of Child and Family Studies, 16*, 660–670.

Dishion, T. J., Nelson, S. E., & Yasui, M. (2005). Predicting early adolescent gang involvement from middle school adaptation. *Journal of Clinical Child and Adolescent Psychology, 34*, 62–73.

Dishion, T. J., & Stormshak, E. (2007). *Intervening in children's lives: An ecological, family centered approach to mental health care.* Washington, DC: American Psychological Association.

Dishion, T. J., & Tipsord, J. M. (2011). Peer contagion in child and adolescent social and emotional development. *Annual Review of Psychology, 62*, 189–214.

Dodge, K. A., Coie, J. D., & Lynam, D. (2006). Aggression and antisocial behavior in youth. In W. Damon (Series Ed.) & N. Eisenberg (Vol. Ed.), *Handbook of child psychology: Vol. 3. Social, emotional, and personality development* (6th ed., pp. 719–788). Hoboken, NJ: Wiley.

Dowell, K. A., & Ogles, B. M. (2010). The effects of parent participation on child psychotherapy outcome: A meta-analytic review. *Journal of Clinical Child and Adolescent Psychology, 39*, 151–162.

Drugli, M. B., Larsson, B., Fossum, S., & Mørch, W.-T. (2010). Five- to six-year outcome and its prediction for children with ODD/CD treated with parent training. *Journal of Child Psychology and Psychiatry, 51*, 559–566.

Dumas, J. E., Arriaga, X., Begle, A. M., & Longoria, Z. (2010). "When will your program be available in Spanish?": Adapting an early parenting intervention for Latino families. *Cognitive and Behavioral Practice, 17*, 176–187.

Dumas, J. E., Begle, A. E., French, B., & Pearl, A. (2010). Effects of monetary incentives on engagement in the PACE parenting program. *Journal of Clinical Child and Adolescent Psychology, 39*, 302–313.

Dumas, J. E., Blechman, E. A., & Prinz, R. J. (1994). Aggressive children and effective communication. *Aggressive Behavior, 20*, 347–358.

Dumas, J. E., Rollock, D., Prinz, R. J., Hops, H., & Blechman, E. A. (1999). Cultural sensitivity: Problems and solutions in applied preventive intervention. *Applied and Preventive Psychology, 8*, 175–196.

Duncan, L. G., Coatsworth, J. D., & Greenberg, M. T. (2009). Model of mindful parenting: Implications for parent–child relationships and prevention research. *Clinical Child and Family Psychology Review, 12*, 255–270.

Durlak, J. A., & DuPre, E. P. (2008). Implementation matters: A review of research on the influence of implementation on program outcomes and the factors affecting implementation. *American Journal of Community Psychology, 41*, 327–350.

Erath, S. A., El-Sheikh, M., & Cummings, E. M. (2009). Harsh parenting and child externalizing behavior: Skin conductance level reactivity as a moderator. *Child Development, 80*, 578–592.

Eyberg, S. M., & Boggs, S. R. (1998). Parent–child interaction therapy for oppositional preschoolers. In C. E. Schaefer & J. M. Briesmeister (Eds.), *Handbook of parent training: Parents as co-therapists for children's behavior problems* (2nd ed., pp. 61–97). New York: Wiley.

Eyberg, S. M., Nelson, M. M., & Boggs, S. R. (2008). Evidence-based psychosocial treatments for children and adolescents with disruptive behavior. *Journal of Clinical Child and Adolescent Psychology, 37*, 215–237.

Fergusson, D. M., & Lynskey, M. T. (1997). Early reading difficulties and later conduct problems. *Journal of Child Psychology and Psychiatry, 38*, 899–907.

Fernandez, M., & Eyberg, S. (2009). Predicting treatment and follow-up attrition in parent–child interaction therapy. *Journal of Abnormal Child Psychology, 37*, 431–441.

Forgatch, M. S., Patterson, G. R., DeGarmo, D. S., & Beldavs, Z. G. (2009). Testing the Oregon delinquency model with 9-year follow-up of the Oregon Divorce Study. *Development and Psychopathology, 21*, 637–660.

Fowler, P., Tompsett, C., Braciszewski, J., Jacques-Tiura, A., & Baltes, B. (2009). Community violence: A metaanalysis on the effect of exposure and mental health outcomes of children and adolescents. *Development and Psychopathology, 21*, 227–259.

Frankel, F., Myatt, R., Cantwell, D. P., & Feinberg, D. (1997). Parent assisted transfer of children's social skills training: Effects on children with and without attention-deficit/hyperactivity disorder. *Journal of the American Academy of Child and Adolescent Psychiatry, 36,* 1056–1064.

Frey, K. S., Nolen, S., Van Schoiack-Edstrom, L., & Hirschstein, M. (2005). Effects of a school-based social–emotional competence program: Linking children's goals, attributions, and behavior. *Journal of Applied Developmental Psychology, 26,* 171–200.

Frick, P. J., Kamphaus, R. W., Lahey, B. B., Loeber, R., Christ, M. A., Hart, E. L., et al. (1991). Academic underachievement and the disruptive behavior disorders. *Journal of Consulting and Clinical Psychology, 59,* 289–294.

Frick, P. J., & Nigg, J. T. (2012). Current issues in the diagnosis of attention-deficit/hyperactivity disorder, oppositional defiant disorder, and conduct disorder. *Annual Review of Clinical Psychology, 8,* 77–107.

Garland, A. F., Brookman-Fraze, L., & Chavira, D. A. (2010). Are we doing our homework? *Clinical Psychology: Science and Practice, 17,* 162–165.

Garland, A. F., Hawley, K. M., Brookman-Fraze, L., & Hurlburt, M. S. (2008). Identifying common elements of evidence-based psychosocial treatments for children's disruptive behavior problems. *Journal of the American Academy of Child and Adolescent Psychiatry, 47,* 505–514.

Griffin, K. W., Samuolis, J., & Williams, C. (2011). Efficacy of a self-administered home-based parent intervention on parenting behaviors for preventing adolescent substance use. *Journal of Child and Family Studies, 20,* 319–325.

Grossman, D. C., Neckerman, H. J., Koepsell, T. D., Liu, P. Y., Asher, K. N., Beland, K., et al. (1997). Effectiveness of a violence prevention curriculum among children in elementary school: A randomized controlled trial. *Journal of the American Medical Association, 277,* 1605–1611.

Hawes, D., & Dadds, M. R. (2005). Callous–unemotional traits are a risk factor for poor treatment response in young conduct problem children. *Journal of Consulting and Clinical Psychology, 73,* 737–741.

Hawes, D. J., Brennan, J., & Dadds, M. R. (2009). Cortisol, callous-unemotional traits, and pathways to antisocial behavior. *Current Opinion in Psychiatry, 22,* 357–362.

Henggeler, S. W., Pickrel, S. G., Brondino, M. J., & Crouch, J. L. (1996). Eliminating (almost) treatment dropout of substance abusing or dependent delinquents through home-based multisystemic therapy. *American Journal of Psychiatry, 153,* 427–428.

Henggeler, S. W., & Schoenwald, S. K. (1999). The role of quality assurance in achieving outcomes in MST programs. *Journal of Juvenile Justice and Detention Services, 14,* 1–17.

Henggeler, S. W., Schoenwald, S. K., Borduin, C. M., Rowland, M. D., & Cunningham, P. B. (2009). *Multisystemic therapy for antisocial behavior in children and adolescents* (2nd ed.). New York: Guilford Press.

Hinshaw, S. P., & Melnick, S. (1995). Peer relationships in children with attention-deficit/hyperactivity disorder with and without comorbid aggression. *Development and Psychopathology, 7,* 627–647.

Hoeve, M., Dubas, J. S., Eichelsheim, V. I., van der Laan, P. H., Smeenk, W., & Gerris, J. R. M. (2009). The relationship between parenting and delinquency: A meta-analysis. *Journal of Abnormal Child Psychology, 37,* 749–775.

Holmbeck, G. N., Devine, K. A., & Bruno, E. F. (2010). Developmental issues and considerations in research and practice. In J. R. Weisz & A. E. Kazdin (Eds.). *Evidence-based psychotherapies for children and adolescents* (2nd ed., pp. 29–43). New York: Guilford Press.

Hoza, B., Johnston, C., Pillow, D., & Ascough, J. C. (2006). Predicting treatment response for childhood attention-deficit/hyperactivity disorders: Introduction of a heuristic model to guide research. *Applied and Preventive Psychology, 11,* 215–229.

Hubbard, J. A., McAuliffe, M. D., Morrow, M. T., & Romano, L. J. (2010). Reactive and proactive aggression in childhood and adolescence: Precursors, outcomes, processes, experiences, and measurement. *Journal of Personality, 78,* 95–118.

Huey, S. J., & Polo, A. J. (2008). Evidence-based psychosocial treatments for ethnic minority youth: A review and meta-analysis. *Journal of Clinical Child and Adolescent Psychology, 37,* 262–301.

Ingoldsby, E. M. (2010). Review of interventions to improve family engagement and retention in parent and child mental health programs. *Journal of Child and Family Studies, 19,* 629–645.

Insel, T. R. (2009). Translating scientific opportunity into public health impact: A strategic plan for research on mental illness. *Archives of General Psychiatry, 66,* 128–133.

Ishikawa, S. S., & Raine, A. (2003). Prefrontal deficits

and antisocial behavior: A causal model. In B. B. Lahey, T. E. Moffett, & A. Caspi (Eds.), *Causes of conduct disorder and juvenile delinquency* (pp. 277–304). New York: Guilford Press.

Jensen-Doss, A., Hawley, K. M., Lopez, M., & Duvivier Osterberg, L. (2009). Using evidence-based treatments: The experiences of youth providers working under a mandate. *Professional Psychology: Research and Practice, 40,* 417–424.

Johnson, E., Mellor, D., & Brann, P. (2008). Differences in dropout between diagnoses in child and adolescent mental health services. *Clinical Child Psychology and Psychiatry, 13,* 515–530.

Johnston, C., Mah, J. W. T., & Regambal, M. (2010). Parenting cognitions and treatment beliefs as predictors of experience using behavioral parenting strategies in families of children with attention-deficit/hyperactivity disorder. *Behavior Therapy, 41,* 491–504.

Kaminski, J. W., Valle, L. A., Filene, J. H., & Boyle, C. L. (2008). A meta-analytic review of components associated with parent training program effectiveness. *Journal of Abnormal Child Psychology, 36,* 567–589.

Kazantzis, N., Whittington, C., & Dattilio, F. (2010). Meta-analysis of homework effects in cognitive and behavioral therapy: A replication and extension. *Clinical Psychology: Science and Practice, 17,* 144–156.

Kazdin, A. E. (1996). Dropping out of child psychotherapy: Issues for research and implications for practice. *Clinical Child Psychology and Psychiatry, 1,* 133–156.

Kazdin, A. E. (2003). Problem-solving skills training and parent management training for conduct disorder. In A. E. Kazdin & J. R. Weisz (Eds.), *Evidence-based psychotherapies for children and adolescents* (pp. 241–262). New York: Guilford Press.

Kazdin, A. E. (2005). *Parent management training: Treatment for oppositional, aggressive, and antisocial behavior in children and adolescents.* New York: Oxford University Press.

Kazdin, A. E. (2008). Evidence-based treatment and practice: New opportunities to bridge clinical research and practice, enhance the knowledge base, and improve patient care. *American Psychologist, 63,* 146–159.

Kazdin, A. E., Holland, L., & Crowley, M. (1997). Family experience of barriers to treatment and premature termination of child therapy. *Journal of Consulting and Clinical Psychology, 65,* 453–463.

Kazdin, A. E., Holland, L., Crowley, M., & Breton, S. (1997). Barriers to Participation in Treatment Scale: Evaluation and validation in the context of child outpatient treatment. *Journal of Child Psychology and Psychiatry, 38,* 1051–1062.

Kazdin, A. E., Marciano, P. L., & Whitley, M. K. (2005). The therapeutic alliance in cognitive-behavioral treatment of children referred for oppositional, aggressive, and antisocial behavior. *Journal of Consulting and Clinical Psychology, 73,* 726–730.

Kazdin, A. E., & Whitley, M. K. (2006). Pretreatment social relations, therapeutic alliance, and improvements in parenting practices in parent management training. *Journal of Consulting and Clinical Psychology, 74,* 346–355.

Kazdin, A. E., Whitley, M., & Marciano, P. L. (2006). Child–therapist and parent–therapist alliance and therapeutic change in the treatment of children referred for oppositional, aggressive, and antisocial behavior. *Journal of Child Psychology and Psychiatry, 47,* 436–445.

Kling, A., Forster, M., Sundell, K., & Melin, L. (2010). A randomized controlled effectiveness trial of parent management training with varying degrees of therapist support. *Behavior Therapy, 41,* 530–542.

Kohen, D. E., Leventhal, T., Dahinten, S., & McIntosh, C. M. (2008). Neighborhood disadvantage: Pathways of effects for young children. *Child Development, 79,* 156–169.

Kolko, D. J., Baumann, B. L., Bukstein, O. G., & Brown, E. J. (2007). Internalizing symptoms and affective reactivity in relation to the severity of aggression in clinically referred, behavior-disordered children. *Journal of Child and Family Studies, 16,* 745–759.

Kolko, D. J., Dorn, L. D., Bukstein, O. J., Pardini, D., Holden, E. A., & Hart, J. (2009). Community vs. clinic-based modular treatment of children with early-onset ODD or CD: A clinical trial with 3-year follow-up. *Journal of Abnormal Child Psychology, 37,* 591–609.

Kumpfer, K. L., & Alvarado, R. (2003). Family-strengthening approaches for the prevention of youth problem behaviors. *American Psychologist, 58,* 457–465.

LaFerriere, L., & Calsy, R. (1978). Goal attainment scaling: An effective treatment technique in short-term therapy. *American Journal of Community Psychology, 6,* 12–20.

Lanza, H. I., & Drabick, D. A. G. (2011). Family routine moderates the relation between child impulsivity and oppositional defiant disorder symptoms. *Journal of Abnormal Child Psychology, 39,* 83–94.

Larson, J., & Lochman, J. E. (2002). *Helping schoolchildren cope with anger: A cognitive-behavioral intervention.* New York: Guilford Press.

Lavigne, J. V., LeBailly, S. A., Gouze, K. R., Binns, H. J., Keller, K., & Pate, L. (2010). Predictors and correlates of completing behavioral parent training for the treatment of oppositional defiant disorder in pediatric primary care. *Behavior Therapy, 41,* 198–211.

Lee, C.-Y. S., August, G. J., Realmuto, G. R., Horowitz, J. L., Bloomquist, M. L., & Klimes-Dougan, B. (2008). Fidelity at a distance: Assessing implementation fidelity of the Early Risers prevention program in a going-to-scale intervention trial. *Prevention Science, 9,* 215–229.

Lee, S. S., August, G. J., Bloomquist, M. L., Mathy, R., & Realmuto, G. M. (2006). Implementing an evidence-based preventive intervention in neighborhood family centers: Examination of perceived barriers to program participation. *Journal of Primary Prevention, 27,* 573–597.

Lee, S. S., August, G. J., Gewirtz, A. H., Klimes-Dougan, B., Bloomquist, M. L., & Realmuto, G. M. (2010). Identifying unmet mental health needs in children of formerly homeless mothers living in a supportive housing community sector of care. *Journal of Abnormal Child Psychology, 38,* 421–432.

Lemerise, E. A., & Arsenio, W. F. (2000). An integrated model of emotion processes and cognition in social information processing. *Child Development, 71,* 107–118.

Lewis, M. D., Granic, I., Lamm, C., Zelazo, P. D., Stieben, J., Todd, R. M., et al. (2008). Changes in the neural bases of emotion regulation associated with clinical improvement in children with behavior problems. *Development and Psychopathology, 20,* 913–939.

Liddle, H. A., & Hogue, A. (2000). A family-based, developmental–ecological preventive intervention for high-risk adolescents. *Journal of Marital and Family Therapy, 26,* 265–279.

Lochman, J. E., Boxmeyer, C. L., Powell, N. P., Barry, T. D., & Pardini, D. A. (2010). Anger control training for aggressive youths. In J. R. Weisz & A. E. Kazdin (Eds.), *Evidence-based psychotherapies for children and adolescents* (2nd ed., pp. 227–242). New York: Guilford Press.

Lochman, J. E., Boxmeyer, C., Powell, N., Qu, L., Wells, K., & Windle, M. (2009). Dissemination of the Coping Power Program: Importance of intensity of counselor training. *Journal of Consulting and Clinical Psychology, 77,* 397–409.

Lochman, J. E., Curry, J. F., Burch, P. R., & Lampron, L. B. (1984). Treatment and generalization effects of cognitive-behavioral and goal-setting interventions with aggressive boys. *Journal of Consulting and Clinical Psychology, 52,* 915–916.

Lochman, J. E., Powell, N. P., Boxmeyer, C. L., Qu, L., Wells, K. C., & Windle, M. (2009). Implementation of a school-based prevention program: Effects of counselor and school characteristics. *Professional Psychology: Research and Practice, 40,* 476–482.

Loeber, R., & Pardini, D. (2008). Neurobiology and the development of violence: Common assumptions and controversies. *Philosophical Transactions of the Royal Society B: Biological Sciences, 363,* 2491–2503.

Lopez, M., Osterberg, L., Jensen-Doss, A., & Rae, W. (2011). Effects of workshop training for providers under mandated use of an evidence-based practice. *Administration and Policy in Mental Health and Mental Health Services Research, 38,* 301–312.

Luebbe, A. M., Bell, D. J., Allwood, M. A., Swenson, L. P., & Early, M. C. (2010). Social information processing in children: Specific relations to anxiety, depression, and affect. *Journal of Clinical Child and Adolescent Psychology, 39,* 386–399.

Lundahl, B. W., Tollefson, D., Risser, H., & Lovejoy, M. C. (2008). A meta-analysis of father involvement in parent training. *Research on Social Work Practices, 18,* 97–106.

Luthar, S. S., Cicchetti, D., & Becker, B. (2000). The construct of resilience: A critical evaluation and guidelines for future work. *Child Development, 71,* 543–562.

Mah, J. W. T., & Johnston, C. (2008). Parental social cognitions: Considerations in the acceptability and engagement in behavioral parent training. *Clinical Child and Family Psychology Review, 11,* 218–236.

Maher, E. J., Marcynyszyn, L. A., Corwin, T. W., & Hodnett, R. (2011). Dosage matters: The relationship between participation in the Nurturing Parenting Program for infants, toddlers, and preschoolers and subsequent child maltreatment. *Children and Youth Services Review, 33,* 1426–1434.

Masten, A. S. (2001). Ordinary magic: Resilience processes in development. *American Psychologist, 56,* 227–238.

Masten, A. S., & Coatsworth, J. D. (1998). The development

of competence in favorable and unfavorable environments: Lessons from research on successful children. *American Psychologist, 53,* 205–220.

Masten, A. S., & Wright, M. O'D. (2009). Resilience over the lifespan: Developmental perspectives on resistance, recovery, and transformation. In J. W. Reich, A. J. Zautra, & J. S. Hall (Eds.), *Handbook of adult resilience* (pp. 213–237). New York: Guilford Press.

McCabe, K., & Yeh, M. (2009). Parent–child interaction therapy for Mexican Americans: A randomized clinical trial. *Journal of Clinical Child and Adolescent Psychology.*

McCart, M. R., Priester, P. E., Davies, W. H., & Azen, R. (2006). Differential effectiveness of behavioral parent-training and cognitive-behavioral therapy for antisocial youth: A meta-analysis. *Journal of Abnormal Child Psychology, 34,* 527–543.

McCay, M., Nudelman, R., McCadam, K., & Gonzales, J. (1996). Evaluating a social work engagement approach to involving inner-city children and their families in mental health care. *Research on Social Work Practice, 6,* 462–472.

McCay, M., Stoewe, J., McCadam, K., & Gonzales, J. (1998). Increasing access to child mental health services for urban children and their caregivers. *Health and Social Work, 23,* 9–15.

McDonald, R., Dodson, M. C., Rosenfield, D., & Jouriles, E. N. (2011). Effects of a parenting intervention on features of psychopathy in children. *Journal of Abnormal Child Psychology, 39,* 1013–1023.

McMahon, R. J., & Forehand, R. L. (2003). *Helping the noncompliant child* (2nd ed.). New York: Guilford Press.

Meichenbaum, D. (1977). *Cognitive-behavior modification: An integrative approach.* New York: Plenum Press.

Meltzer, L. J. (Ed.). (2007). *Executive function in education: From theory to practice.* New York: Guilford Press.

Mendez, J. L., Carpenter, J. L., LaForett, D. R., & Cohen, J. S. (2009). Parental engagement and barriers to participation in a community-based preventive intervention. *American Journal of Community Psychology, 44,* 1–14.

Mikami, A. Y., Lerner, M. D., Griggs, M. S., McGrath, A., & Calhoun, C. D. (2010). Parental influence on children with attention-deficit/hyperactivity disorder: II. Results of a pilot intervention training parents as friendship coaches for children. *Journal of Abnormal Child Psychology, 38,* 737–749.

Miller, G. E., & Prinz, R. J. (2003). Engagement of families in treatment for childhood conduct problems. *Behavior Therapy, 34,* 517–534.

Miller, S., Loeber, R., & Hipwell, A. (2009). Peer deviance, parenting, and disruptive behavior among young girls. *Journal of Abnormal Child Psychology, 37,* 139–152.

Miller, W. R., & Rollnick, S. (2002). *Motivational interviewing: Preparing people for change* (2nd ed.). New York: Guilford Press.

Mitchell, P. F. (2011). Evidence-based practice in real-world services for young people with complex needs: New opportunities suggested by recent implementation science. *Children and Youth Services Review, 33,* 207–216.

Moadab, I., Gilbert, T., Dishion, T. J., & Tucker, D. M. (2010). Frontolimbic activity in a frustrating task: Covariation between patterns of coping and individual differences in externalizing and internalizing symptoms. *Development and Psychopathology, 22,* 391–404.

Moffitt, T. E., & Caspi, A. (2001). Childhood predictors differentiate life-course persistent and adolescent-limited antisocial pathways among males and females. *Development and Psychopathology, 13,* 355–375.

Morawska, A., Sanders, M. R., Goadby, E., Headley, C., Hodge, L., McAuliffe, C., et al. (2011). Is the Triple P-Positive Parenting Program acceptable to parents from culturally diverse backgrounds? *Journal of Child and Family Studies, 20,* 614–622.

Moretti, M. M., Catchpole, R. E. H., & Odgers, C. (2005). The dark side of girlhood: Recent trends, risk factors, and trajectories to aggression and violence. *Canadian Child and Adolescent Psychiatry Review, 14,* 21–25.

Morrissey-Kane, E., & Prinz, R. J. (1999). Engagement in child and adolescent treatment: The role of parental cognitions and attributions. *Clinical Child and Family Psychology Review, 2,* 183–198.

Mrug, S., & Windle, M. (2009). Mediators of neighborhood influences on externalizing behavior in preadolescent children. *Journal of Abnormal Child Psychology, 37,* 265–280.

Nigg, J. T., & Huang-Pollock, C. L. (2003). An early-onset model of the role of executive function and intelligence in conduct disorder/delinquency. In B. Lahey, T. Moffett, & A. Caspi (Eds.), *Causes of conduct disorder and juvenile delinquency* (pp. 227–253). New York: Guilford Press.

Nix., R. L., Bierman, K. L., McMahon, R. J., & the Conduct Problems Prevention Research Group. (2009). How attendance and quality of participation affect treatment response to parent management training. *Journal of Consulting and Clinical Psychology, 77,* 429–438.

Nock, M. K., & Ferriter, C. (2005). Parent management of attendance and adherence in child and adolescent therapy: A conceptual and empirical review. *Clinical Child and Family Psychology Review, 8,* 149–166.

Nock, M. K., & Kazdin, A. E. (2005). Randomized controlled trial of a brief intervention for increasing participation in parent management training. *Journal of Consulting and Clinical Psychology, 73,* 872–879.

Odgers, C., Moffitt, T. E., Broadbent, J. M., Dickenson, N., Hancox, R. J., et al. (2008). Female and male antisocial trajectories: From childhood origins to adult outcomes. *Development and Psychopathology, 20,* 673–716.

Ollendick, T. H., Grills, A. E., & King, N. J. (2001). Applying developmental theory to the assessment and treatment of childhood disorders: Does it make a difference? *Clinical Psychology and Psychotherapy, 8,* 304–314.

Ollendick, T. H., Jarrett, M. A., Grills-Taquechel, A. E., Hovey, L. D., & Wolff, J. C. (2008). Comorbidity as a predictor and moderator of treatment outcome in youth with anxiety, affective, attention-deficit/hyperactivity disorder, and oppositional/conduct disorders. *Clinical Psychology Review, 28,* 1447–1471.

Ostrov, J. M., & Crick, N. R. (2007). Forms and functions of aggression during early childhood: A short-term longitudinal study. *School Psychology Review, 36,* 22–43.

Patterson, G. R. (1975). *Families: Applications of social learning to family life* (rev. ed.). Champaign, IL: Research Press.

Patterson, G. R., Capaldi, D., & Bank, L. (1991). An early starter model for predicting delinquency. In D. Pepler & K. H. Rubin (Eds.), *The development and treatment of childhood aggression* (pp. 139–168). Hillsdale, NJ: Erlbaum.

Patterson, G. R., & Chamberlain, P. (1994). A functional analysis of parent resistance during parent training therapy. *Clinical Psychology: Science and Practice, 1,* 53–70.

Patterson, G. R., Reid, J., Jones, R., & Conger, R. (1975).

A social learning approach to family intervention: Families with aggressive children. Eugene, OR: Castalia.

Pelham, W. E., & Fabiano, G. A. (2008). Evidence-based psychosocial treatments for attention-deficit/hyperactivity disorder. *Journal of Clinical Child and Adolescent Psychology, 37,* 184–214.

Pepler, D. J., Jiang, D., Craig, W. M., & Connolly, J. (2010). Developmental trajectories of girls' and boys' delinquency and associated problems. *Journal of Abnormal Child and Adolescent Psychology, 38,* 1033–1044.

Podell, J. L., & Kendall, P. C. (2011). Mothers and fathers in family cognitive-behavioral therapy for anxious youth. *Journal of Child and Family Studies, 20,* 182–195.

Prinz, R. J., Blechman, E. A., & Dumas, J. E. (1994). An evaluation of peer-coping skills training for childhood aggression. *Journal of Clinical Child Psychology, 23,* 193–203.

Prinzie, P., Onghena, P., Hellincks, W., Grietens, H., Ghesquiere, P., & Colpin, H. (2004). Parent and child personality characteristics as predictors of negative discipline and externalizing problem behavior in children. *European Journal of Personality, 18,* 73–102.

Prochaska, J. O., & DiClemente, C. C. (1986). Toward a comprehensive model of change. In W. R. Miller & N. Heather (Eds.), *Addictive behaviors: Processes of change* (pp. 3–27). New York: Plenum Press.

Raaijmakers, M. A. J., Smidts, D. P., Sergeant, J. A., Maassen, G. H., Posthumus, J. A., van Engeland, H., & Matthys, W. (2008). Executive functions in preschool children with aggressive behavior: Impairments in inhibitory control. *Journal of Abnormal Child Psychology, 36,* 1097–1107.

Resnicow, K., Soler, R., Braithwait, R. L., Ahluwalia, J. S., & Butler, J. (2000). Cultural sensitivity in substance abuse prevention. *Journal of Community Psychology, 28,* 271–290.

Reyno, S. M., & McGrath, P. J. (2006). Predictors of parent training efficacy for child externalizing behavior problems—a meta-analytic review. *Journal of Child Psychology and Psychiatry, 47,* 99–111.

Robin, A. L., & Foster, S. L. (1989). *Negotiating parent–adolescent conflict: A behavioral–family systems approach.* New York: Guilford Press.

Rohrbach, L. A., Grana, R., Sussman, S., & Valente, T. W. (2006). Type II translation: Transporting prevention interventions from research to real-world practice settings. *Evaluation and Health Professions*, 29, 302–333.

Rubia, K., Halari, R., Smith, A. B., Mohammed, M., Scott, S., Giampiètro, V., et al. (2008). Dissociated functional brain abnormalities of inhibition in boys with pure conduct disorder and in boys with pure attention deficit hyperactivity disorder. *American Journal of Psychiatry*, 165, 889–897.

Rubin, K. H., Hymel, S., & Mills, R. S. (1989). Sociability and social withdrawal in childhood: Stability and outcomes. *Journal of Personality*, 57, 237–255.

Ruttle, P. L., Shirtcliff, E. A., Serbin, L. A., Ben-Dat Fisher, D., & Schwartzman, A. E. (2011). Disentangling psychobiological mechanisms underlying internalizing and externalizing behaviors in youth: Longitudinal and concurrent associations with cortisol. *Hormones and Behavior*, 59, 123–132.

Sanders, M. R. (1999). Triple P-Positive Parenting Program: Towards an empirically validated multilevel parenting and family support strategy for prevention of behavior and emotional problems in children. *Clinical Child and Family Psychology Review*, 2, 71–90.

Sanders, M. R. (2008). Triple P-Positive Parenting Program as a public health approach to strengthening parenting. *Journal of Family Psychology*, 22, 506–517.

Sanders, M. R., Markie-Dadds, C., & Turner, K. M. T. (2000). *Practitioner's manual for Standard Triple P*. Brisbane, Queensland, Australia: Families International.

Sanders, M. R., Pidgeon, A. M., Gravestock, F., Connors, M. D., Brown, S., & Young, R. W. (2004). Does parental attributional retraining and anger management enhance the effects of the Triple P-Positive Parenting Program with parents at risk of child maltreatment? *Behavior Therapy*, 35, 513–535.

Sandler, I. N., Schoenfelder, E. N., Wolchik, S. A., & MacKinnon, D. P. (2011). Long-term impact of prevention programs to promote effective parenting: Lasting effects but uncertain processes. *Annual Review of Psychology*, 62, 299–329.

Sauter, F. M., Heyne, D., & Westenberg, M. (2009). Cognitive-behavior therapy for anxious adolescents: Developmental influences on treatment design and delivery. *Clinical Child and Family Psychology Review*, 12, 310–335.

Schaeffer, C. M., Petras, H., Ialongo, N., Masyn, K. E., Hubbard, S., Poduska, J., et al. (2006). A comparison of girls' and boys' aggressive–disruptive behavior trajectories across elementary school: Prediction to young adult antisocial outcomes. *Journal of Consulting and Clinical Psychology*, 74, 500–510.

Schoenwald, S. K., Sheidow, A. J., & Chapman, J. E. (2009). Clinical supervision in treatment transport: Effects on adherence and outcomes. *Journal of Consulting and Clinical Psychology*, 77, 410–421.

Seguin, J. R., & Zelazo, P. D. (2005). Executive function in early physical aggression. In J. Archer, R. E. Tremblay, W. W. Hartup & W. Willard (Eds.), *Developmental origins of aggression* (pp. 307–329). New York: Guilford Press.

Semple, R. J., Lee, J., Rosa, D., & Miller, L. F. (2010). A randomized trial of mindfulness-based cognitive therapy for children: Promoting mindful attention to enhance social–emotional resiliency in children. *Journal of Child and Family Studies*, 19, 218–229.

Seng, A. C., & Prinz, R. J. (2008). Parents who abuse: What are they thinking? *Clinical Child and Family Psychology Review*, 11, 163–175.

Serketich, W. J., & Dumas, J. E. (1996). The effectiveness of behavioral parent training to modify antisocial behavior in children: A meta-analysis. *Behavior Therapy*, 27, 171–186.

Shimokawa, K., Lambert, M. J., & Smart, D. W. (2010). Enhancing treatment outcome of patients at risk of treatment failure: Meta-analytic and mega-analytic review of a psychotherapy quality assurance system. *Journal of Consulting and Clinical Psychology*, 78, 298–311.

Silverman, W. K., Ortiz, C. D., Viswesvaran, C., Burns, B. J., Kolko, D. J., Putnam, F. W., et al. (2008). Evidence-based psychosocial treatments for children and adolescents exposed to traumatic events. *Journal of Clinical Child and Adolescent Psychology*, 37, 156–183.

Silverman, W. K., Pina, A. A., & Viswesvaran, C. (2008). Evidence-based psychosocial treatments for phobic and anxiety disorders in children and adolescents. *Journal of Clinical Child and Adolescent Psychology*, 37, 105–130.

Silverthorn, P., & Frick, P. J. (1999). Developmental pathways to antisocial behavior: The delayed-onset pathway in girls. *Development and Psychopathology*, 11, 101–123.

Simpson, H. B., Maher, M., Page, J. R., Gibbons, C. J., Franklin, M. E., & Foa, E. B. (2010). Development of a patient adherence scale for exposure and response prevention therapy. *Behavior Therapy*, 41, 30–37.

Snell-Johns, J., Mendez, J. L., & Smith, B. H. (2004). Evidence-based solutions for overcoming access barriers, decreasing attrition, and promoting change with underserved families. *Journal of Family Psychology, 18,* 19–35.

Snyder, J., Schrepferman, L. S., McEachern, A., Barener, S., Johnson, K., & Provines, J. (2008). Peer deviancy training and peer coercion: Dual processes associated with early-onset conduct problems. *Child Development, 79,* 252–268.

Spring, B. (2007). Evidence-based practice in clinical psychology: What it is, why it matters, what you need to know. *Journal of Clinical Psychology, 63,* 611–631.

Springer, C., & Reddy, L. A. (2010). Measuring parental treatment adherence in a multimodal treatment program for children with ADHD: A preliminary investigation. *Child and Family Behavior Therapy, 32,* 272–290.

Stadler, C., Grasmann, D., Fegert, J. M., Holtmann, M., Poustka, F., & Schmeck, K. (2008). Heart rate and treatment effect in children with disruptive behavior disorders. *Child Psychiatry and Human Development, 39,* 299–309.

Sterrett, E., Jones, D. J., Zalot, A., & Shook, S. (2010). A pilot study of a brief motivational intervention to enhance parental engagement: A brief report. *Journal of Child and Family Studies, 19,* 697–701.

Stormshak, E. A., & Dishion, T. J. (2009). A school-based, family-centered intervention to prevent substance use: The Family Check-Up. *American Journal of Drug and Alcohol Abuse, 35,* 227–232.

Szapocznik, J., & Williams, R. A. (2000). Brief strategic family therapy: Twenty-five years of interplay among theory, research, and practice in adolescent behavior problems and drug abuse. *Clinical Child and Family Psychology Review, 3,* 117–134.

Thomas, R., & Zimmer-Gembeck, M. J. (2007). Behavioral outcomes of parent–child interaction therapy and Triple P-Positive Parenting Program: A review and meta-analysis. *Journal of Abnormal Child Psychology, 35,* 475–495.

Trentacosta, C. J., Hyde, L. W., Shaw, D. S., Dishion, T. J., Gardner, F., & Wilson, M. (2008). The relations among cumulative risk, parenting, and behavior problems during early childhood. *Journal of Child Psychology and Psychiatry, 49,* 1211–1219.

Tuvblad, C., Zheng, M., Raine, A., & Baker, L. A. (2009). A common genetic factor explains the covariation among ADHD, ODD, and CD symptoms in 9–10 year old boys and girls. *Journal of Abnormal Child Psychology, 37,* 153–167.

Urquiza, A. J., & Winn, C. (1999). *Treatment of abused and neglected children: Infancy to age 18.* Washington, DC: Clearinghouse on Child Abuse and Neglect Information.

Vanderbilt-Adriance, E., & Shaw, D. S. (2008). Conceptualizing and re-evaluating resilience across levels of risk, time, and domains of competence. *Clinical Child and Family Psychology Review, 11,* 30–58.

Van Lier, P. A. C., van der Ende, J., Koot, H. M., & Verhulst, F. C. (2007). Which better predicts conduct problems?: The relationship of trajectories of conduct problems with ODD and ADHD symptoms from childhood into adolescence. *Journal of Child Psychology and Psychiatry, 48,* 601–608.

Warzak, W. J., & Floress, M. T. (2009). Time-out training without put-backs, spanks, or restraint: A brief report of deferred time-out. *Child and Family Behavior Therapy, 31,* 134–143.

Waschbusch, D. A., Carrey, N. J., Willoughby, M. T., King, S., & Andrade, B. F. (2007). Effects of methylphenidate and behavior modification on the social and academic behavior of children with disruptive behavior disorders: The moderating role of callous/unemotional traits. *Journal of Clinical Child and Adolescent Psychology, 36,* 629–644.

Webster-Stratton, C., & Hancock, L. (1998). Training for parents of young children with conduct problems: Contents, methods, and therapeutic processes. In G. E. Schaefer & J. M. Breismeister (Eds.), *Handbook of parent training* (pp. 98–152). New York: Wiley.

Weisman, A. G., Okazaki, S., Gregory, J., Goldstein, M. J., Tompson, M. C., Rea, M., et al. (1998). Evaluating therapist competency and adherence to behavioral family management with bipolar patients. *Family Process, 37,* 107–121.

Weisz, J. R. (2004). *Psychotherapy for children and adolescents: Evidence-based treatments and case examples.* Cambridge, UK: Cambridge University Press.

Weisz, J. R., Chorpita, B. F., Palinkas, L. A., Schoenwald, S. K., Miranda, J., Bearman, S. K., et al. (2012). Testing standard and modular designs for psychotherapy treating depression, anxiety, and conduct problems in youth. *Archives of General Psychiatry, 69,* 274–282.

Weisz, J. R., & Kazdin, A. E. (Eds.). (2010). *Evidence-based psychotherapies for children and adolescents* (2nd ed.). New York: Guilford Press.

Wiggins, A., Sofroonoff, K., & Sanders, M. R. (2009). Pathways Triple P-Positive Parenting Program: Effects on parent–child relationships and child behavior problems. *Family Process, 48,* 517–530.

Wills, C. E., & Holmes-Rovner, M. (2006). Integrating decision making and mental health interventions research: Research directions. *Clinical Psychology: Science and Practice, 13,* 9–25.

Winters, K. C., & Leitten, W. (2007). Brief intervention for drug-abusing adolescents in a school setting. *Psychology of Addictive Behaviors, 21,* 249–254.

Woodward, C. A., Santa-Barbara, J., Levin, S., & Epstein, N. (1978). The role of goal attainment scaling in evaluating family therapy outcome. *American Journal of Orthopsychiatry, 48,* 464–476.

Zelazo, P. D., & Müller, U. (2002). Executive function in typical and atypical development. In U. Goswami (Ed.), *Handbook of childhood cognitive development* (pp 89–105). Oxford, UK: Blackwell.

Index